Health Reforms in Central and Eastern Europe

Health Reforms in Central and Eastern Europe

Options, Obstacles, Limited Outcomes

James Warner Björkman & Juraj Nemec

eleven international publishing

Published, sold and distributed by Eleven International Publishing
P.O. Box 85576
2508 CG The Hague
The Netherlands
Tel.: +31 70 33 070 33
Fax: +31 70 33 070 30
e-mail: sales@budh.nl
www.elevenpub.com

Sold and distributed in USA and Canada
International Specialized Book Services
920 NE 58th Avenue, Suite 300
Portland, OR 97213-3786, USA
Tel: 1-800-944-6190 (toll-free)
Fax: +1-503-280-8832
orders@isbs.com
www.isbs.com

Eleven International Publishing is an imprint of Boom uitgevers Den Haag.

ISBN 978-94-6236-063-1
ISBN 978-94-6094-769-8 (E-book)

Printed in The Netherlands

Table of Contents

Foreword

Reforms of health systems resemble the classic task of Sisyphus because no organizational algorithm can perfectly balance the allocation of access to health services versus their cost and quality. As form is repeatedly reformed, these changes (or the lack thereof), as well as their consequences, must be mapped. The purpose of this book is to examine selected national systems of health care in Central and Eastern Europe, as well as proposals to reform them.

Each chapter provides contextual information and data on the empirical realities of a specific country at five-year intervals since 1990 plus the organizational framework of its health care system. It then explores the historical thread of reforms attempted and their current state of implementation by addressing criteria for reforming national health systems such as cost, effectiveness, efficiency, equity and feasibility. Chapters stress country-specific policy elements like roles of actors, the shadow economy, access, cost containment, centralization and decentralization.

While no blueprint is offered, intriguing patterns emerge across the cases that the concluding chapter identifies along with observations about 'next steps' in the unfolding process of health reforms in Central and Eastern Europe. One finding is that health reforms in Central Europe deliver results on a limited scale; another is that public policy and governance in the region fall short of international standards. Finding the balance between market incentives and government regulation within different conditions remains a major challenge.

Support for comparative research on health system reforms came from several sources. As the prime association for public administration in the region, the Network of Schools and Institutes of Administration in Central and Eastern Europe is an arena for East-East collaboration through assisting, mediating and facilitating joint research, educational and training programs as well as through discussions among instructors, civil servants, trainers, public sector managers and politicians. By promoting training programs as well as the discipline of public administration in post-Communist countries, NISPAcee fosters the development of professional public management, public policy and governance by assisting political and economic transition through effective public service. Annual conferences between 2008 and 2011 featured special panels on health reforms and their implementation in order to compare processes and outcomes of health reforms in the region, including explanations for successes and failures.

With financial assistance from the Brian Mitchell Charitable Settlement (UK), the International Political Science Association's Research Committee on Comparative Health Policy helped to organize these panels. During these panels, participants were challenged to explore health reforms in their respective countries through systematic comparison of empirical data since 1990 with careful attention to country-specific issues. Likewise, analysis of the appropriateness of market instruments in health care in the region was financed by the Czech Grant Agency (GACR Project P403/12/0366). The editors gratefully acknowledge all these sources of support.

Finally, the book has been greatly enhanced through internal reviews by Professor KGH Okma (USA/Belgium) and Professor Frantisek Ochrana (Czech Republic). The editors are grateful for their comments and suggestions. The editors also attribute to one another any errors of omission or commission but collectively accept responsibility for them. The Sisyphean task continues.

James Warner Björkman
The Hague, The Netherlands

Juraj Nemec,
Brno, Czech Republic and Banska Bystrica, Slovakia

List of Abbreviations

ADB	Asian Development Bank
AIPRG	Armenian International Policy Research Group
AMD	Armenian Drams (currency)
APSREP	Armenia Public Sector Reform Project
BBP	Basic Benefits Package
CIA	Central Intelligence Agency
CIS	Commonwealth of Independent States
DFID	Department for International Development
DRG	Diagnostic Related Groups
FSU	Former Soviet Union
GDP	Gross Domestic Product
HC	Health Centers
HCL	Health Care Law
HFA	Health For All
HIF	Health Insurance Fund
HIL	Health Insurance Law
HMIS	Health Management Information System
HMLTP	Health Management and Leadership Training Program
HSDP	Health Systems Development Program
IMF	International Monetary Fund
IMR	Infant Mortality Rate
IT	Information Technology
LA	Loan Agreement
MCs	Medical Centres
MDGs	Millennium Development Goals
MHI	Mandatory Health Insurance
MKD	Macedonian Denar (currency)
MoH	Ministry of Health
NGO	Non-Governmental Organization
NIS	Newly Independent States
OECD	Organization for Economic Co-operation and Development

OG	Official Gazette
OPE	Out-of-Pocket Expenditure
OPP	Out-of-Pocket Payment
PADCO	Planning and Development Cooperative International
PHC	Primary Health care
PFB	Poverty Family Benefits
PRSP	Poverty Reduction Strategy Paper
PSRC	Public Sector Reform Commission
SEA	State Employment Agency
SHA	State Health Agency
UN	United Nations
UNDP	United Nations Development Project
UNICEF	United Nations Children's Fund
USAID	United States Agency for International Development
US$	United States Dollar (currency)
VHI	Voluntary Health Insurance
VMRO-DPMNE	Internal Macedonian Revolutionary Organization, Democratic Party for Macedonian National Unity
WB	World Bank
WFP	World Food Program
WHO	World Health Organization

1 Health Reforms in Central and Eastern Europe since 1990: Comparative Context and Concerns

James Warner Björkman

Modern systems of social protection provide access to health care for citizens as a right. The legitimacy and viability of nation-states are partly based on the provision of publicly financed health services, but spiraling costs of providing care and growing demand for services are major factors for the rise in public deficits and for associated financial instability. Therefore, promises regularly appear to reform the health sector by lowering costs, expanding access and/or improving the quality of care.

As a specialized subsystem of society, however, no national health system can be self-sufficient. It depends on external supports for several types of inputs. In cultural terms, its legitimacy is based on what a health system and its practitioners are allowed to do that is considered proper, acceptable, desirable or needed by the population. Its performance is grounded in techniques of knowledge in the art and science of medicine; consequently it requires personnel ranging from skilled professionals through paramedical technicians to ancillary staff. And its environment includes access to essential resources such as land, capital, infrastructure, instruments and drugs as well as subsidies, transfer payments and generation of revenue. With the exception of knowledge techniques that, once developed, can be used again and again without diminution, supply of these external supports is always limited and problematic. Because it absorbs limited resources – particularly in trained manpower and economic wealth, a health system necessarily competes with other subsystems in society such as education, investments, communications, defense and other non-health expenditures.

Despite these contextual limitations, the term 'health reform' trips teasingly off tongues of politicians and professionals who solemnly seek to resolve the dilemmas of national systems that try to deliver health care. Yet reform is a complex process embedded in empirical realities of power and privilege as well as economic constraints. Reform requires changes in form that is already entrenched in standard operating procedures as well as in habitual expectations and behaviors that are both well rooted and resilient. The chapters in this volume demonstrate a chronic gap between proclamation and implementation, between intent and result, between promise and performance in terms of access, quality and cost of health services.

This volume explores experiences with health reforms in selected countries of Central and Eastern Europe – all once members of the former Soviet Union (FSU) or its orbit. After the fall of the Berlin Wall in 1989 and dissolution of the USSR in 1991, nations in the region engaged in extensive social and economic reforms that included major changes in their health care systems. Most reforms were examples of 'panic policies' that sought to expunge the communist legacy and, given external pressure from international donors, to move towards a market-based system without testing of what such a model entails. The authors of the following chapters examine the institutional legacies of their respective national health care systems and their health reform efforts during the past two decades. In the policy-making arena, the authors describe the prevalent ideas, basic institutions and vested interests of their particular country as well as the role of external advisors during attempts to implement formal reforms. The chapters reveal that 'policy' includes not only formal statements of intentions but also efforts at implementation and the more or less permanent process of 'after reform' maintenance.

Based on categories outlined in the attached appendix, each chapter in this comparative study of health care reforms provides information and data at five-year intervals since 1990. For comparative enquiry, reform was defined as major shifts in decision-making power over the allocation of resources and in the distribution of financial risks in funding between as well as within public and private sectors (Björkman 2009; Okma and Crivelli 2010). As examples, such shifts include changes in selective contracting of health care providers, in authority over capital investments, in entitlements of public health insurance and in restrictions on medical decision-making imposed by practice guidelines. Decision-making power and financial risks can shift from the national level to regional and local governments (or vice versa), or from governments to individual insurers and patients. All chapters address criteria for reforming national health systems such as effectiveness, efficiency, equity, cost and feasibility.

The case-study countries share institutional legacies of three erstwhile empires – Russian, Ottoman and Austro-Hungarian – that ended in World War I. In many ways, post-imperial experiences of their successor states continue to shape contemporary behavior. Six of the countries are members of the European Union since 2004 – Hungary, Slovenia, the Czech Republic and Slovakia – and Bulgaria and Romania since 2007. Two countries – Macedonia and Slovenia – were constituent republics of federal Yugoslavia. And two – Armenia and Russia – are within the loosely structured Commonwealth of Independent States (CIS). Of the three countries in the 'classical' core of central Europe, two are successor states of Czechoslovakia that peacefully split in 1993. Most countries in this volume are, therefore, relatively young European nations with old political and institutional legacies.

Income levels range from middle income (Slovenia and the Czech Republic) to relative poverty (Armenia and Macedonia). Demographics vary in terms of population size and urbanization as well as life expectancy and rates of maternal mortality. Russia has over twice the number of inhabitants than the other eight countries combined, yet it ranks second lowest in both life expectancy and government spending allocated to health – and has the highest rate of maternal mortality.

As a percentage of Gross Domestic Product (GDP), government expenditure on health in all nine countries averages 4.8 within a range of 2% to 7%. All face severe fiscal and budgetary pressures aggravated by expanding demand for health services and the dominant position of the medical profession that controls access to health care. Whatever else characterizes national health systems, their design and reform necessarily entail cost-control measures accompanied by mechanisms to secure the cooperation of health professionals (Freddi and Björkman 1988). During the past quarter century, the cost of providing health care has escalated throughout the world – and no less so in central and eastern Europe.

Table 1.1 Comparative Context of Countries (1990-2011)

Country	Populations (Millions)		Population Density/km^2		% Urban	Per capita GDP (US$)	
	1990	2011	1990	2011	2008	1990	2011
Armenia	3.5	3.0	124	105	64	637	3 033
Bulgaria	8.7	7.1	79	67	70	2 377	7 202
Czech Rep	10.4	10.2	134	134	74	3 748	20 444
Hungary	10.4	10.0	115	107	65	3 186	14 050
Macedonia	1.9	2.1	75	80	59	2 342	5 016
Romania	23.2	21.4	101	90	55	1 651	8 863
Russia	148.3	138.7	9	8	73	3 485	12 993
Slovakia	5.3	5.5	110	111	57	2 211	17 644
Slovenia	2.0	2.0	99	101	51	8 699	24 533

Source: <http://data.worldbank.org>, <www.unfpa.org>, <www.globalhealthfacts.org>, <www.cia.gov> (various years).

Table 1.2 Comparative Data on Health Statistics

Country	Government Expenditure (% of GDP)	Government Expenditure Allocated to Health (%)	Government Expenditure on Health (% of GDP)	Life Expectancy (Years at Birth)		Maternal Mortality Per 100 000 Live Births
Year	**2010**	**2010**	**2010**	**1990**	**2011**	**2010**
Armenia	28	6	2	68.5	69.1	29
Bulgaria	38	10	4	71.6	73.1	13
Czech Rep	44	15	7	71.4	77.2	8
Hungary	49	10	5	69.3	74.8	13
Macedonia	35	13	5	71.6	74.7	9
Romania	40	11	4	69.7	72.5	27
Russia	39	8	3	68.9	70.3	39
Slovakia	40	14	6	70.9	71.5	6
Slovenia	50	14	7	73.3	77.3	18

Source: WHO 2012: <www.globalhealthfacts.org>.

In several ways, the pathways of health reforms in Central and Eastern Europe resemble those of industrialized nations. At its core, any proposal for reform seeks to modify the way arrangements are currently organized. Reform seeks to change 'form' and, in so doing, to re-arrange the distribution of costs, benefits and valued resources. In the health sector, three issues regularly appear among proposals for reform – cost, access and quality; phrased otherwise, there are proposals for reforms in financing (revenue as well as expenditure), reforms in services (who gets what, when, where, how) and reforms in assurance that professionals are delivering competent care. Decades of experience suggest that reform is not necessarily a good thing but reform, like beauty, is often in the eye of the beholder. Because attempts at reform are inevitable as long as health care delivery systems remain problematic, this volume explores experiences with reforms in selected countries of Central and Eastern Europe.

Reform has been on the international agenda for decades as approaches to reform evolved in fields well beyond health care (Whyte 2004). The 1950s and 1960s were characterized by 'institution building', an approach that focused on individual organizations. Institutions were modeled on – if not directly transferred from – so-called 'developed' countries. During these decades, many public sector institutions were initiated, including state-owned enterprises with a strong emphasis on state-based delivery of social services. By the late 1960s and early 1970s, the emphasis on institution building had softened into concern for strengthening institutions that already existed. This shift to 'institutional strengthening' sought to provide tools that would improve performance rather than to initiate wholesale change.

During the 1960s and 1970s, great reliance was placed on the role of government agents, particularly civil servants, for achieving strategies intended to reach neglected target groups and to improve delivery systems in order to reach such targets. In the 1980s, development was increasingly focused on people rather than on institutions and the key sectors were education and health care. Structural adjustment appeared as a composite of policy reforms that were based on requirements or 'conditionalities' of economic and social changes by the recipients of donor funds. Capacity building broadened to include private as well as associational efforts in addition to government action, and there was greater attention to the environment as well as national economic behavior. In the 1990s, a paradigm of 'governance' emerged that reunited public administration with political participation. The decade was also characterized by reassessments of technical cooperation and its limitations, plus the emergence of local ownership as a vital factor for sustainability.

In the first decade of the 21st century, internationally endorsed Millennium Development Goals (MDGs) became a key driver for change based on results-oriented management and long-term investments. The age of the 'quick fix' has been replaced by an appreciation of the 'long slog'. Emphasis is on knowledge-based networks that emphasize continual learning as well as on synergistic adaptation through participation by non-government actors in building capacity. A striking feature of the new forms of public-private collaboration is the focus on private entrepreneurship and modern management techniques based on high expectations about the benefits of information technology.

For several decades, public sector reforms had been premised on the assumption that improving the ability of government to manage its business will lead to improved social and economic progress. The first generation of reforms sought to cut public expenditures and to revive the private sector. Measures included budget cuts, tax reforms, limited privatization, liberalization of prices and, most conspicuously, efforts to downsize the public sector – the latter being almost invariably described as 'bloated' and in need of surgery followed by a strictly enforced diet.

It quickly became evident that the transformation of government would require a long time and that the savings from reduced bureaucratic costs would be insufficient to provide even basic levels of public services. A second generation of public sector reforms then sought to improve the efficiency and effectiveness of government. While the first generation reforms stressed downsizing, contracting and improved control over budgeting and public expenditures, second generation reforms advocated decentralization to subnational levels, the creation of semi-autonomous agencies in the central government, and reforms of human resource management (recruitment, selection and training).

More recently, the agenda for reform has refocused yet again as a third generation of reforms seeks to improve social outcomes through better service delivery. This strategy emphasizes sector-wide approaches, particularly in health and education, in order to produce a coherent program for delivery of services that involves both governmental and non-governmental organizations. While these generations of reforms are overlapping rather than strictly sequential, all reforms have been driven by a combination of external and internal agencies. Multilateral and bilateral aid entails conditionalities that require a (commitment to) change in governmental behavior before money can be transferred. In turn, national planning commissions and ministries of finance require line agencies to adopt reforms that may include a combination of these generations.

Public sector reforms range across a repertoire of policy instruments: streamlined budgets, staff reductions, raised tariffs, contracting out and other forms of privatization. Reform of the health sector has focused on four main options, none of which is mutually exclusive, and all of which may occur at the same time. These are the establishment of autonomous organizations, the introduction of user fees, contracting out of services, and the enablement and regulation of the private sector.

Most countries share basic goals in health policy: universal (or near-universal) access to health services, equity in sharing the financial burden of illness, and good quality health care. Given the growing share of public money in funding health care, governments have become concerned about efficiency and cost control. Patient satisfaction, patient choice and the autonomy of professionals are important goals too. Yet despite the similarity in policy goals, national arrangements for financing health care vary widely. The sources of financing for health care are general taxation (in the United Kingdom, Scandinavia and until recently most countries in Central and Eastern Europe), social health insurance (*e.g.*, Germany, France, Japan and increasingly in Central Europe) and private health insurance (employment-based health insurance in the USA, and higher income groups in Germany and Australia that opt out of the public system). Direct cash payments are important, too, through out-of-pocket expenditures and through co-payments or deductibles. Governments often mitigate the effects of user fees by exempting specific groups such as the elderly and chronically ill patients or low-income families. In low-income countries external aid supplements national resources.

Variations in funding and contracting models in health care can be traced to country-specific historical developments, but two events in Europe have been crucial as models for policy. The first was the introduction of mandatory social health insurance for industrial workers and their families in Germany in 1883. Several countries in Europe, Asia and Latin America followed the German example of state-sponsored (but not state-administered) mandatory social insurance to protect the family income of industrial workers against the risks of illness, disability, unemployment and old age. Mandatory membership enforced by social insurance meant that the so-called 'sickness funds' had stable revenue streams and could create wider pools of shared risk. In the 20th century, these non-governmental funds became core actors in the public policy arena by sharing responsibility for social policy-making but under ever-greater government regulation.

The second major innovation in the funding of health care was the establishment in 1948 of Britain's National Health Service (NHS). The NHS extended the German insurance model by providing coverage to the entire population with costs paid out of general taxation. While hospitals were nationalized, family physicians remained independent as practitioners. During the first half of the 20th century, many European countries followed the German example by establishing separate income protection schemes for certain groups in society (*e.g.*, disability and unemployment benefits for industrial workers). Only after World War II did the full range of modern welfare state programs appear, including old age pensions, disability and unemployment benefits, health insurance, sickness pay and child support. In the first decades of post-war reconstruction, there was popular support for this expansion of state-sponsored schemes. By the end of the 20th century, funding for health care in most countries had become hybridized – *i.e.*, by adopting elements from both the British and German models. Employment-based arrangements for certain categories of workers were combined with population-wide and tax-based universal schemes.

After the oil crises during the 1970s, economic, demographic and ideological factors contributed to reshaping the popular notion of the welfare state from being a solution for social problems to being an economic burden and a cause of economic stagnation (Wilensky 2002). Economic stagflation with persistently high levels of unemployment meant that state revenues stagnated or declined while public expenditures continued to grow. Moreover, as the end of the post-war baby boom became visible, demographers had to revise their earlier demographic projections downward – and future pension outlays upwards. In addition, ideological views about the role of the state had gradually changed. On both the left and right of the political spectrum, critics agreed that state powers had become too intrusive in the lives of individuals. Growing discontent over fiscal burdens and disappointing results of public programs, rising consumerism and patient advocacy groups claiming a stronger say in the allocation and organization of health care – all challenged existing arrangements for providing welfare.

Governments sought alternative models of governance to reduce the dominant role of the state and to decentralize decision-making with more room for individual choice and entrepreneurial ideas (Cutler 2002). Some countries took hesitant steps to introduce market competition in health care by reducing state control over the funding and planning of health care services. They also sought to broaden patients' choice of provider and health plan. Other countries turned to traditional tools of controlling public expenditure by setting strict budgets, reducing the scope of public insurance and increasing direct patient payments.

As chapters in this volume illustrate, health sector reforms have a significant parallel with civil service reforms. In most cases, reforms have been stimulated by economic recession and by severe fiscal problems in the state treasury rather than by an ideologically driven taste for reform. Declining budgets have adversely affected service delivery, even in countries that previously had reasonably well performing public health services. Central Ministries of Finance and Planning initiated reforms, and Ministries of Health struggled to respond to policy directives outside of their control. Economic realities of recession and fiscal crises affect not only the types of policies being implemented but also reactions to them by the users, beneficiaries and citizens. Given endemic economic crises, the stage of raising revenue through the introduction of user fees in order to supplement budgetary resources is critical for governments. But the success of the policy, no matter how logical in theory, has been constrained by the dwindling capacity of citizens to pay for health care. Furthermore, the administrative cost of collecting user fees and of monitoring exempted categories of users often exceeds the revenue collected. The initial reform, however well intended, had not considered inevitable transaction costs.

While reforms have been widely espoused in international arenas as well as by technical experts, their implementation has been much more limited. It is difficult to assess the real potential for reforms in the health sector because more time is needed for assessment. Rather ironically, too, countries with the most radical reform agenda appear to be those with the least capacity to implement them; as Caiden and Wildavsky (1980) commented caustically some decades ago about planning and budgeting, the smaller the capacity, the greater the ambition, and vice versa. Perniciously the depth of the economic recession in such contexts requires a radical approach in terms of policy pronouncements, yet reduces ability to implement such a radical agenda.

Proposed reforms face other barriers, too. One important constraint is the lack of skilled and motivated staff to provide services or administrative support. Organizations that traditionally favor hierarchy and command over initiatives and team development are unlikely to act on newly acquired formal autonomy. While New Public Management emphasizes the importance of linking performance to rewards, parallel informal systems often undermine the formal reward systems. For example, promotions in traditional patrimonial systems are often based on patronage and favors rather than on objective assessments of performance and merit. Management information systems frequently fail to function effectively. Another significant obstacle is the lack of incentives for individuals within the health sector to plan or to monitor their work in terms of the information that is produced. In other words, there is almost no feedback system for self-correcting action.

A further sign of weak capacity is poor coordination among different actors (Akukwe 1999). Governments experience great difficulty in translating broad policy statements into concrete strategies for implementation. As a consequence, there are problems in specifying and then enacting the details of decentralization policies. It is not clear, *e.g.*, as to the level of government at which financial rights and responsibilities lie. Likewise, it is not clear which organization should report which data to whom. These are all simple but disastrous problems in coordination.

Some of the constraints on capacity are, of course, rooted in the broader public sector rather than only within the Ministry of Health or similar agencies. Until recently, *e.g.*, in many countries all revenues generated from user fees had to be returned to the national treasury – thus providing little incentive for their collection. Such a disincentive more or less ensured that such fees had zero impact upon the quality of health care. In contrast, when local hospitals are allowed to keep the user fees that they collect rather than returning them to central coffers, not only do those hospitals have a better record for collection of fees but also they re-invest the surplus in such long-term benefits as higher quality equipment, more reliable stocks of pharmaceuticals and medical supplies, and even lower (or exempted) fees for the truly destitute (Björkman and Mathur 2002).

Both internal and external pressures for change encourage national governments to seek solutions and new ideas. This search fueled the growth of cross-national studies in the field of health policy. International organizations and consultancy firms became carriers of widespread but often ill-tested ideas. While comparative studies aim to analyze processes of health reform across the globe, a common problem is the facile assumption that policy as stated in law or formal government documents is the same as policy actually implemented. For many reasons, the outcomes of reform often differ greatly from the original policy intentions and statements. Faced with public discontent over unintended results, governments feel pressured yet again to adjust their policies and the cycle continues.

Empirical experience with goals and means for health reform indicate potential global convergence on patterns of performance, but countries implement change within their own institutional legacies and within the restraints of existing national institutions and political boundaries. The timing and speed of change of the health reform processes vary as well. In some countries, governments implement major change rapidly. In other countries characterized by strong opposition by organized stake-holders, reform efforts are adjusted, delayed or even abandoned.

Combinations of core elements – funding, contracting (including payment modes) and ownership – determine the allocation of financial risks and decision-making power among the main players in health care. Government ownership and tax-funded services require strong government influence whereas private funding (insurance and direct patient payments) combined with legally independent providers restricts the role of the state even though governments can – and often do – impose rules to protect patients or safeguard the quality of and access to health care.

These terms help to characterize features of health care systems and policy-making but they do not explain the causes or effects of policy change. In order to understand why countries embark on particular reform paths, one must investigate not only external and internal pressures for change but also structural features of social policy-making that enable politicians and policy entrepreneurs to change the system. However, institutional legacies and popular support for existing policy arrangements create powerful barriers to change.

In order to get reforms in the health sector on a sustainable track, structural changes need to be enforced. Such a track has to lead to outcomes that ensure minimum care for all citizens. Unfortunately, public hospital care in many countries has become unaffordable for the poor due to steep user fees. Additional hidden costs complicate this situation – 'under the table payments' to doctors being just one type. Subsidizing such a system, instead of reforming it, will only channel additional funds to the wrong (non-poor) recipients. Indeed, health sector reforms have been used as crutches to pretend that one is changing the system but basically staying the course or even regressing. The issue is not whether people should share the costs because the people always end up paying. The real issue is who is to pay more and who is to pay less or nothing at all.

The next nine chapters examine arrangements for the delivery of health care services in selected countries of Central and Eastern Europe and efforts to reform them. Each chapter provides contextual information on the empirical realities of a specific country since 1990 as well as the organizational framework of its health care system. It then explores the historical thread of reforms attempted and their current state of implementation. While most countries keenly embraced recommendations of the World Bank, the World Health Organization and other international agencies or private organizations, few paid attention to the feasibility of such reforms. There were some policy innovations but also repetitions of mistakes that had occurred elsewhere. The cases reveal similarities of attempts during the post-communist era: high hopes and expectations followed by frustration and disillusionment. In reality, few nations abandoned existing institutions. Instead the new policy models added a layer of governance to old structures that did not disappear. While no blueprint is offered, intriguing patterns emerge across the selected cases that the concluding chapter identifies along with observations about the feasibility of 'next steps' in the unfolding process of health reforms in Central and Eastern Europe.

APPENDIX

Categories for collecting data and information in a comparative study of national health reforms through structured multi-country research; empirical data for systematic cross-country comparisons were sought at five-yearly intervals between 1990 (base-year) and 2010 (or the most recent year available)

1. *Demographic characteristics*
   - Geographic area (km^2)
   - Population
   - Population density (population/km^2)
   - Urban (%)
   - Life expectancy at birth (male and female)
   - Infant morality rate
2. *Economic data* (normalized with 1990 as base-year and converted into US dollars)
   - Total GDP
   - GDP per capita
   - GDP growth rate (1980-1990, 1990-2000, 2000-2010)
   - Inflation rate
3. *Health care expenditures*
   - Outlays at all levels of government (audited)
   - Public outlays as percentage of total intergovernmental budgets
   - Private out-of-pocket outlays (estimates)
   - Total health expenditures (public and private)
   - Total health expenditures as percentage of GDP

4. *Health resources* (public, private, total)
   - Physicians
   - Physicians/100,000 population
   - Other health professionals
   - Other health professionals/100,000 population
   - Hospital beds
   - Hospital beds/100,000 population
5. *Normative issues* (descriptive assessment)
   - Cultural orientations (solidarity-individualism continuum; sectarianism)
   - Welfare principles (role of state: collectivist/residual; income protection)
   - Dominant values in health policy (by political party or faction)
6. *Governance of health sector* (descriptive assessment)
   - Main funding sources (taxes, private out-of-pocket, public/private insurance)
   - Contracting and payment models (integrated, competitive, selective)
   - Ownership mix (public, private, municipal, sectarian, self-employed)
   - Administration (degree of government control, centralized/decentralized, regulated, stake-holder involvement, public/private partnerships, neo-corporatism)
7. *Major political positions, postures and trends* (contextual and historical features)

2 Health Reforms in Armenia, 1990-2010

Lianna Mkhitaryan

After its independence in 1991, the Republic of Armenia took the path from a centralized system of governance towards a market economy. During the course of reforms, radical changes aimed at structural and regulatory changes in the centralized and inefficient health care system inherited from the Soviet era. These changes focused on decentralization, devolution and privatization, new mechanisms of finance, and reforms for effective management. The 1996 Law on Local Self-government transferred responsibility for the provision of health care services as well as the ownership of facilities to local governments (for primary health care) and regional governments (for hospitals). Financial responsibility was devolved to facility level.

Subsequent adoption of relevant legislation enabled privatization of hospitals and health care facilities in the pharmaceutical and dental care sectors. New approaches to health financing focused on diversifying revenues for the health sector, improving financial management and sustainability, and linking financing to the quality and volume of services provided. Measures on optimizing the health system's effectiveness were undertaken to rationalize the system through restructuring, reorganization of functions, and redistribution of resources. However, these measures did not provide sufficient stimuli to increase cost-effectiveness or the quality of services. At present, the country has gaps in the distribution of human and technological resources, low remuneration of personnel, and lack of strategic planning. The emphasis of current reforms is on improved state budget financing and more efficient use of resources.

This chapter analyzes national policies, processes and outcomes of health reforms in Armenia during 1990-2010. It presents a socio-economic profile of the country including demographic characteristics and economic data, health care resources, expenditures and normative issues. It describes the health sector governance system as well as contextual and historical features of major political positions, postures and trends. It sketches the history of reforming health system in Armenia and the changes that have occurred in the decision-making power over the allocation of resources and the distribution of financial risks in health care funding between and within public and private sectors. It examines short- and medium-term reforms, including analysis of real achievements and remaining issues with particular focus on economy, services accessibility and quality. And it summarizes the problems in policy-making and implementation, internal and external successes and failures, and country-specific reforms.

Reforms were implemented in the Armenian health care system because health services can no longer be provided free and on demand for the entire population. Efforts to establish a cost-effective, equitable and sustainable health system brought overall improvements in primary health care and maternity services; however, they did not meet all of the objectives of health care policies. State expenditures on health care remain low, which necessitates direct out-of-pocket payments for funding the system.

The measures implemented have improved the state of Armenia's health system with positive impacts on key indicators. Raising the role of private providers produced more revenue and increased provider income but it failed to ensure equal access of population to qualitative health care. The government of the Republic of Armenia seeks to improve the situation by supporting the poor and by targeting social groups to receive medical care and drugs free of charge. However, there is need to resolve the problem of price regulation, to reduce shadow operations, and to improve governance, including decision-making in social policy, distribution of resources and implementing more effective financial protection mechanisms.

During the Soviet era, Armenian health care was organized as a public system that guaranteed free medical assistance and access to a complete range of public health care services for the entire population. Although Armenia had one of the best health care systems among the Soviet republics (USAID 2010), the system as a whole was inefficient. It emphasized quantitative indicators and had excess physical capacity, excess medical staff and too many hospital beds. While the principle of universal coverage of population ensured equitable access to primary, secondary and tertiary health care services, the system was highly centralized with strong vertical management. Allocation of finances for the system was based on five-year central plans emanating from Moscow. The state determined the level, composition and mechanisms for allocation of public spending based on national norms in order to ensure the provision of health care services in compliance with certain standards. Strict top-down control over expenditures of public resources characterized the system.

During the economic transition after independence in 1991, the country experienced political and social transformations. A severe economic crisis, sociopolitical problems and a dramatic decline in the level of health care expenditures undermined the public health achievements of the socialist era, dramatically affected the status of health care service provision and, eventually, caused the collapse of public health activities. Available public financing failed to sustain the inherited system characterized by expensive tertiary curative care rather than primary and preventive medicine. Due to inadequate clinical and managerial skills of health care providers, overstaffed facilities in disrepair, obsolete equipment and insufficient supplies (USAID 2010), there were long periods of non-payment of wages to medical personnel. Private payments by the population became the main source of financing for health care services. However, impoverishment of the population led to an inability to pay for basic health care that, in turn, led to a decline in the utilization of health care services and ultimately damaged the health status of the population by increasing mortality and morbidity rates.

In the mid-1990s, Armenia began to implement health reforms in the initial phase of public sector reforms. The reforms were supported by international financial institutions and bilateral agencies like the World Bank, the World Health Organization, USAID and the UK Department for International Development. Health reforms sought to increase the utilization of sustainable, high-quality primary health care services, optimize and modernize hospital networks to improve the quality and efficiency of services, and strengthen the capacity of the Ministry of Health to implement effective health sector policies.

2.1 Profile of Armenia

Armenia is a landlocked mountainous country located in the South Caucasus between Europe and Asia. The country borders Georgia on the north, Iran and Azerbaijan (Nakhichevan) on the south, Azerbaijan on the east, and Turkey on the west. The country covers 29,743 km^2 that, for administrative purposes, are divided into ten *marzes* (regions) which include 48 urban and 878 rural communities. Of the country's 3.2 million inhabitants, approximately 1.3 million reside in the capital city, Yerevan (Statistical Yearbook of Armenia 2011). Nearly 65% of population lives in urban areas; population density is about 104 persons per square kilometer (UN 2010). In the early 1990s, Armenia experienced a decline in population growth. Continuing emigration, seasonal migration and trends in reproductive behavior among Armenians affect the country's demography. The government plans to introduce new policies to increase the birth rate, protect childhood and motherhood, increase life expectancy, decrease the mortality rate, halt emigration and encourage immigration. It forecasts 0.3% annual population growth of the country through 2015.

Life expectancy at birth in Armenia was the highest among the Soviet republics – in 1986 an average of 73.3 years (70.5 for males; 75.7 for females). Since then the country has experienced war and a severe economic crisis, including a 60% fall in real Gross Domestic Product (GDP) during 1991-1993, as well as pervasive poverty since the beginning of the transition period. The level of public expenditures for health care is the lowest in the region so both quality and utilization of the health care services deteriorated dramatically. Sociopolitical problems coupled with drastic declines in the utilization of health care services (Demirchyan and Thompson 2001) caused the health status of Armenians to deteriorate. In 1991 life expectancy fell to an average of 70.4 years (67.4 for males; 73.3 for females) and only returned to its previous level (73.4 years) in 2004.

During the past two decades, health indicators related to mortality and life expectancy improved (Table 2.1). Since 1990, life expectancy has increased by 2.0 years among females and 2.2 years among males. In 2010 this indicator was estimated to be 74.1 years (70.6 for men; 77.2 for women). These official indicators compare favorably to countries with similar or even higher levels of income. Average life expectancy in European countries is 78.8 years; in Central Asian countries it is 69.1 years. Life expectancy in Armenia is noticeably higher than the average of 68 years in the Commonwealth of Independent States (CIS) (WHO 2009).

However, there are great discrepancies between data reported nationally, data from surveys and data estimated by WHO. Taking into consideration the quality of data, life expectancy may be lower than official figures suggest (Shuhrcke *et al.* 2007:17). While figures for reproductive behavior indicate a decline in the birthrate over recent decades, survey data are not available on reproductive behavior in the early 1990s. It is not clear how much the reproductive rate has changed since the onset of the transitional period.

Table 2.1 Selected Health Status Indicators

	1990	1995	2000	2005	2009	2010
Female life expectancy at birth (years)	75.2	75.9	75.7	76.5	77.0	77.2
Male life expectancy at birth (years)	68.4	68.9	70.9	70.3	70.6	70.6
Infant mortality (per 1 000 live births)	18.5	14.2	15.6	12.3	10.2	11.4
Under-five mortality rate (per 1 000 live births)	56.0	39.7	36.0	27.3	23.6	26.5
Adult Mortality Rate (15-59) per 1 000 population		64.6	47.9	56.6	54.9	52.4
Aggregate birth rate per 1 000 population[1]	22.5	15.0	10.6	11.7	13.8	13.8

Sources: UNICEF Social Monitor 2009; Statistical Yearbooks of Armenia.

1 Birth rates for 1990-2000 were calculated by the National Statistics Committee on the basis of the total number of population re-estimated as per the 2001 Population Census results.

Rates of infant, child, and maternal mortality have all declined. Infant mortality declined by about half since 2000 due to the improvements in primary health care interventions. The recent figure for infant mortality compares well with other transition countries. The estimated under-five-year child mortality rate (hereafter, U5MR) was 23.6 deaths per 1,000 live births in 2009, which was the lowest level of U5MR for the group of Southern Caucasus[2] and Central Asian countries[3] and approximately double the rate for Russia.[4] While the 2009 U5MR spiked to 42 in rural Armenia compared to an average 5.7 in Western European countries, indicators of mortality rates should be treated with a degree of caution (Hayrapetyan and Khanjian 2004:3). Among countries formerly in the Soviet Union, there are significant discrepancies between official infant mortality rates (IMR) and rates calculated from alternative sources (UNICEF 2001:9). These variations are explained by such factors as the definition of "live birth" and the non-registration of births. The adult mortality rate (ages 15-59) was 64.6 per 1,000 populations in 2006 and 52.4 for 2010. Non-communicable diseases such as cardiovascular disease, cancer, and accidents are the major causes of death among adults.

During the transition period, significant changes occurred in Armenia's demographic profile because high unemployment initiated a wave of migration from the country. An estimated 700,000 people left Armenia during the 1990s (Hovhannisyan *et al.* 2001). Due to the combined effects of emigration and a decline in the birth rate the population of the country 'aged' rapidly. The 2010 total fertility rate was 1.7 children per 1,000 females of reproductive age (15-49) compared with 1.5 the previous year. Both figures are significantly lower than the threshold of 2.1 births per 1,000 females of reproductive age required in order to maintain a stable population (Armenia Demographic and Health Survey 2010:8). Having small families has become a major trend in reproductive behavior in Armenia. Because fewer teenagers are now entering adult reproductive age due to the drastic post-1990 decrease in fertility, future growth of the population will be negatively affected.

During 1990-1994, the country experienced a dramatic drop (53%) in Gross Domestic Product (GDP) due to sharp decrease of industrial production combined with the inflation of prices. The greatest decrease in the volume of GDP was recorded in 1992 (42 percentage points), which was six times higher than in other CIS countries. In 1994 an increase in GDP was recorded, and since then, Armenia has had stable GDP growth for more than a decade. During 1994-1998, the GDP growth rate grew by 31.7% or 6.3% annually. However, by 1998 the level of GDP had approached only 61% of its 1990 level. During 2000-2007, GDP has increased 43% with an average annual growth rate of 11.75%.

2 Corresponding figures for Georgia and Azerbaijan are 29 and 34, respectively.

3 Central Asian average equals 43.

4 The corresponding figure for Russia is 12.

Table 2.2 Selected Economic Data

	1990	1995	2000	2005	2008	2009	2010
Total GDP[5] (US$ billions)	2.3	1.5	1.9	4.9	11.9	8.7	9.4
Total GDP[6] (US$ billions)	N/A	4.5	9.9	13.7	17.2	15.4	16.8
GDP per capita[7] (US$)	636	1 227	1 951	3 903	5 808	4 983	5 357

Sources: Total GDP CIA – The World Fact Book; IMF 2011. World Economic Outlook.

Since the global financial crisis and economic downturn that began in 2008, the rate of GDP growth has again declined. Moreover due to rising external debt in recent years and reliance on foreign remittances (estimated at 14% of GDP in 2007), Armenia faces considerable challenges. The decline in revenues from external sources has caused a major budget deficit. In 2008 Armenia's economic growth rate dropped to 6.8%. Instead of the World Bank's projected 11% decline of real GDP, a 14.4% downturn was observed in 2009 that has pushed the country 'into its worst recession since just after independence' (ADB 2010:106). As Table 2.2 indicates, by 2010 (<www.usaid.gov/our_work/environment/climate/country_nar/armenia.html>) – top Armenia's economy showed a slow recovery and ranked 130 in the world in GDP per capita (US$5,179).

Before the crisis, due to stable economic growth during the previous decade, Armenia had joined the group of middle-income economies. Economic growth had brought an increase in real wages, stabilized employment, and increased consolidated budget spending on social sectors. Combined with a growing inflow of private transfers, these measures contributed to significant poverty reduction in the country. However, the crisis caused rising unemployment. In 2009 the unemployment rate was 10% (CIA – The World Fact Book). Combined with the adverse effects of soaring food and fuel prices in 2008, it worsened economic prospects for those who were already poor.

Table 2.3 Rates of GDP Real Growth and Average Inflation

	1991-1995	1996-2000	2001-2005	2006-2007	2008	2009	2010
Average GDP real growth	−20.8	5.4	12.2	13.7	6.9	−14.4	4.7
Average inflation rate	1 261.5	44.6	4.1	4.4	8.4	6.5	6.9

Sources: CIA – The World Fact Book; IMF 2011. World Economic Outlook.

5 Estimated at market prices.
6 Estimated at purchasing power parity.
7 Estimated at purchasing power parity.

According to a recent study on the impacts of the financial crisis, the economic decline in Armenia had particularly serious consequences for poor and vulnerable groups and erased its achievements in poverty reduction during previous years (UNDP 2010). From the second quarter of 2008 to the second quarter of 2009, the level of extreme poverty nearly doubled from almost 4% to about 7%; the number of extremely poor individuals increased by over 107,000 (WFP 2010:99). Another 172,000 people fell below the poverty line between 2009 and 2010. The overall estimated number of the poor is currently 906,000 of whom 297,000 are extremely poor (UNDP 2010). Correspondingly, the incidence of poverty in 2009 was 34.1% compared to 27.9% in 2008 (Statistical Yearbook of Armenia 2010). The proportion of population living below the international poverty line (US$1.25 per day) was estimated to have reached 27% in 2009 (CIA – The World Fact Book). The share of the extremely poor in 2009 was 3.6% compared to 1.6% in 2008 (Statistical Yearbook of Armenia 2010). Consequently, the general population was forced to decrease private consumption. About 43% of the surveyed households in Armenia reduced food consumption, reduced or stopped medicine purchases and reduced or stopped visits to health services (Guerschanik Calvo 2010:29). The hardest hit were the households experiencing income shocks since reduction of expenditures was made in ways that increased their vulnerability.

According to WHO, government spending on health as a share of a country's GDP should not be less than 6%-9%, but budgetary expenditures on health care in Armenia plunged from about 2.7% of GDP in 1990 to 1.3% in 1997, and below 1% until 2000. Since then, spending channeled from the state budget to the health sector has been rather low (Table 2.4).

Table 2.4 Selected Health Care Expenditures (US$)

Expenditure Type	1990	1991	1995	2000	2005	2008	2009	2010
Private out-of-pocket outlays (estimates)	N/A	N/A	94.6	92.7	89.3	over 60	over 65	over 50
Total health expenditures (public + private), millions	N/A	15	34	252	645	below 410	below 330	below 320
Total health expenditures as percentage of GDP	2.7	N/A	2.4	1.9	1.4	1.55	1.8	1.72
Total health expenditures per capita	152[8]	N/A	27	39	72	98	86.4	103.8

Source: Developed by author based on information provided by the Ministry of Health.

8 Estimated in USSR rubles rather than converted to US$ because, during the USSR's final year, both official and real exchange rates varied greatly.

In 2000, public health care expenditure amounted to 4.4% of the state budget or about 1% of GDP; corresponding expenditures from the state budget for health care were nearly US$ 37 million (around AMD 21 billion). The situation began to improve in 2003 as strong economic growth enabled the country to reduce poverty rates with potential positive effects on health care access and equity. In 2005 the state health budget allocations increased to 7.4% of the state budget and comprised 1.4% of the GDP.

Although the state health budget in Armenia had been growing and was 1.8% of GDP in 2009, it decreased to 1.6% of GDP in 2010. However, these figures are lower than the average of 3-4% in low to middle income countries. Those indicators for other NIS countries are 4% in Belarus, 6.3% in Moldova and 5.4% in Azerbaijan. The increase was attributed to the high priority of health care in the allocation of funds across sectors of state budget. The government introduced budgetary policy that projected health care to reach 10% of the state budget by 2008 and 12% by 2015. The global economic crises, however, postponed implementation of state programs in Armenia and tested the resiliency of the country's reforms (Brainerd 2010).

Per capita public expenditures in the health sector can be compared with expenditures in other countries. WHO recommendations indicate that the minimal level of per capita financial resources should not be less than US$ 15 annually. Average health expenditures in Western Europe comprise 8-10% of GDP and annual expenditure per capita exceeds the recommended standard by more than 100 times. Armenia does not reach this standard and spends much less. During 1998-2002 per capita expenditures on health services were US$6-9.5 compared with US$2,000-2,500 in Europe, US$1,785 in Canada and US$4,235 in the USA (Tonoyan 2005:20). Even in low-income countries this figure was US$12.

While expenditures on health as percent of GDP are rising, the overall level remains low. In 2004, 53% of expenditures in health care were allocated to hospitals. Simultaneously, private expenditures on health care were higher than public expenditures – 4.6% versus 1.3% of GDP respectively.

During the Soviet era, government payments to hospitals were based on the number of beds, so Armenia built excess capacity in hospital beds. Together with low effectiveness of health care management and financing, oversupply as well as general socio-economic status of the population not only diminished demand but also caused under-consumption of services (Tonoyan 2004:11). In 2000, hospital bed occupancy rates fell more than 200% while home visits by doctors declined by over 30%. The implementation of optimization measures during the past two decades has substantially reduced the number of hospital beds in the country.

Table 2.5 Selected Health Care Resources

	1990	1995	2000	2005	2008	2009	2010
Physicians	14 630	12 657	12 270	12 307	12 929	13 177	13 591
Physicians per 100,000 people	410	337	323	382	399	406	417
Other health professionals	35 250	31 324	22 632	18 364	18 594	18 526	18 649
Others per 100,000 people	982	833	595	570	574	570	572
Hospital beds	32 500	28 711	20 795	14 353	12 358	12 068	12 160
Beds per 100,000 people	860	762	547	446	381	371	373

Source: Statistical Yearbooks of Armeni.

Between 1990 and 2002, the number of physicians fell but then increased. However, the number of other health professionals showed a stable decline over the two decades. Although the number of physicians per capita is nearly twice as large in Armenia as in western countries, physicians are not evenly distributed. In 2010, the number of physicians per 100,000 people in urban areas was 650, while it varied between 14 and 32 in rural areas.

2.2 Normative Issues

As a set of values and beliefs with learned behaviors shared within society, culture provides a sense of identity and belonging. Armenians are proud of being the first nation to adopt Christianity in the early fourth century. The Armenian alphabet invented in the fifth century by Mashtots gave Armenians a cultural and religious identity as well as the means to survive as a nation despite the efforts of larger and more powerful neighbors to subsume or exterminate them. Having an alphabet allowed Armenia to change its cultural orientation from the Iranian East towards the Christian Mediterranean West and to develop its own scholarly institutions and literature within a century (Gewertz 2005). Armenians became independent, almost self-sufficient, and impervious to attempts by powerful empires to re-impose their culture on them. Armenians' cultural orientation influences them as individuals, families, community members and professionals as well as shapes their organizational culture. On a daily basis it influences how they interact with others within and across regional and national borders. Consequently, some stereotyped cultural perceptions exist that are caused by the country's current or historical relations with other countries.

The history of the Armenian people was wrought during centuries of exposure to dominant cultures based on a constant tension with the more powerful ruling majority. This fact had lasting effects on the development of Armenian cultural orientations. Living under dominant cultures, the Armenian community was forced to focus on strengthening internal community and family ties that served to preserve their national identity. Though the Armenian community spent much more time under the rule of the Ottoman Empire, the social and cultural effects of exposure to communism are omnipresent in the country. Soviet values about the functioning of the state still influence the consciousness of political leaders of the country, while corruption and the lack of enforcement of the rule of law permeate society (Ohanian 2007). The struggle between values perceived in Armenian society as European (the rule of law, civil rights, freedom of the press, women's rights) and the lasting effect of Soviet suppression of ideas, beliefs and values has left the country striving towards progressive goals that cannot be reached due to incompatible cultural mentalities. With the opportunity for self-government as a completely free polity came the responsibility of breaking down the cultural impediments that have perpetuated a value system characterized by dangerous precedents and obstacles to universally progressive and just concepts.

Armenia has a traditional patriarchal culture in which the women and men have different status and standards of behavior to which they are held. Females usually keep a lower social profile and practise discretion in public (*e.g.*, not smoking in public or drinking in bars) in order to avoid developing an undesirable reputation. To be accepted as professionals and to gain the professional respect of colleagues in the workplace, female professionals have to work harder than their male counterparts. Since respect comes with age in Armenia, younger professionals have to work harder than their older colleagues.

Investigation by cross-cultural researchers and international consultants to analyze and identify basic values prevailing in Armenian society revealed cultural values that constitute a permanent part of Armenian mentality. Based on Hofstede's studies, Armenian cultural values place the country among the countries with high power distance that indicates importance of hierarchy in the society. Avoidance of uncertainty, which is in direct proportion to the degree of freedom in the country, displays high need among Armenians to control uncertainty. On both values Armenia has a rating close to France and India. Consequently, political discussions are usually handled with great care and some of an individual's personal beliefs may best remain undisclosed.

Armenian cultural values were long based on the family unit, the Church, and a collectivity principle. Correspondingly, Armenia falls into the group of countries with a collective mentality in which the group is valued over the individual and the individual's responsibility to the group overrides the individual's rights. In this type of culture characterized by high power distance and strong collective mentality, employees expect an autocratic management style, offset by the support given to the subordinate's family. High power distance, combined with high avoidance of uncertainty, gives rise to a pyramid-shaped bureaucratic structure that is both formal and centralized. Work procedures and relationships among individuals are formally established through strict regulations and laws or custom and tradition. Group solidarity in Armenia is very important with priority to protect achievements rather than take risks in an uncertain future.

During recent decades, income inequality in Armenia increased dramatically, which has led to polarization in society and contributed to an increased gap in the quality of health care provided to the poor and the better-off. The income of Armenians derives from various sources. The main source for all groups is income received for work performed although the share of wages in total income has fallen sharply. Earned income is not adequate to maintain a proper level of welfare because it forms less than the half of total income of population. Remittances from abroad and other profits have become much more important sources of income than before the transition.

Pensions are another source of income that plays a critical role in supporting the poorest households in Armenia. As there are no private pension funds, welfare issues concerning the elderly are significant in Armenia. Pensioners number about 18% of the population and the low pensions are an important factor contributing to inequality. In order to improve the state pension system, the government increased the level of contributions for certain income groups and increased the amount of the minimal monthly pension. However, pensions remain low relative to average wages[9] and are the lowest among NIS countries (Tonoyan 2005:17). Almost 97% of pensioners need constant medication and 41% need home care (Information Agency Regnum).

The system of state social assistance was gradually improving to provide targeted funds to the poorest population groups that allowed the state to reduce the social risks related to the low and inconstant incomes of vulnerable groups and to ensure that they receive a minimum level of welfare. Until 1997, state social assistance in

9 Under the state pension system the average pension in January 2010 was AMD24,617 while the minimal salary was AMD30,000. The Republic of Armenia does not formally define the minimum pension, but informally it equals the amount of the basic pension, which at present is AMD8,000.

Armenia followed the former Soviet Union (FSU) approach of benefits provided to certain population groups (the elderly, children, people with disabilities and those citizens who had completed a special service to the state such as participants in the Great Patriotic War or heroes of labor) under a defined system of state privileges. In 1997, a shift occurred from the system of privileges to a system of monetary compensations for privileges provided to certain groups (children, people with disabilities, pensioners) defined by corresponding legislation. However, this monetary compensation was allocated without taking into account the level of the household's welfare so it caused an ineffective distribution of scarce state budget funds available for social assistance. On the other hand, after the destructive earthquake in 1988, Armenia received humanitarian assistance that was either targeted on certain population groups or provided to people whatever their level of vulnerability. Neither approach ensured equity or effectiveness of distribution.

In order to ensure equity and effectiveness of social assistance, a shift was implemented towards targeted social policy based on a system of Poverty Family Benefits (PFB). To define the level of assistance for each registered household, a system called 'Paros' for assessing household vulnerability was introduced in 1994. In 1999, the PFB system replaced the system of state compensation and humanitarian assistance distribution in the sphere of social assistance. Based on the principle of voluntary involvement and targeted on the neediest, PFB recognizes the targeted household subject to state social assistance and defines:

- the vulnerability level of the household based on a set of socio-economic indicators;
- a certain marginal score for the level of welfare of the household that serves as a basis for allocating state social assistance; and
- the amount of the benefit depending on the size, composition or level of vulnerability of the household.

The following social programs currently exist in Armenia:

- Basic programs of PFB and lump sum financial assistance,
- Social pensions,
- Child allowance for children under two years of age,
- Lump sum childbirth allowance (funded by the state Social Insurance Fund),
- Provision and repair of free compensatory aids and rehabilitation devices for the disabled,
- Residential care for old people and children without parental care,
- Home care for the elderly and the disabled living alone,
- State assistance for young people leaving care institutions,
- Benefit for work that provides temporary employment.

In addition to state programs of social assistance, humanitarian aid and separate charity programs are implemented through international donor organizations and local non-governmental organizations based on household vulnerability scores.

Implementation of targeted social assistance programs has had a positive impact by reducing extreme poverty. However, the high level of unemployment, general poverty of the population, and the existence of a hidden economy as well as selective taxation allow the PFB system to satisfy only the needs of those below the poverty line (nearly one-third of the population). During recent years, the authorities focused on increasing the size of benefits and improving the targeting of the system. However, their efforts have not yet solved the problem. Currently, 110,000 families in Armenia receive the PFB that total AMD 35 billion (US$400 million).

The 2004 Law on Minimum Consumer Basket and Minimum Living Standards Budget provided the legal basis to compute and approve a minimum consumer basket and minimum living standards as well as to regulate activities related to state social policy implementation. The Ministry of Health is responsible for compilation of the minimum food basket, and the Ministry of Labor and Social Issues is responsible for calculation of the non-food part of the minimum basket based on the results of households' living standards surveys implemented by the Republic of Armenia's National Statistical Services. The minimum consumer budget serves as a basis for defining the amount of minimum salary, pension, and state social assistance.

Currently, to avoid pushing the great majority of the country's population into poverty, the government borrows externally to implement public programs in the social sphere and to improve the targeting of pro-poor protection programs. The 2011 State Budget allocates additional tax revenues towards the settlement of social problems. Estimated at US$200 million this insufficient amount calls for implementation of other more efficient state mechanisms.

Like other countries that emerged after the collapse of the Soviet Union, Armenia displays both democratic and autocratic characteristics with poor quality of governance as well as lack of transparent and democratic political leadership. Political parties have rigid structures with top-down internal management styles heavily dependent on the personality of the party chair and top leaders (USAID 2005). Powerful oligarchs, well-established informal institutions,[10] and high inequality of income and property limit inclusion of the general public in political and economic life.

10 In 2010, of the 178 economies in the world, Armenia ranked 123rd on Transparency International's Perception of Corruption Index.

Health care reforms were based on an understanding that free health services could no longer be provided to the whole population. Most people had to pay the full cost of medical services. Although government tried to provide free medical care to vulnerable groups of the population through state-guaranteed programs, under-financing of the health sector necessitated partial payments by even the persons included in these groups. Moreover, the low priority given to health by the government limited the available public resources. Furthermore, since the poor consume relatively more PHC services, allocation health budgets to secondary and tertiary care violated the principle of equity in health care in terms of access, finance, expenditure and outcomes. Therefore, poor consumers were affected by both the quality and price of care. Correspondingly, the poor tended to seek publicly subsidized care much less frequently than the well-off. This imbalance led to an increase of morbidity with regard to chronic pathologies, length of illnesses as well as initial diagnosis (Tonoyan 2004:13).

The situation began to improve in 2003 as the state health budget allocations gradually increased year by year. Thus, in 2006 there was a 21% increase in the government budget for the health sector, most of which was spent on primary health care. The main focus in arrangements for health care was on the development of an ambulatory-polyclinic system through forming the family medicine system and ensuring an adequate volume and quality of free ambulatory polyclinic services.

Major components of the second stage of reforming the health care system reform process started in 2004. These involved infrastructure development, provision of modern equipment to health facilities in rural areas, and upgrading of PHC service providers' knowledge and skills in order to increase geographical and financial access of the most vulnerable population to basic health services. The main tasks of the health system reforms were to improve access to state-guaranteed free medical care, to balance social and market values in the sector, to reorient health services towards a balanced partnership between primary and hospital care, to promote health and prevent disease through tackling the determinants of health and to shift from the narrow biomedical model towards a social, multi-professional, and multi-sectoral approach to health and health care. In order to ensure the hygiene and epidemiological security of the population, it was planned to intensify activities aimed at preventing infectious and mass non-infectious diseases. The main direction in drug and technological policy was identified as the improvement of their accessibility, safety, and rational use. Actions are taken to improve the state system of drug quality assurance, to introduce new prescription forms, and to ensure affordability of drug prices.

In order to improve health care in Armenia, one government priority has been to increase public funds allocated to the health sector. The Poverty Reduction Strategy adopted for the period of 2004-2015 envisages an average annual growth of 1% in public expenditures. Thus, public expenditure in the health sector as a percentage of GDP is planned to reach 2.5% of GDP in 2015. The main sources of such growth will be the collection of revenues from domestic sources and projects financed by foreign sources. The increase in budget allocations is targeted to raise salaries of PHC medical personnel, to allocate capital spending to improve buildings, and to supply modern equipment, medicines and medical materials. Having grown throughout the period from 2003 to 2010, the share of PHC care in total health expenditures is expected to increase to half of total sector expenditures in 2015.

2.3 Governance of the Health Sector

Currently, the Ministry of Health of the Republic of Armenia manages the health budget while the State Health Agency (SHA) is responsible for purchasing a defined Basic Benefits Package (BBP) for the population. The BBP has been widely used throughout NIS as state health systems transform themselves from one in which all expenses are covered by the state towards a mixed system in which state budget transfers are augmented by formal patient copayments and, in case of Armenia, subsidies from the World Bank to pay some of the transaction costs (PADCO 2002).

The health care system is financed from national and international sources. National sources are the state budget and direct out-of-pocket payments (OPPs) by the population. Apart from international sources, the main formal financing source is the state budget that generates its funds from general tax revenue. No health funds exist; there is no mandatory health insurance and very little voluntary health insurance. The pension system is separated from the health care system. Households must cover health care costs that remain uncovered by the state. A single provider may receive funding from one or more national sources: the national budget through the Ministry of Health, local budgets through regional or local government levels, and payments out of pocket by patients.

The 1996 Medical Care Act created a legal environment enabling a public-private mix to finance health care. This law stipulated that the public budget was no longer the sole authorized financing source and legalized alternative financing mechanisms. Direct OPPs were introduced in 1997 for the majority of health care services beyond the BBP and payable by non-vulnerable and non-targeted groups of the population. Health providers were allowed to mobilize funds from various sources, including local budgets, external aid, health insurance payments and private payments out of pocket.

Incorporation of direct payments by patients into the funding system undermines the principle of equity in the provision of the health care services with respect to access, fairness and equality, and imposes financial risk on many Armenians. According to some experts direct payments by the population in 2002 were about three times more than budget funding (Hakobyan *et al.* 2006). Moreover, a study funded by the World Bank demonstrated that real financial flows to the hospital sector (including direct payments for drugs, food and medical personnel services) were from 3.5 to 4 times greater than funds allocated from the state budget. In 2008, as a share of total health expenditures, household out-of-pocket expenditures comprised 50%, which was the highest in the region (USAID 2010). The survey results indicated that some of the services covered by BBP were still paid by households out of pocket (USAID 2008). According to estimates by the World Bank, the 'shadow market' of paid medical services attributed to 'informal' payments of patients in the health sector in Armenia is the highest among CIS countries – 91% compared to 74% in Russia (WB 2000, cited in Tonoyan 2004:23). In 2002, the government of Armenia planned to raise access to health care for poor and vulnerable groups by 2009 (National Policy on Population Health Protection of the Republic of Armenia).

Currently, out-of-pocket payments comprise at least half of Armenian health care expenditures and, at least 80% of those are informal payments that exceed acceptable levels by European standards where 'direct' payments are only 5%-7% of medical funding. Such a high level of an inequitable source of financing greatly undermines the degree of population protection. Unsurprisingly, according to WHO, Armenia is among the top ten countries in Europe with the highest share of out-of-pocket payments and has one of the lowest positions in financial protection rankings (Yeghiyan 2010). WHO predicted that the global financial crisis would greatly affect the health systems of low and middle income countries that primarily rely on general taxation and direct payments. Consequently, the decrease in economic activities within the country negatively impacts the effectiveness of general taxation schemes in health care financing and so the recent progress observed in Armenia in reduction of OPPs might not be sustainable.

International funding sources include humanitarian aid, donations of medical supplies, equipment and project-specific support through credit or grant programs financed by foreign governments, international donor organizations or multilateral agencies. Grants and credit projects constitute the dominant form of external support that is coordinated by the Ministry of Health.

During the course of reforms contracts were standardized and a provider payment methodology was developed. Health care contracts defined the relationship between consumers or purchasers and health care providers. Contracting is implemented through the State

Health Agency that is a part of the government acting as a third purchasing party. Payment can go to the service provider (physician) directly or to the facility. However, overlaps in coverage and unclear specification of the BBP still hinder the potential benefits of the purchasers' purchasing power (Yeghiyan 2010).

Mechanisms of financing health care were changed. Hospital payment systems based on per diem per patient financing was replaced with case-based financing. Ambulatory care payment systems based on per visit mechanism changed to per capita financing. A global budget mechanism was introduced to the inpatient and outpatient emergency care system. Transition to new financing mechanisms had some positive results; however, reduction in the budget allocations for health care taken place in 1998-2000 caused serious problems in the delivery of health care services. In addition, a major part of budget allocations were channeled to hospital services instead of redistributing them to PHC facilities. The situation began to improve in 2003 as state health budget allocations comprised 1.4% of GDP; nearly 56% of corresponding expenditures from the state budget for health care was distributed to inpatient care, 34% to primary care, 3% to hygienic and anti-epidemic services and 8% to other services and programs (Tonoyan 2004:21).

The goal of financial reforms in health care is financial improvement of the sector, including the efficient use of budgets, reduction of unofficial turnover, introduction of objective criteria for counterpart payments, establishing clinical-economic standards, and reimbursement for provided services as well as ensuring transparency. Policy objectives include 'shifting to cost containment and efficiency' (Langenbrunner 2003:186). Therefore, the next generations of payment incentives are coming into service such as developing hospital global budgets and capitation beyond per diem and per case systems. In order to improve cost efficiency, it is planned to practice selection-based placement. Distinct steps in that direction include execution of an experimental method of specific financing mechanism including compensation co-payment for services provided within state order (for BBP hospital services), which is piloted in four medical centres (MCs) in Yerevan starting from July 2010.

To improve technical equipment of service providers, medical equipment acquired through budgetary allocations and international grants is provided first to PHC facilities with preference given to regional medical institutions. Then, on a competitive basis, it is provided to second- and third-level medical institutions that provide accessible medical care to vulnerable groups.

Of the 82 hospitals in Armenia, 59 are public under the management of the Ministry of Health or regional governments, while 23 are private. Of the 467 PHC facilities,

380 facilities are physician-based in the public sector, 69 are physician-based in the private sector and 18 are under other governmental bodies or departments. There are 638 non-physician-based PHC clinics in the public sector, almost all of which are distributed around the *marzes* of the country. There are no private non-physician-based PHC facilities in Armenia (WHO 2009:6).

A series of reforms were aimed at progressive decentralization and strategic prioritization of the health care system focused on development of PHC and access to health care for vulnerable groups. Due to institutional changes in the governance of the health care sector the Ministry of Health was substantially reduced in size. The Ministry remained responsible for policy formulation, overseeing implementation of reforms, monitoring population's health status and health care provision, determining the terms of medical education, licensing, regulation and setting standards (PADCO 2000). The responsibility for financing was transferred to the State Health Agency that distributes the state allocation to health care facilities and takes full responsibility for management of state financial resources.

The Armenian health system is subject to state control. Until recently, it was deprived of any competitive forces since PHC facilities were state-owned and directly managed by health authorities. Changing the status of secondary health facilities from economically dependent state enterprises to state-owned closed joint-stock companies gave health care facilities managerial and budgetary autonomy and rights to establish contacts with public and private providers. Approval in 2000 of the concept paper "On the Privatization of Healthcare Facilities" paved the way for the beginning of privatization. Since then many hospital services and some PHC services have been privatized. The State Health Agency assumed a strategic purchasing role. Service providers are able to contact the SHA for the services included in the BBP, but they are not allowed to decide on the volume or price of these services. Service providers also negotiate and sign contracts with private enterprises to provide health services.

The changed policies affected stakeholder groups in different ways depending on their relationships to the sector by making them compromise on degrees of control and influence over the reform process. Due to the change in the country's administrative-territorial division in 1996, a split occurred among national, regional and local levels of health care that substantially weakened the mechanisms of quality control and management in the health care system. In the course of the reforms, the Ministry of Health had six ministers who in turn changed their working groups, modified the direction of the reform process and brought their own visions of the health system that caused a degree of instability in the sector. Although the government adopted several health policy reform documents, those documents did not ensure sustainability of each reform or its implementation (Tonoyan 2004:10).

Politics in Armenia occurs within the framework of a presidential representative democratic republic. The President ensures compliance with the Constitution, the normal operation of the legislative, the executive and the judiciary, and serves as the guarantor of sovereignty, territorial integrity and security of the Republic. The President is the Head of Government and of a multi-party system. Executive power is exercised by the government. Legislative power is vested in both the government and Parliament. The unicameral Parliament (*Azgayin Zhoghov* or National Assembly) is currently controlled by a coalition of four political parties: the conservative Republican Party, the Prosperous Armenia Party, the Rule of Law Party and the Armenian Revolutionary Federation.

2.4 HISTORY OF HEALTH REFORMS IN ARMENIA

As a part of Soviet health care, the Armenian health system guaranteed free medical assistance and access to a complete range of public health care services to the entire population. The principle of universal coverage ensured equity and access to of primary, secondary and tertiary health care services. However, the system as a whole was inefficient and emphasized quantitative indicators that led to over-capacity, too many hospital beds and excess medical staff. The system was highly centralized through strong vertical management with strict top-down control over expenditures of public resources. The state budget was the primary funding source for health care. Allocation of financing of the system was based on five-year central plans from Moscow. The state determined the level, composition and mechanisms for allocation of public spending based on national norms, and ensuring the provision of health care services in compliance with certain standards.

Each administrative district of the country had 'a hospital and associated polyclinic providing ambulatory and primary care' (Hovhannisyan *et al.* 2001) to its residents. In rural areas services were 'provided with health posts (with inpatient units), ambulatories and feldsher stations. As health professionals trained in nursing and midwifery with extended training in clinical diagnosis and pharmacology, feldshers were authorized to provide basic treatment and to prescribe a restricted number of drugs at feldsher-accoucher posts/stations with no assigned doctor. Local governments were directly responsible for financing district health facilities.

Primary care was also provided in corresponding 'occupational health care facilities (Balabanova *et al.* 2004) for those employed in specific sectors of the economy'. Facilities attached to large enterprises, such as factories, received considerable subsidies from their associated enterprises. PHC facilities were maintained for the defense forces, for the KGB and for the Communist Party elite under the supervision of a corresponding subdivision of the Ministry of Health, which received substantially higher levels of funding.

Investments in the sector were predominantly allocated for developing a hospital system that provided specialized secondary health care. This strategy brought chronic technological underdevelopment and underutilized PHCs located at urban ambulatory-polyclinic facilities and rural feldsher stations that provided basic services to population of rural areas. Substantial disparities existed in the quality of health care between urban and rural localities as well as between the capital Yerevan and other urban areas that caused patient flows from the regions to the capital city. Access to technically sophisticated modern health care varied in different localities since the failing Soviet economy could not provide the increasingly technical model of health care emerging in the West. Due to inadequate managerial capacity, even limited available financial resources were used inefficiently. Most health facilities were in poor physical condition and had outdated medical equipment and supplies. However, the system still managed to provide universal basic health care and within it an effective system of immunization programs, an achievement that in many of the newly independent states did not survive the break-up of the Soviet Union (Balabanova *et al.* 2004).

When its economic transition began in the early 1990s, Armenia experienced deep political and social transformation. Severe economic crisis and sociopolitical problems affected the status of health services and undermined the public health achievements of the socialist era. Government revenues were no longer able to sustain the inherited system (Shishkin 1999, cited in Balabanova *et al.* 2004), which caused a dramatic decline in the level of health expenditures and, eventually, the collapse of public health activities. Long periods of non-payment of wages to medical personnel as well as lack of financing to maintain health facilities and equipment and to ensure adequate supplies undermined the quality of health services. In addition, the influx of refugees and injured persons due to the Nagorno-Karabakh conflict put a strain on the health care system. By 1997, the main source of financing for the health care system had become private payments out of pocket. Increased poverty meant most of the population was unable to pay for basic health care that, in turn, led to a decline in the utilization of health services, a resurgence of communicable diseases associated with poverty (WHO 2005) and damaged the health status of Armenians. Patients with chronic diseases suffered considerably while rates of mortality and morbidity increased, especially among adults. A major concern of authorities became enhancing accessibility and affordability to PHC services for vulnerable population groups and ensuring overall sustainability of health care provision.

The initial steps of Armenian health reforms were taken after the collapse of the Soviet Union in 1991, but achieved their full scale only after the adoption of the Constitution in 1995. Reforms were incorporated in the initial phase of overall public sector reforms associated with the transition towards market economy principles and liberal democracy.

The rationalization of the system with its excess of personnel and facilities and the reallocation of savings on complementary inputs were major challenges. 'To reallocate expenditures most effectively, the government needed to decide what kind of healthcare system they want, including who provides what and who pays for what' (WB 2001:87). Health reforms introduced by the government 'were based on the assumption that healthcare cannot be provided free of charge' (Selimyan and Daniyelyan 2005:4) and the need to ensure health services for vulnerable groups. Given the inherited system of inefficient health care with its imbalanced structure of services, the reforms focused on three areas: decentralization, devolution and privatization; alternation of financing mechanisms; and effective management.

Adoption of corresponding legislation and implementation of structural and functional reforms of territorial government allowed a decentralization of the health care sector that prioritized developing and strengthening the PHC system. In the 1996 Law on Local Self-government, responsibility for provision of health services and ownership of facilities transferred from central government to local governments (PHC facilities – polyclinics, rural ambulatory facilities, health posts and feldsher stations) and regional governments (hospitals); financial responsibility was devolved to facility level. Adoption of relevant laws enabled privatization of hospitals as well as pharmaceutical and dental health facilities. Decentralization expanded the institutional autonomy, administrative rights and responsibilities of service providers who were allowed to sell their services to the Ministry of Health. However, the top-down approach in the decentralization process considerably weakened vertical and horizontal administrative links between the Ministry, local/regional governments and service providers who deliver different levels and types of health care services.

During the initial stage of devolution in the mid-1990s and until the establishment of the State Health Agency in 1998, local and regional authorities had a degree of independence from the Ministry of Health with respect to their functions. These included negotiating contracts with regional and local providers of health care, monitoring service quality and amending regional and local health care budgets. However, the Ministry retained responsibility for setting prices and defining the coverage of services. With the establishment of the State Health Agency, the Ministry of Health retained responsibility for tertiary-level institutions but responsibility for managing state health care financial resources as well as the authority to reimburse service providers for the public package of services was transferred to the State Health Agency. The latter performs the functions of a social health insurance fund (HIF), is publicly owned and has a high degree of control over assets. While the State Health Agency makes payments to health facilities on behalf of the poor, the payments to hospitals and polyclinics covers only part of the health services provided to the poor and vulnerable groups.

The legal status of the state-owned health care facilities was changed several times and 'remained poorly defined' for a certain period of time (PADCO 2002). At first state-owned health care facilities were given the legal status of state enterprises and financed in accordance with the volume of services they provided. Following the adoption in 1996 of the Law on Joint-stock Companies, the status of those facilities was changed in 1998 to state-owned joint-stock companies owned either by state or by corresponding regional and local governments. Thus, hospitals and polyclinics were delegated responsibilities for managing their financial resources, setting prices for those services that were not included in the BBP, making decisions on staffing issues as well as setting terms and conditions of services delivered. They were allowed to retain profits and invest surplus income at their discretion. For provision of services included in the BBP, separate facilities contracted with the State Health Agency in accordance with the levels of volume and price established by the Ministry of Health. Although facilities were permitted to negotiate and sign contracts with insurance companies and/or enterprises wishing to purchase health care, this did not happen in practice. Members of vulnerable groups were allowed free health care services at hospitals while the rest of public paid fees (with exceptions for emergency cases and diseases of social significance).

The BBP was introduced in 1997 after adoption of a government decree on 'Provision of Services Free of Charge to the Population' that enabled the state to cope with budgetary constraints by reducing its obligations for providing health care. The BBP is reviewed annually for changes indicated by the economic situation. However, given the lack of financing, this process was formalized only in 2004. At first the BBP defined some population groups (three categories of disabled, orphans under 18, veterans, families of war victims, families with more than three children, and children under 18 with one parent) and some diseases of social significance (oncological, mental diseases, sexually transmitted diseases, tuberculosis and malaria) as eligible to receive specific health care services and medicines free of charge. For members of those vulnerable groups and diseases of social significance, the government provided guaranteed full or partial subsidies for services and medicines. Initially, BBP covered mostly primary care with secondary care only for the poor. Subsequently, to improve accessibility to health care services by the poor, the government extended eligibility for the free BBP program to beneficiaries of the family poverty benefit system starting from 2001. At present, universal coverage is provided for primary and outpatient services; selected secondary services are available only to the poor.[11] Basic health services and lab tests at polyclinics are free of charge for everyone. However, state allocations remain too

11 It should be mentioned that eligibility for state programs includes those classified according to a proxy means test. However, the eligibility threshold for the poverty family benefit program is lower than for qualification under the health program. Therefore, notable gaps still exist in targeting the poor and ensuring accessibility of health services by the poor.

low to meet the costs of the BBP. Moreover, lack of awareness among vulnerable groups[12] about services under BBP and differences in the quality of services provided pose important issues about access and financial protection in Armenia's health care system.

PHC facilities (polyclinics) were freed from hospital administrative supervision, although this approach to devolution has a trial-and-error character. Gradually the share of basic PHC services in the budget was increasing. Thus, in 2005, basic PHC services represented 65% of the Ministry's PHC budget, and virtually the entire population was considered to be a potential beneficiary. Since late 2006, PHC services (including lab tests) were provided at no charge for whole population. And Yerevan-based polyclinics and hospitals were merged into MCs.

After establishment of the Public Sector Reform Commission (PSRC) by government decree, reforms of the public sector began within the framework of the Armenia Public Sector Reform Program (APSREP). During 1996-2003, international development partners and donor organizations provided both technical assistance and financial support. The World Bank and the United Kingdom's DFID provided methodological guidance for reforms of the Armenian public sector by working with government authorities, state institutions and the PSRC. Reforms of central government included the reorganization and restructuring of ministries. During 1999-2001, two levels of management (line ministries and three types of bodies below them: agencies, inspectorates and state noncommercial organizations) were established. Deconcentration across the government enabled separate functions of policy development, inspection and service provision 'to redesign purpose and scope of functions, rationalize them and introduce new activities' (Hovsepyan and Khudaverdyan 2006:13). A functional remit given to the Ministry of Health allowed it to concentrate on strategic policy matters and to ensure vertical hierarchy of sector governance. The adoption of the Law on State Non-commercial Organizations in 2002 stipulated reconstitution of public health care services and provided facilities to state non-commercial organizations.

The initial phase of privatization of enterprises through open subscription for capital stocks began in 1995. In the course of privatization of health care facilities during 1996-1997, 116 facilities were privatized – mostly pharmacies, medical equipment services and dental polyclinics – through the transfer or sale of government facilities to for-profit

12 Among mentioned population groups included in state order programs in the BBP financed by the SHA, the rationale for disabled categories II and III needs closer scrutiny. Current disability certification process for obtaining the status of category II or III does not allow including people necessarily deserving subsidized health care than the average individual or household. Total spending on these two groups is estimated at about 5% of the total health budget (WB 2011b).

or non-profit-making persons or legal entities licensed by the Ministry of Health to provide health care services. Adopted in 2000, a document entitled "Concept of the Strategy of Privatization of Health care Facilities" set out policy objectives for the privatization of health care facilities. Those objectives are to:

- improve transparency of financial flows,
- attract additional financial resources through private investments,
- enhance the effectiveness and efficiency of used resources,
- increase the quality and diversity of services and providers, and
- expand choice for health care users and facilitate a competitive environment.

This document prohibited the privatization of some health care services and providers, including most urban and rural PHC facilities, services of the State Health Agency, national blood services, infectious disease hospitals and forensic medicine commissioner departments.

In 2003, privatization of other health care facilities was implemented in Yerevan that involved secondary and tertiary health care facilities with nearly 1,300 hospital beds. Private inpatient hospital beds are 9.2% of all hospital beds in Armenia compared to 4.0% in the ten states that joined the European Union in May 2004 and 22% in the 15 countries that belonged to the EU before May 2004 (WHO 2005). Data are, however, difficult to compare because of differences in definitions of what is considered to be a 'private' inpatient bed.

At this stage, the decentralization and privatization steps 'were not accompanied by strengthened regulation and supervision arrangements raising concerns about possible financial mismanagement and the fulfillment of social functions' since the government had not managed to regulate the market for the provision of health care properly as well as to ensure health care access, quality and safety (USAID 2010). Because the privatization of hospitals is often associated with corruption, in order to eliminate incidents of 'fraudulent activity and political patronage in the sensitive social sector' (Hakobyan *et al.* 2006), the process of privatization ended in 2003. Built on international guidelines, the 2002 Law on Protection of Economic Competition prohibits anti-competitive agreements and the abuse of a dominant position, defines concentration and, above a certain threshold, creates a notification obligation. However, the impact of activities to combat corruption has been minor due to weak enforcement of corresponding legislation and implementation gaps.

Changes in financing mechanisms included diversification of sector revenue sources, improving financial management and linking the financing of health care to the quality and volume of services provided. Although hospitals were allowed 'to sell health services to the public and generate revenues since 1993' (Tonoyan 2004), the legal framework for introducing other means to finance health care, including user-charges, appeared in 1996 in the Law on Medical Aid and Services to the Population. The law identified the responsibility of the state for developing and implementing of health programs and stipulated the right to receive medical aid and services free of charge within the framework of state health target programs, guaranteed by the state, and beyond the framework of state programs. To ensure competition among service providers and to promote the improvement of service provision quality, the Law introduced an open enrollment mechanism that established the right for patients to select health care providers of their choice. This mechanism presupposed engagement of ethical, patient-focused, and clinically and managerially skilled health care professionals in the PHC system. The law also specified financing sources for health care services as the state budget, insurance contributions, direct payments, and other sources not prohibited by law.

In 1997, the government of Armenia adopted the Decree on Health Target Programs that introduced official user-charges for health care services. However, the low level of medical personnel salaries contributed to the institutionalization of a system of informal payments throughout the state-funded health care system. While entrepreneurs were allowed to establish private practice in the health care sector, the legislation poorly regulated the status, structure and provision of services by private providers. In this situation of increased financial autonomy, the change of financing mechanisms had not ensured increased quality and cost-effectiveness of services provided. In the great majority of cases, patients faced the necessity of paying both types of fees: officially established and unofficial. Correspondingly, after the privatization of health care facilities and the changed financial mechanisms, health care services became unaffordable for most Armenians. Access to health care became increasingly dependent on whether a household could afford the 'informal' payments to doctors. A 2003 survey in Armenia by the Institute of Advanced Studies within the European Union's Copernicus Program found that 77.5% of Armenian households with the fewest assets could not afford health care services. The same study found 56% made an out-of-pocket payment. More than half of hospital beds had not been used for years while self-sustaining medical institutions had been unable to pay wages to their staff (Tonoyan 2004). Moreover, informal payments made to medical personnel rather than their institutions as well as lack of funding had adverse impacts on investments in the assets of medical institutions.

The Ministry of Health is the highest executive authority that elaborates and implements the policies of Armenian government in the health care sector. The Ministry is responsible for the sustainable provision of services to the population. The authority of the Ministry is based on decisions of the government of Armenia such as laws, orders and decrees of the President. To enhance accessibility of health services, increase efficiency and ensure sustainable management and operation of the sector, the Government of Armenia approved a number of laws and normative documents in order to regulate relationships within the sector. Adopted in 1995, the Program for Development and Reform of the Healthcare System of the Republic of Armenia for 1996-2000 identified the areas of reform, including management, infrastructure, finance and medical education. Other important laws that facilitated implementation of sector reforms were:

- 1992: Law on Sanitary-Epidemic Safety for the Population,
- 1995: The Constitution that set out the right of individuals to health protection and affirmed protection of family, maternity and childhood by the state,
- 1997: Decree on Provision of Services Free of Charge to the Population that stipulated introduction of the first state Basic Benefit Package,
- 1997: Decree on Health Target Programs and State Order of the Republic of Armenia that introduced official user-charges, and
- 1998: Law on Pharmaceuticals that addressed all aspects of the procurement and supply of pharmaceuticals in Armenia.

Based on the 1997 Decree, the SHA was established in 1998 as purchaser of publicly financed health care services and made responsible for national budgets and expenditures. Financing of the system is based on fees for services covered under BBP and capitation taxes. The SHA is responsible for reimbursing health care service providers. A provider payment methodology was developed, contracts were standardized, and the SHA pays hospitals and polyclinics on behalf of the poor. However, according to estimates (WB 2003), state payments to health care providers in 2002 covered only 45% of the cost of services. Informal payments finance the balance.

The Strategy of Healthcare System Development in Armenia 2000-2003 formulated objectives and goals to increase the quality and accessibility of services delivered in both ambulatory and inpatient settings, and to improve organization and management of the system. This document outlined the directions to achieve goals of promoting PHC and to balance social and market values in the health care sector as well as changes in the institutional and regulatory frameworks and government policies. Since 2006, BBP provides universal coverage for PHCs. The government of Armenia adopted the concept of PHC development for 2008-2013 that envisages technical equipment of polyclinics with primary attention to regional facilities. It plans to repair 50 ambulatories and 110 feldsher stations, retrain 150 doctors and nurses every year as well as increase the salary of medical personnel by 30%. The concept paper anticipates increasing budget allotments to 30%-35% annually (from AMD 19 billion in 2008 to AMD 47 billion in 2011) and providing pregnant women with certificates for free obstetric care in order to pay for childbirth (Qushqyan 2010).

Since public spending remains insufficient to cover the health costs of the whole population, the Ministry of Health seeks alternative financing mechanisms to shift some share of payments out of pocket to Mandatory Health Insurance (MHI). It developed a concept paper on the Introduction of Medical Insurance that was approved by the government of Armenia. At present, the optimization of the health care system and the introduction of medical insurance are at the centre of attention in the Ministry of Health. However, only 33,000 Armenian citizens have medical insurance, 99% of whom have insured their health in the framework of corporate contracts (ArmInfo 2011).

After 1997, support by donors enabled authorities to implement a series of projects aimed at improving quality and efficiency of the PHC system. Resources were provided to outpatient care, establishing family medicine and strengthening the health financing system. Hundreds of health professionals were trained and retrained as the Ministry of Health promoted the use of family doctors in PHCs. In order to overcome public perception that doctors at primary health facilities are less qualified than those in hospitals and to improve their credibility, training was provided to PHC doctors. Technical assistance was provided to design indicators and benchmarks for monitoring service performance improvements, including a plan to legalize and regulate private payments to health care personnel. Practice guidelines were introduced to achieve the goal of PHCs to detect, diagnose and prevent sickness as early as possible through screening and diagnostic procedures, medical case management, practice management, and reporting to national and local health authorities. Infrastructure and equipment in selected PHC facilities were improved. A Health Management Information System (HMIS) was introduced with new medical and financial reporting forms, automation of data collection, payments and accounting.

Since 2004, the country had been engaged in the second stage of reforming the health care with emphasis on improved state budget financing and more efficient use of the resources. The reform process was implemented in the framework of Armenia Health System Modernization Projects (AHSMP1) aimed at system modernization to ensure better access of the population to quality health services and reduce the differences in utilization of essential health care services between the poorest and richest income groups of population. In the first phase of the modernization process (2004-2010) the geographical and financial access of Armenia's most vulnerable population to quality basic health services increased. Due to extensive upgrading service providers' knowledge and skills, infrastructure development and provision of modern equipment to health facilities in rural areas nearly 82% of the country's population was covered by retrained family medicine providers (WB 2011a). The principal hospital networks in the regions were turned into a high quality health care providers' network.

At present, the country is engaged in the second stage of reforming the health care system to overcome a gap in the distribution of human and technological resources, lack of strategic planning, a need for effective capacity building, etc. On going reforms are implemented in the framework of AHSMP2 that was launched in 2007 and expected to end in December 2012. The framework of the AHSMP2 is envisaged to:

- Scale up the implementation of PHC reforms based on family medicine through re-training nurses and family physicians, improving the PHC infrastructure (beyond the communities supported under the AHSMP1), and developing PHC guidelines relevant for family medicine (including primary and secondary prevention of avoidable mortality).
- Support public hospital efficiency and quality improvement program piloted in selected hospital network institutions through development and implementation of strategic restructuring plans for selected hospital networks (four in Yerevan and one per region) which will include: relocation of services through consolidation of infrastructure and services; essential medical equipment; modernization of management structures and improving management capacity; strengthening accountability arrangements; IT equipment for financial management systems; introducing quality assurance systems; improving management of health care waste; and
- Strengthen the capacity of the Ministry of Health and its key agencies to perform their functions of policy development, monitoring of implementation, regulation and oversight of the health sector. It is also expected to strengthen governance and management of health care provider institutions and the oversight function of marz structures on regional level, to strengthen the legal and regulatory environment, to improve supervision, accountability and management of public hospitals, and to improve public expenditure management in the health sector.
- Future plans of the government of Armenia are to continue upgrading health facilities as outlined in the optimization plans in all regions, improve the quality of training of family practice teams as well as of health professionals in secondary and tertiary specialty areas, support institutional strengthening, such as an introduction of performance-based payment of providers, and improve governance and regulatory arrangements (WB 2010).

2.5 Short-Term and Medium-Term Reforms Outcomes

The introduction of radical reforms in a health care system no longer able to provide free on-demand health care to the entire population and the reliance on payments out-of-pocket directly by the population undermined the principle of equity with respect to access, quality and financing. The transfer of decision-making authority from the central level to the local implemented in the course of decentralization process was not accompanied by the transfer of consistent funding for health care services to local governments (Cardno 2010:3). Chronic underfunding of the system coupled with blurring of roles and responsibilities had detrimental effects on the provision of health care provision (Bobak *et al.* 2004). Insufficient public funds, the low quality of medical staff and informal payments hindered access by poor patients to adequate health services. The lessons learned indicated that in a system with substantial excess capacity of hospital beds, the introduction of provider autonomy, contracting and changes in provider payment mechanisms produced neither efficiency gains nor rationalization.

Although the government initially ensured the BBP for the most vulnerable groups of population, funding fell short of targets and necessitated patient co-payments even in the case of these targeted groups. Consequently, there was a drop in health care utilization rate among the most vulnerable groups between 1996 and 1999 – *e.g.*, a 21% drop in the rate of utilization among families with four or more children. Moreover, the privatization of health care facilities that began in 1997 plus the change in financial mechanisms through the transfer of a considerable part of financial risks to the private sector not only worsened accessibility of the most essential services for socially vulnerable groups but even 'exacerbated the medical poverty trap' (Tonoyan 2004). Likewise a sharp decline in timely referrals to doctors caused an increase of morbidity. At that stage the promotion of PHC had not been sufficiently prioritized, and a modern system of health care standards and quality control had not been introduced.

The outcome of the projects implemented during the first stage reforms in 1997-2003 ensured sustainable and substantial impact on institutional development. Those reforms 'reduced the state's role in healthcare delivery' (Staines 1999:46) and promoted market mechanisms through introduction of user-fees. However, they failed to introduce compulsory health insurance system in the country while the plans to replace tax-based health financing with a national compulsory social health insurance were unsuccessful since the feasibility of doing so was constrained by economic circumstances (HSDP 2007:9). According to the World Bank, health care financing in Armenia 'was moved off budget and out of the control of the treasury system before other accountability measures were developed. The lack of accountability and clearly defined financial flows rapidly led to suspicions of corruption, which were soon confirmed. Site visits revealed that no government funds had reached most health care facilities for more than nine months after the State Health Agency was established as an autonomous off-budget fund and became responsible for allocating government health care funds and purchasing services' (Staines 1999:46).

More efforts were needed to fund essential services in order to place the interest and rights of each patient at the centre of attention. On one hand, measures were needed to concentrate resources on selected providers and improve the perceived quality and accessibility of health care services by the population. Correspondingly, the efficiency of allocation and use of public expenditures on health through rationalization of inputs on the supply side needed to be improved. On the other hand, the regulatory framework for family medicine had to be amended so that target medical personnel could be trained clinically to practice their new skills and family medicine concept. While the government of Armenia demonstrated a commitment in 1999 to engage in 'multisectoral strategies to tackle the determinants of health, ensuring the use of health impact assessment', very little has been done since then to reform training of health professionals (Hayrapetyan and Khanjyan 2004). Provider accountability, quality assurance and appropriate service delivery reforms matured to achieve the expected provider performance and efficiency as well as increasing transparency and performance in public hospitals through introduction of better management and fiduciary practices and performance-based payment mechanisms.

At that stage the main challenge in Armenia's health system was to ensure better access of the population to quality health services, reduce informal payments, reallocate the health budget towards development of more cost-effective PHC system, and rationalize health service provision, including the optimization of excess capacity in the hospital sector. Differences in utilization of essential health care services between the poorest and richest income groups of population needed to be reduced. Increasing utilization of essential health services closer to international benchmarks for countries with similar demographic and epidemiologic profiles, and improving health-related MDGs, mainly in infant mortality, maternal mortality, and prevention and control of public health threats (such as HIV/AIDS and tuberculosis amenable to health sector interventions) were on the agenda of the next generation reforms to be implemented in the country.

Although the effects of reform were tangible, they were insufficient to compensate for the lack of state health funding needed to assure guaranteed free services for vulnerable population groups. Thus, reallocation of the state health budget towards development of more cost-effective PHC system, rationalization and optimization of service provision in the hospital sector, and reduction of informal payments are still the main challenges in Armenia's health system.

However, 'the separation of functional accountability and scope of responsibilities, especially at community level, remained vague'. Therefore, capacity building of local authorities, improvement of accountability mechanisms at local level to identify health care priorities, and securing financial commitment of local decision-makers to allocate appropriate funding to address health care services in regional, city, and village municipalities became a primary concern of central authorities. In addition, many administrators continued to adhere to old management styles that did not meet the requirements of new environment. Moreover, the low level of salaries and the 'lack of effective capacity building of medical personnel to provide for health care sector administrators with the necessary skills' hindered implementation of execution of delegated functions.

Health System Performance Assessment reports demonstrated the positive impact of the government's health reforms on improving the quality of, and access, to health services for the population. These reports presented important information on the sources and volumes of financial flows in the sector that, in turn, enabled decision-makers to assess and review the results and make essential policy adjustments. Lessons learned from the project supported scaling up high-impact activities (*i.e.* family medicine development), investing in infrastructure to leverage difficult policy and structural reforms (*i.e.* hospital optimization and modernization), and improving institutions and governance through better regulations and skills development (*i.e.* strengthening government capacity to develop and monitor effective health sector policies).

The second phase of modernizing the health care system is aimed at scaling up the implementation of family medicine based PHC reforms, improving public hospital efficiency and quality, and strengthening the capacity of the Ministry of Health. The government continues to upgrade health facilities in all *marzes*, improve the quality of training of family practice teams, and train health professionals in specialty areas. Institutional strengthening is expected to ensure sustainability of reforms, introduce performance-based payment of providers, and improve governance and regulatory arrangements. Financial commitment by local decision-makers to support funding to address and to resolve health care issues is being strengthened.

According to the 2010 Assessment of the Accomplishment of the Healthcare Program and the National Healthcare Report prepared with support of the World Bank and WHO, child mortality was decreased, while the efficiency of the hospital sector, overall utilization of services, and the average duration of life increased (Qushqyan 2010). However, because of the economic crisis, the programs of modernization of regional hospitals and ambulance services were postponed. Nonetheless, the government implemented measures in the health sector by maintaining a budget system for dispensing medical care and approving programs targeted at ensuring health services for vulnerable population groups. The government order was based on proposals by state and private health care facilities. Since the problems of health care are impossible to resolve through the state budget, the introduction of additional sources of financing through an insurance-based system is considered to have positive impact on the overall health care system of the country. During the

1990s, Armenia twice attempted to introduce medical insurance but, unlike many other transition countries, was not successful due to socio-economic factors that hindered the implementation of Mandatory Medical Insurance (MMI). A decline in subsidized health services and in visits for medical aid led to an increase in the length of illness and chronic pathology. At present, most people are too poor to afford Voluntary Medical Insurance (VMI). Therefore, the Ministry of Health is 'just examining possibility of introduction of the MMI' (Qushqyan 2010). To introduce the latter, the Ministry 'created a working group that collaborates with the experts from Central Bank of RA to figure on all calculations needed for the creation of the basis of MMI system in the country'.

Since July 2010, a pilot project to introduce co-payment mechanisms for health care services has been implemented in Yerevan's four MCs. Co-payment anticipates payment of the difference between the cost of state-guaranteed health care and the real amount estimated by facilities. This approach enables a forecast of expenditures by patients. At the same time it seeks to legalize informal payments out of pocket and direct these financial flows towards increased salaries of medical personnel. At present copayments mechanisms only apply to two major state order programs: emergency and gynecology. Copayments level is high enough and ranges from 40% to 60% of the total cost. Patients from vulnerable groups are not subject to co-payment; their treatment is implemented through the framework of the Basic Benefit Package.

To ensure active participation and direct involvement of both public and private sectors, communities and civil society and to coordinate their activities, the creation of a special council is envisioned that includes representatives of the Ministry of Health, NGOs, auditing companies and the management of health care facilities. These councils will elaborate all important issues about medical facilities from service provision to development issues.

2.6 Summary and Conclusion

The Government of Armenia introduced radical reforms in Armenian health care in order to establish a more cost-effective, equitable and sustainable system. The reforms were based on an assumption that health care can no longer be provided free and on demand for the entire population. Implemented measures improved the state of Armenia's health system over two decades and had a positive impact on key indicators that are better now than at the beginning of the transition period. Market mechanisms raised the role of private providers, enhanced revenue and increased provider income. Considerable improvements were achieved in primary health care (PHC) and maternity services throughout the country. Important achievement in terms of allocative efficiency was observed in sustaining equal balance between inpatient and outpatient care (WB 2011b). While these measures improved the state of Armenia's health system, they did not meet all of the objectives of health care policies. They failed to ensure equal access of population to qualitative health care including state-guaranteed health services.

To a great extent, successes achieved could be attributed to targeted projects addressed to concrete issues of specific groups of population. Although implemented projects sought to provide financing for the health system in Armenia over two decades, state expenditures on health care remained at 1.6% of GDP in 2010 – well below the average of 4.0% in low/middle income countries. Since 'state health expenditures are not sufficient to support the core system and to meet the health needs of the population' (Qushqyan 2010), health care provision remains largely based on out-of-pocket payments and a high level of informal payments. Health professionals are still expected to provide services for very low salaries and, therefore, tend to supplement scanty wages by means of informal payments out of pocket by patients. In 2010, payments out of pocket contributed 'nearly 65% of the revenues in the sector' (Qushqyan 2010), which undermines the principles of equity and access to health care and strongly affects the poorest and the most vulnerable. Although the government of Armenia ensured the availability of BBP to vulnerable groups, its funding fell short of targets and required patient participation in financing even in the case of the targeted groups.[13] The high level of out-of-pocket payments by patients – many of which are in the form of unofficial payments – is considered a sign of poor governance (Lewis 2008). Consequently, Armenia's health care system still has substantial room for improvement in governance to improve decision-making in social policy, decrease existing gaps in the distribution of human and technological resources and effective mechanisms of financial protection, low remuneration of personnel, and lack of strategic planning.

The lack of access to health care services created a psychological barrier among the population, as a result of which many Armenians do not give serious consideration to their health and try, to the extent possible, not to use services provided by the health care system. Thus, overall rates of health care utilization in Armenia, whether measured as outpatient contacts per person or acute care hospital admissions per thousand of population, are about half the levels observed in Western and Eastern Europe or the CIS (WB 2011b). Consequently, 'relatively weak financial protection against high out of pocket and informal payments for health resulted in the poverty headcount is several percentage points higher

13 Notable gaps exist in targeting the poor and ensuring accessibility of health care services by the poor. To a certain extent this is caused by the fact that qualification eligibility threshold under the health program is much more restrictive than the one for the family poverty benefit program. Consequently, equalizing eligibility criteria for both programs should be considered as a short-term priority policy issue. This reform will require increasing health care expenditures that are estimated at 0.1% of GDP (WB 2011b). This rise in expenditure might be offset by restructuring the disability program for category II and category III disability groups and by expanding coverage of the poor.

than it would be in the presence of adequate risk-pooling arrangements' (WB 2011b). In order to improve population health outcomes and households against high out-of-pocket payments for health care there is need to ensure that people do not face medical expenditures that either drive them below the poverty line (facilitate impoverishment) or exceed some threshold of household resources as a result of an episode of ill health.

The economic crisis that began in 2008 has increased the level of poverty in the country. To a great extent the crisis undermined recent achievements in the health care sector and led to lower implementation of reform programs. At present, the country faces a challenging post-crisis economic environment characterized by a gradually declining share of the government budget allocated to health. Thus, budget allocations from nearly 8% in 2005 were decrease to about 6% in 2010-2011. Although the economy began to recover in 2010 with 2.1% growth, and picked up to 4.6% growth in 2011, the government of Armenia sought additional international assistance to counteract lower capital inflows and fiscal revenues. Due to external borrowing, the external-debt-to-GDP ratio reached 35% in 2010 compared to 13.7% in 2007 (ADB 2011). In spite of these measures, the country still has to deal with underfunded health services 'suffering from weak administrative, technical and logistical capacity; inadequate financial investment; inappropriately skilled and poorly motivated health personnel; and poor population health awareness' (USAID 2010). Consequently, sectoral public expenditure policies need to better balance sector-specific objectives and population expectations with the imperative of a sustainable fiscal adjustment. This means 'ensuring value for money and efficiency of spending within the available expenditure envelope' (WB 2011b).

The country preserved many features of the Soviet-style health system encompassing universal coverage and delivery of a comprehensive range of medical services through the system of PHC facilities. Significant progress was made in hospital consolidation, oversupply diminished and a sharp reduction in the number of hospital beds produced savings. However, hospital mergers still remain on the agenda. With approximately 125 hospitals in Armenia, the number per 100,000 of population is about twice as high as the corresponding figure for most of Western European countries. Many of the surplus facilities are relatively small, in poor condition, and in many cases located in remote rural areas. Strong hospitals are available in the cities, but clinics in rural areas are poorly maintained. Therefore, many Armenians are reluctant to use local, but frequently low quality, health facilities. Although the introduction of the institute of family doctors considerably improved the availability and accessibility of a range of health services in some rural areas, there are still too many specialist doctors and not enough general practitioners. Due to their current condition hospitals in rural areas do not have large operations and maintenance costs. Therefore, surplus hospitals could be closed and access of the local population to health care services could be assured through making necessary investments in the PHC system.

The introduction of co-payment mechanisms was seen as a significant health financing reform to address informal barriers to access. It was accompanied by new stipulations on how revenues should be distributed to salaries within hospitals. According to the World Bank, higher spending levels are needed in order to ensure financial protection against high out-of-pocket and informal payments for health care. Therefore, co-payment mechanisms will not ensure long-term solutions to major health care challenges. They can only serve as a transitional arrangement until a future date when the benefit package can be more adequately funded and expanded. Such changes will require close monitoring as well as keeping population informed about how the program works.

Access to affordable medicines and medical care is important issue for the whole population in Armenia due to their high price as well as unavailability of low-cost drugs and medical care items. Expenditures on pharmaceuticals account for nearly 45% of total out-of-pocket payments in health care. The share of total health expenditures spent on drugs comprises nearly 30%. Corresponding figure among most OECD countries is about 15%. High levels of health expenditures on drugs are due partly to high levels of population self-treatment, since this enables people to avoid paying out of pocket at health facilities. The government should make better use of its purchasing power to negotiate prices for certain families of drugs and/or include them in the basic benefit package. Moreover, taking appropriate measures to improve prescribing behavior of physicians might ensure better access to drugs and lower levels of out-of-pocket payments. Corresponding measures to implement general drug price regulation policies would inevitably help to improve the situation and ensure the availability of core generic pharmaceuticals at reasonable cost.

Local authorities in Armenia lack financial resources to ensure the health of community residents. They cannot provide sufficient financing for operational and maintenance costs of health care facilities within their administrative boundaries or provide facilities with basic medical supplies, drugs, equipment, etc. Enabling local authorities to support health care facilities would have positive impact on the principle of equity and access to health care services.

The development of law enforcement mechanisms, the introduction of mandatory health insurance, and complementary private insurance focused on tertiary health services would contribute to a more adequate allocation of financial resources in health care. In combination with state coverage, private medical insurance could make expensive types of medical services (such as oncology and cardiology) more affordable to the general public. Since the government is planning to introduce a mandatory system, the Ministry of Health should pay special attention to the basics of an effective and socialized model of health insurance that would combine consumer choice and decrease social inequality in the access to health care.

While the Government of Armenia seeks to improve the situation within the framework of the Poverty Reduction Strategy Paper, current reforms emphasize improvement of state budget financing and more efficient use of resources. But there is need to resolve the problem of price regulation and to reduce shadow operations in the health care sector. Correspondingly, implementation of the second phase of health system modernization under strong leadership is an essential pillar in the process of reforms to remove informal payments, to decrease the gap between the rich and the poor, to ensure access, to reduce health inequity, and, therefore, to become a modern, effective and customer-oriented system able to improve the overall health status of Armenians.

3 Health Reforms in Bulgaria

T. Kostadinova, G. Manliev, M. Vladimirova and N. Feschieva

Bulgaria faces a demographic crisis. Within its 110,944 km^2, its population has steadily declined from 8,669,269 people in 1990 to 7,351,234 in the 2011 census. According to projections, the country's population will decline by another quarter million to 7,137,000 in 2020. In addition to high emigration, the fertility rate in 2009 was only 1.57 children per woman of childbearing age – well below replacement. Bulgaria's population is also rapidly ageing. People aged 60 and above comprise 22.8% of the population, an age group that is predicted to increase to 27.6% in 2020 and 38.6% in 2050. The older population is itself ageing. The oldest old (*i.e.*, persons aged 80 years or over) constitute the fastest growing segment of the population; by 2050 one-fifth of the older population will be aged 80 or over. Currently, the oldest old constitute 3% of the population in Europe and 2.1% in Bulgaria. In 2050 one-tenth of Europeans and 7.4% of Bulgarians are projected to be 80 or over (Feschieva *et al.* 2011).

The increase in life expectancy in Europe is related to the improved survival rates, but Bulgarians lag behind EU populations of the same age. Compared with the 15 EU countries with high life expectancies at age 65, life expectancy for Bulgaria's older population is seven years lower. While the rate of infant mortality is decreasing, it is not yet at the level of Western Europe.

During 2008-2010, GDP was stable at 67 billion Bulgarian leva or €34 billion. According to the National Statistical Institute, Bulgarian GDP per capita was €4,500 in 2008 compared to €1,500 in 1999 although, based on Purchasing Power Parity, GDP per capita in 2008 could be calculated to be €10,100. However, from 1995 to 2000 Bulgaria experienced

Table 3.1 Demographic Characteristics

	1990	1995	2001	2005	2010
Population (thousands)	8 669	8 384	7 891	7 771	7 351
% Urban	67.2	68.1	68.2	69.0	71.5
Life expectancy (male)	68.0	70.0	71.7	69.3	70.0
Life expectancy (female)	74.7	76.6	78.4	76.4	77.0
Infant mortality rate	15.9	17.5	14.4	10.4	9.4

Source: Bulgarian National Statistical Institute (NSI) <www.nsi.bg>.

Table 3.2 Key Health Indicators for Bulgaria, 1990-2010

Year	Birth Rate Per 1,000	Crude Death Rate Per 1,000	Population Growth (%)	Infant Mortality Rate Per 1,000 Live Births	Total Fertility Rate Per Woman
1990	112.1	12.6	(−) 0.22	14.8	1.8
1995	8.6	14.7	(−) 0.70	14.8	1.23
2000	9.0	14.1	(−) 0.51	13.3	1.27
2005	9.2	14.6	(−) 0.54	11.6	1.31
2010	10.0	14.6	(−) 0.46	9.4	1.49

Source: National Statistical Institute and National Centre for Health Informatics <www.nsi.bg>.

negative growth; *i.e.*, its economy contracted. The inflation rate also declined from 11.3% in 2000 to 4.5% in 2010 with an average rate of 7.5% during 2000-2010.

Volatility of GDP occurred during the transitional period from a centrally planned to a market economy. During 1991-1997, Bulgaria entered a series structural, fiscal and debt crises. The country introduced a currency board to stabilize the money supply in order to open a way to sustainable growth. The annual growth rate reached 5% for the period 2000-2008. After 2009, as a consequence of the global crisis, the growth rate declined to about 2%.

Employment data show stable development. From 40% in 2000, the employment rate rose to 64% in 2009-2010 that approximates the mid-level of EU countries. The urban employment rate is higher than in rural areas; likewise male employment is higher than for

Table 3.3 Employment Rate in Bulgaria, 2000-2010 (%)

	1995	2000	2003	2008	2010
employment	41.7	39.7	42.4	50.8	46.7
• urban	46	45	49	55	51
• rural	31	29	36	40	35
• male	46	44	47	57	51
• female	38	36	38	46	42
unemployment	12.8	16.0	12.7	9.1	11.2

Source: <www.nsi.bg>.

Table 3.4 Economic Data

	1990	1995	2000	2005	2009	2010	2011
GDP (billion US$)	8.1	13.1	13.6	24.1	47.1	50.3	53.5
GDP per capita (US$)	943	1 559	1 718	3 101	6 215	6 797	7 229
Inflation rate (%)	438	62	11.3	6.5	0.6	4.5	4.2

Source: National Statistical Institute of Bulgaria <www.nsi.bg>.

females. The unemployment rate followed cyclical changes. During the last five years, the rate was in the range of 7%-12%.

3.1 Health Expenditures

Finance for Bulgaria's health care system has been based on general taxation from state and municipal budgets. In addition, health care financing includes a private out-of-pocket (OOP) component, a significant portion of which involves under-the-counter payments. With its 1998 Health Insurance Law (HIL), Bulgaria introduced a compulsory and a voluntary health care system as an alternative to central budgeting. Funding for the health care system is financed through the National Health Insurance Fund, state and municipal budgets, voluntary HIF, local and foreign legal bodies, individuals and co-payments.

According to the Law on National Health, state and municipal budgets cover free of charge emergency care; psychiatric care; blood transfusions; obligatory immunizations; epidemiological activities (control); health programs and projects of national, regional, and local importance; state sanitary control; construction, basic repair, modernization, improvements and reconstruction of health institutions; health administration; national centres and institutes with no direct treatment activity; expensive treatments beyond the range of the obligatory health insurance (if ordered by the Minister of Health); expenses related to public health care; expertise of permanent working incapacity and professional diseases. The Ministry of Health funds specialized health institutions at national and regional levels as well as the public health system. Life-saving consumables for hemodialysis, cardiology, and other activities as well as drugs for cancer patients and expensive treatment of other severe diseases are also secured out of the budget of the Ministry of Health – all paid by the National Health Insurance Fund (NHIF).

Every Bulgarian citizen is supposedly insured to receive a package of health care services, determined and paid by the NHIF in accordance with the National Framework Contract.

Since July 2000, outpatient facilities have been funded entirely by the NHIF through its regional divisions. Since July 2001, the NHIF has participated in funding inpatient facilities, initially covering about 20% of all hospital expenditure while the municipalities continue to fund hospitals in their territory (with the exception of regional hospitals funded by the Ministry of Health). Thus far, voluntary health insurance has a limited role in financing health care; it applies to high-income groups and some private and public companies. Out-of-pocket spending constitutes an estimated 20% of total health care expenditure. Informal payments, common in the 1980s under the previous regime, increased during the past decade in order to obtain drugs in hospitals, access to high quality services and a variety of outpatient services. Throughout the country co-payments have been introduced with a fixed fee as a proportion of the minimal monthly salary.

In 2000, the Ministry of Health distributed 292 million Bulgarian leva (about 30% of total health care expenditures) in order to finance health and health care establishments. In the same year, the NHIF spent 126 million leva on outpatient care – 30% directed to primary care, about 20% to specialized care, 10% to dental care and about 30% for pharmaceuticals. In 2009-2010, the budget of Ministry of Health was almost 600 million leva so support for medical care has doubled.

Estimation of health care expenditures requires identification of their sources that include the budgets of the government, the National Health Fund and the municipalities as well as private expenditures. The government budget for health includes the Ministry of Health plus regional health units that monitor the quality of local health services. It covers three items: staff and other costs for maintaining the Ministry, its executive agencies and 28 regional health units; capital expenditures for public and municipal hospitals; and medicaments for specific diseases like cancer and oncologica. According to the "Annual

Table 3.5 Funding for Health Care as Percentage of GDP

	1995	2000	2003	2004	2005	2006	2007	2008
State Budget	4.1	2.4	2.3	2.0	2.0	1.5	1.5	1.3
National Health Fund	-	1.2	1.9	2.3	2.6	3.5	3.9	4.5
Municipalities	-	0.8	0.5	0.3	0.2	0.2	0.2	1.2
Voluntary Health Funds	-	-	0.1	0.2	0.4	0.6	0.8	1.0
Household Expenditures	1.3	1.3	1.2	1.2	1.2	1.2	1.2	1.2
Total Percentage of GDP	5.4	5.7	6.0	6.0	6,4	7.0	7.6	9.2

Source: Annual Report of the Minister of Health 2009; <www.mh.government.bg>.

Report for Health of Nation 2009", Table 3.5 presents the funding of health care in Bulgaria in terms of sources.

During 2003-2004, EU member states spent an average of 8.2% of GDP on health expenditures while public expenditures for health care in Bulgaria amounted to 6.1%. In recent years Bulgaria increased health care expenditures, mainly for funding general practitioners (GPs) and hospital treatment. Bulgaria is moving closer to the average funding level for health care in new EU member states. In 2000, the average public cost for medical expenditure per capita was US$81; it then increased gradually to US$300 in 2009. Although there are no official data for 2009-2011, government budget outlays for health have increased and are estimated to be 4.3% of GDP. Additionally, there is a trend of increases in household payments for medical services from 3.2% of an average household budget in 1999 to 5.6% in 2009. According to estimates for 2010-2011, household medical expenditure has reached more than 2% of GDP (Delcheva 2011).

3.2 Health Resources

Until 1990, the number of medical staff per 100,000 Bulgarians was good: 329 physicians, 70 dentists, 621 nurses and 87 midwives. In 2010, the numbers were 378 physicians and 88 dentists. There are regional differences in the number of physicians – *e.g.*, 471 in Sofia versus 238 in Razgrad – and the number of nurses has declined. The physician-nurse ratio

Table 3.6 Human Resources in Health Care (1997-2009)

	1997	2000	2003	2006	2009
Physicians	28 655	27 526	28 128	28 111	27 198
Physicians per 100,000	346	338	361	366	370
General Practitioners	NA	5451		5127	4786
GPs per 100,000	NA	67	69	67	65
Dentists	5 240	6 778	6 475	6 512	6 493
Dentists per 100,000	63	83	83	85	86
Nurses	47 434	31 479	29 650	31 599	31 966
Nurses per 100,000	573	386	380	411	423
Other health staff	11 811	7 289	5 800	5 997	5 823
Other staff per 100,000	71	45	37	38	38

Source: Annual Report of Minister of Health 2009, <www.mh.government.bg>.

is 1:1.2 compared to 1:2.3 in the EU. In 2010, Bulgaria had 4761 GPs or 65 GPs per 100,000 Bulgarians compared to an average of 99 in the EU. GPs in Bulgaria comprise 18% of all medical staff, which is lower than the EU average of 29%. Yet the average age of human capital in Bulgaria has increased; in 2009 physicians averaged 51 years of age.

Compared with other EU states, Bulgaria has a middle position. After its accession to the EU the numbers of physicians and nurses migrating to other EU member-states have been increasing due to higher salaries, better quality of life and better conditions for professional development. The country has six medical universities that prepare medical staff: physicians, dentists and pharmacologists. Currently entrance numbers are approximately 2700 students annually.

Primary health units include medical centres for medical and dental services, clinical labs and diagnostic-consultative centres. In 2011, the number of hospitals rose to 340 of which 88 or about one-fourth are private. In 2010, there were 735 beds per 100,000 inhabitants. Emergency services are organized in 198 units with 392 health teams located in different territorial areas.

3.3 Normative Issues

Bulgaria's health system is in the process of development. Some envisaged reforms have been achieved in, *e.g.*, primary health care, while reforms are pending in the financing of hospital care. Despite the implemented reforms, the health insurance model has not yet acquired the characteristics that correspond to European requirements in order to ensure

Table 3.7 Health Care Institutions and Beds (2000-2010)

	2000		2008		2010	
Location	**Number**	**Beds**	**Number**	**Beds**	**Number**	**Beds**
Hospitals	244	52 712	305	45 712	312	45 832
• Multi-profile	140	38 279	157	32 559	164	32 576
• Specialized	102	14 113	148	13 153	148	13 256
Dispensaries	49	4 272	46	4 154	34	3 102
Primary Health Units	1 190	367	1 678	961	1 716	938
Other Medical Units	159	4 720	179	4 282	189	4 570

Source: <www.nsi.bg>; Annual Report of the Minister of Health for 2009, <www.mh.government.bg>.

quality of service to patients. The vision of a future health system should be debated, analyzed and evaluated by all stakeholders in the system. To sketch the long-term development of universal mandatory health insurance in Bulgaria, the following conditions are required: accelerated economic development to support the development of health care; development and accumulation of administrative capacity for health insurance; sufficiently high levels of personal income to secure stable cash flows into the health insurance system; effective structure of labor markets to provide revenue for insurance; adequate condition of health infrastructure including an integrated information system that serves health services as well as provides complete information about the health condition of patients; effective control of funds, suppliers and individual medical professionals, including strict sanctions for violation of the rules.

One key component of health reform in Bulgaria is the development of a comprehensive policy for long-term care (LTC). Because Bulgaria's population is ageing rapidly, the need for LTC will continue to rise. Currently many acute care hospitals are burdened with long-term care patients. Scaling up long-term care facilities, strengthening social services and improving home care would allow acute-care hospitals to focus on core activities and thus contribute to a more efficient hospital sector overall (World Bank 2007).

3.3.1 Welfare Principles

Health policy is oriented to provide health care to those who need it. Emergency services are a public good delivered free of charge to all citizens. Funding is through the national budget. Primary health care and hospital services are based on solidarity principles with payment of health insurance fees to the National Insurance Fund. All employees pay compulsory health contributions according to their salary level. The government pays health contributions for civil servants, soldiers, policemen, school children, students, registered unemployed and retired people. The number of citizens in these groups is over half of the country's population, which means a strong paternalistic position of the state. There are specific regulations for treating groups with special health needs such as free delivery of medicines for people suffering cancer, diabetes and other diseases. In this way, the government alleviates pressure on the family budget for many people (Dimova *et al.* 2007).

The government established a 'special social fund' to support hospital care of citizens with low income and those outside the health insurance system. The fund covers the cost of treatment for vulnerable groups. The law on health care introduced 'user charges' for medical services in two cases. For medical check-ups by GPs, the fee is 1% of the minimal salary (€1.25 in 2010). In 2008, the government decided that user charges for retired people are to be half of a regular charge. Another charge is for hospital care not longer than ten days at a rate of 2% of the minimal salary per day (€2.50) (Atanasova *et al.* 2010).

In general, Bulgaria's health system is welfare oriented. It provides medical care for socially weak persons and families, even for free riders. It is characterized by:

- emergency care free of charge,
- primary and hospital care through compulsory payment of health contributions to the National Health Fund by the employer and the employee or by the self-employed, and 100% by the government for civil servants, children, pupils, students, registered unemployed and retired people,
- user charges for specific medical services,
- social Fund to cover hospital care for poor people,
- co-payment by uninsured patients for their choice of a doctor's team for treatment, and
- private payment by companies and persons who seek better services, hospital care and personal choice (Vekov 2009).

From 2012, the government plans to introduce co-payment by patients regarding choice of a doctor's team for hospital treatment. The co-payment is fixed for different options and amounts between €150 and €500. Although an additional support for the hospital budget, the main argument for introducing this measure is to eliminate corrupt practices among doctors.

3.3.2 Dominant Values of Health Policy

Since 2000, the Bulgarian health care system has operated on the principles of solidarity, equity, accessibility and plurality as well as universal access to medical services – all approved by the Bulgarian parliament in the HIL. Solidarity refers to the methods of calculating and collecting the health insurance premium proportionate to salaries and wages. Working people are legally obliged to pay health care contributions to the NHIF on a monthly basis; the Fund pays for those who need primary or hospital care. The government covers the health insurance for civil servants, army and police servants, unemployed and retired people, children, pupils and students. The Ministry of Health funds hospitals for buying modern equipment and modernizing specific treatments such as heart disease, transplantation and other diseases with high costs. In practice, the solidarity principle is seriously undermined by 'free riders'. Because approximately one million citizens (1/7th of the population) do not pay health insurance contributions, there is great financial pressure on funding, especially for hospital treatment (Atanasova *et al.* 2010).

In terms of universal access and equity, no Bulgarian has been denied medical care at any level of service – primary, specialized and hospital care – whatever ethnic, cultural and social differences. The current referral system streamlines the transfer of patients from smaller, general facilities to specialized units, depending of the severity and urgency of the case. Although many Bulgarians do not pay their insurance premiums, they receive urgent and elective medical care at all levels as needed at high cost, thus causing significant congestion and shortages of funds.

As for plurality, both public and private facilities are partners on an equal basis with the National Insurance Fund. They provide relevant medical services and have access to public funds. Patients are permitted to change their health care providers and switch from private to public practitioner without restrictions.

The challenge of keeping health expenditures in Bulgaria in balance is made more difficult by the high levels of out-of-pocket spending for health services in all levels of the system. Expenditure on drugs is a particularly significant problem. Figure 3.1 illustrates the extent to which out-of-pocket expenditures are driven by spending on drugs, a pattern that is particularly detrimental to ensuring access to priority drugs for the poor.

In order to gain access to high quality services in hospitals, illegal payments are widespread. Sometimes hospitalized patients have to buy drugs themselves. Although there are no reliable estimates of the size of unofficial payments, a 2006 survey by the Open Society Institute (2008) indicates the magnitude of the informal payments to be mainly in cash and totaled over 160 million leva. In addition to the immediate challenge of ensuring sustainability of the drug budget, the medium-term pharmaceutical reform agenda must address inappropriate prescribing patterns. The introduction by the government of less rigid contracting models for pharmaceutical procurement (*e.g.*, that move beyond price alone) would be a

Table 3.8 Public Perceptions of Corruption in Health Care (%)

	2006	**2008**
Hospital – daily care	29	21
Hospital – childbirth assistance	40	37
Hospital – surgical operations	48	46
Specialized Outpatient Care	20	16
Primary Care	10	8

Source: Open Society Institute 2008.

Figure 3.1 Out-of-Pocket Health Spending on Drugs (by quintile)

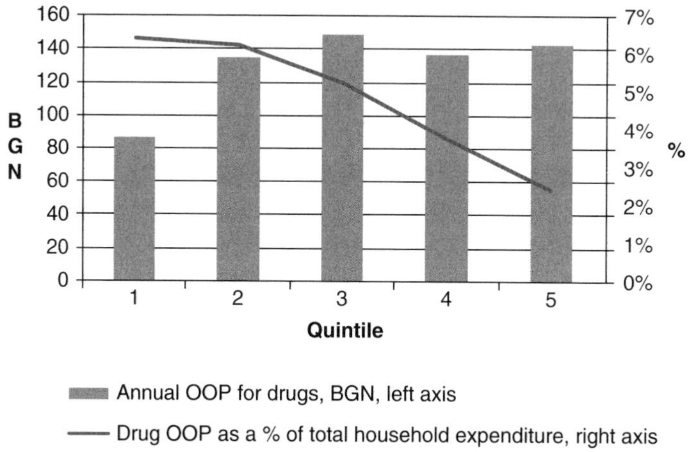

Source: World Bank 2007.

positive step to counteract this tendency. Overall, addressing the present weaknesses in the pharmaceutical sector could have a major impact on the population's satisfaction with the health system (Vekov 2011).

3.4 Governance of the Health Sector

The main institution responsible for governing health care in Bulgaria is its Ministry of Health, which is involved in the development of health policy and the budget for health care together with the Council of Ministries and the Parliament. For implementation, 28 regional inspectorates for health care have been established that monitor the quality of health care services. The regional inspectorates existed until 2011 to promote and control public health. In early 2011, as a result of administrative reform in all ministries, they merged with the regional centres for health care. This step is one response by the Bulgarian government to the challenges of the economic crises.

The NHIF is the basic financial institution for primary, specialized and hospital care. Its budget is formed from the compulsory contributions by employed persons and the payments by the state for special groups. The problem is that more than one million citizens do not pay health insurance fees, which significantly decreases the NHIF budget. The NHIF distributes the revenues among primary and hospital care as well as funds for consumption of medications.

Several laws have shaped health policy in Bulgaria: laws for public health, health establishments, drugs and pharmaceuticals, health insurance as well as other acts with specific importance. Private HIFs were created at the beginning of health reforms in 2000 in order to cover a voluntary package of health and mainly hospital services. Due to lack of clear distinction between the coverage of treatment by the NHIF and private health funds, the role of private insurance funds is not very significant. Debate about their transformation has been open since 2009 (Annual Report 2009).

There is a free access to the emergency care in Bulgaria for every citizen, insured and uninsured. Those who regularly pay their health contributions have access free of charge to primary and hospital services. The government, together with the Union of Bulgarian physicians, developed an updated version of compulsory 'national medical standards' that are intended to ensure quality of care in all levels and sectors – primary, specialized and hospital care. The National Council for Accreditation of Health Establishments provides accreditation according to national standards for health services and for education (for university hospitals). After accreditation, special commissions conduct audits of quality in hospital services (Kerekovska *et al.* 2007).

In January 2010, a new governmental institution was created – the Executive Agency 'Medical Audit' – whose mission is to work for continuous improvement of health care quality and safety. EAMA monitors activities of health care providers and of both compulsory and voluntary HIFs. It motivates them to improve their professionalism. During its first six months the institution elaborated checklists and inspected the performance of 97 health establishments to assess the compliance with medical standards. It has developed and maintained registers for complaints by patients; it also organized two roundtables to discuss quality issues in health care and the future collaboration with the other health care stakeholders. The most important result of its activity is that fear and mistrust of the health care professionals from the establishment of a new institution were replaced by gratitude and appreciation because the aim of EAMA is not to punish but to guarantee access to health care of good quality and safety, to protect the rights of patients and to disseminate good practices. Among the strategic goals of EAMA are to:

- develop a system for total quality management at a national level,
- initiate the legislation for quality management,
- avoid the dissemination of corrupt health care practices,
- develop data base in the field of health care quality,
- develop a reporting system for medical errors.

New amendments to the Law on Health Care Establishments have been approved by Parliament that will change the organization and management of the system after 2011. The development of national and 28 regional 'health maps' will specify the number of health care establishments needed to guarantee access by the population to the necessary health care services. Accreditation of health care establishments is a voluntary process. Only health care establishments that undertake training will receive compulsory accreditation. The Ministry of Health prepared national and regional health maps in order to optimize the number of hospitals and increase quality of care. E-health services have been developed as well. Personal e-dossiers have been introduced, gradually covering an increasing part of the population.

3.5 Major Political Positions, Postures and Trends

Political life in Bulgaria is stable. Three political groups influence the course of health reforms. The political rightwing (Union of Democratic Powers) prepared the strategy and started substantial reforms in 1998-2000. At that time the health insurance model was introduced; GPs began their practices for primary health care; clinical pathways were introduced in hospital care as a treatment and financing instrument; dental care was privatized; and a door to private initiatives in health care was opened.

Since 2003, the impact of political parties on health reforms has been weak. The political left wing (Socialist party) seeks to maintain high levels of access to and state support for health care. It opposed proposals for market-oriented reforms and higher percentage of health contributions. In 2005, the Socialists prepared a national strategy for health of the nation that was adopted in 2008 without political consensus. Although the Socialist party governed the country during 2005-2008, it did not make significant steps in terms of health care reforms. Two parties emerged in political life that became significant during 2002-2006 and 2009-2011. One party (National Movement Simeon Second) did not make any reforms; rather it froze them. The second party – 'Citizens for European Development of Bulgaria', currently governing the country – has no alternative. The health reforms were inevitable, due to delay and serious problems.

The stagnant economic situation in the country caused irregular financing of health care providers and reduction of financial resources by 20%. This process causes very low rates of satisfaction among health care professionals and among the population. The problem with clinical pathways as a financial mechanism is again on the table for discussion. All hospitals are to be inspected in order to assess compliance with medical standards, a process required according to amendments of the Law on Health Care Establishments. Thus, a decision about restructuring of hospital care must be made.

Table 3.9 SWOT Analysis of Health Care in Bulgaria

Strengths	**Weaknesses**
Highly qualified medical personnel	Lack of integrated information system
Negotiations between health care providers and the NHIF	Insufficient communication and collaboration between all institutions involved in health policy development
Free choice of health care provider	Lack of costing of health services
Quality assessment through accreditation of health care establishments	
Well-developed network of health care establishments of different type	Insufficient coordination between the emergency health care and the other pillars of the system
Sustainable and qualified system for higher education in medicine, dental medicine, pharmacy and nursing	Insufficient number of GPs specialized in general medicine
Introduced market elements in health care: competition between health care providers, negotiation of health care services, etc	Insufficient number of nurses
	Population not well-informed about the rights of patients
	Insufficient financial resources for health promotion and disease prevention
	Large number of uninsured citizens
	Bureaucracy and corruption
	Difficult access to health care in regions with unfavorable conditions
Opportunities	**Threats**
To encourage civil participation in the health sector through co-payment for health services	Increasing poverty – many households have a living standard below average
Encouraging the development of voluntary health insurance	Ageing population and growing need for social assistance and health care services
Access to EU funds and projects	Increasing the social and health inequalities
International assistance and cooperation	Emigration of labor force, particularly highly qualified – decrease in the number of medical staff with EU accession
Implementation of e-health	Insufficient financing of health care
Better opportunities for continuous education of health care providers	Reduced staff due to shortage of nurses and doctors in some specialties
Development of the medical tourism	Negative demographic trends

Source: Own construction.

The Ministry of Health drafted a new proposal for health care – specifically for restructuring the hospital sector. The serious problems and postponed reforms lead to discussions and even scandals in political life. For example, the idea for the implementation of official co-payment of health care services of approximately 20% without its preliminary agreement at political level was a reason for the resignation of the second Minister of Health in less than a year.

3.6 HISTORY OF HEALTH SYSTEM REFORMS

With the HIL a system of compulsory and voluntary health insurance was introduced in Bulgaria that has been implemented in phases since July 2000. Compulsory health insurance is implemented by the NHIF and its territorial divisions (Regional Health Insurance Funds); these undertake risk pooling and medical care purchasing functions on behalf of the population. Voluntary health insurance is optional and is conducted by shareholder companies registered according to commercial law. Compulsory health insurance in Bulgaria is carried out in compliance with the following basic principles:

- obligatory participation to the contributions' collecting,
- solidarity of insured persons in the use of accumulated funds,
- basic package of medical services guaranteed by the NHIF's budget,
- equity in using the guaranteed package of medical services,
- free choice of medical care provider,
- responsibility of insured persons for their health,
- participation of state, insured persons and employers in the management of NHIF,
- contracting with providers of medical care,
- equality of all health care providers in concluding contracts with the NHIF,
- transparency in the activity of the NHIF and public control over its expenses.

Currently, Bulgaria's health system is financed through two sources: insurance premiums and taxes. Premiums for mandatory health insurance amount of 8% of income; the employer pays half of the contribution and the employee contributes the other half. Central and local budgets cover the unemployed, the poor, pensioners, students, members of the military and civil servants. Taxes are allotted for health care services as per law. Other sources include voluntary health insurance contributions, subscriptions by employers for specified health services, cash payments by citizens, and co-payments by patients.

Administered by the NHIF, social health insurance in Bulgaria does not envision exclusion from the obligatory system. However, 15% of the population lacks health insurance rights due to unpaid contributions and only 1.8% of the population has contracted voluntary private health insurance. GPs control access to specialized outpatient and hospital care. Public and private for-profit hospitals coexist. Care is provided through general hospitals, specialized hospitals, hospitals for aftercare, long-term care and rehabilitation, and psychiatric care hospitals.

3.6.1 *Hospital Administration and Management*

The management of hospitals depends on who owns them. There are several models of ownership for health establishments in Bulgaria. All must be registered as enterprises under the Trade Law. University hospitals and national centres are owned 100% by the state; managed by a Board of Directors with an Executive Director, the main principal is the Minister of Health. Regional hospitals are owned by the state (51%) and by local municipalities (49%). These are managed by Boards of Directors as representatives of the local authority. Municipal hospitals are limited liability companies owned 100% by the municipalities. Since January 2006, all hospital activities are fully financed by the NHIF on the basis of 325 clinical pathways that are supposed to include all diagnoses (Dimova *et al.* 2007).

Outpatient health care receives per capita plus fee-for-service from the NHIF. Every patient also pays 1% of minimal salary for every visit to a GP or specialist. All public hospitals have signed contracts with the NHIF to be financed on the basis of GPs. In addition, hospitals get 2% of the minimum monthly salary for each day of stay in a hospital, but for no more than 10 days per year. Some hospitals have signed contracts with the NHIF for high-specialized activities that are paid by fee-for-service. The Ministry of Health finances psychiatric hospitals for activities provided (number of patients treated), hemodialysis, transplantations, emergency care, expensive drugs, etc. Private hospitals also have signed contracts with the NHIF on the basis of clinical pathways as well as highly specialized activities. The hospital's owner finances its investments.

In 2005, there were 128,653 health care and social assistance employees who comprise 6% of national employment. In 2004, the number of practitioners included 27,423 physicians, 5,100 GPs, 10,001 outpatient specialists and 5,659 dentists. There are opportunities for hospital physicians to work in outpatient settings as well. Outpatient physicians generate revenues and income. Hospital physicians are salaried employees. According to contracts with the NHIF, remuneration of hospital staff cannot exceed 40% of revenues from the clinical pathways.

The current contribution rate of 8% is insufficient to cover health expenditure despite discussions in parliament about plans to extend coverage of all services and to raise the rate of health insurance to 10%. Although the health system has aimed to provide free and accessible comprehensive health care, in practice during the last decade, patients have increasingly paid out of pocket for many health services. Despite good intentions of achieving universal and equal access to health care, several factors cause substantial inequalities in access to health services. The lowest-income households, dominated by rural populations and ethnic minority groups, are the most disadvantaged in terms of restricted access to health care. In 2002, a survey of health expenditures by households found that over one-third of all Bulgarian households has a very low monthly income – less than €200. Total health expenditures do increase with household income but the lower the income level, the higher the relative share spent on health services (Atanasova *et al.* 2010).

3.6.2 Organization of Providers

Before 1999, primary and secondary (specialized) outpatient care had been provided in freestanding district or hospital-attached polyclinics. Patients were allocated by address to four types of district-based primary care physicians: internists, pediatricians, gynecologists and dentists. After consulting one of these, patients were referred to a specialist based in a polyclinic or hospital. Patients could also obtain direct access to specialists in case of medical need. In 1997, cost sharing by patients was introduced for these cases.

A major feature of reform in the outpatient sector is a radical change in the form and ownership of the establishments and in their legal status, which has led to equal status among all types of institutions, whether state-owned, municipal or private. The reform involved the creation of new types of outpatient institutions that embrace single and group practices for primary health care; single and group practices for specialized medical and dental care; medical, dental or medical-dental centres; independent medical-diagnostic and medical-technical laboratories, and independent diagnostic-consultative centres. Practices are assigned in accordance with the National Health Map, an instrument for structural reform that specifies minimum and target numbers for institutions and health care professionals by region.

Most polyclinics have been transformed into diagnostic-consultative centres and registered as trade companies in accordance with the law. These new institutions for specialized outpatient care are housed in former polyclinic buildings owned by the municipalities. Single and group practices for primary and specialized outpatient care have the right to acquire ownership of the premises and medical equipment, or to rent consulting rooms from the municipalities. Single practices in primary and specialized medical and dental care are the property of the respective physicians and dentists. Group practices for primary and specialized health care, medical, dental and medical-dental centres, diagnostic-consultancy centres, independent medical-diagnostic and medical-technical laboratories and the hospices are established as trade companies, co-operative, or limited liability companies by the state, by municipalities or jointly with other persons. Outpatient doctors have the legal status of independent contractors rather than civil servants. Outpatient care providers contract with the NHIF in order to participate in statutory provision; providers that do not sign contracts can provide private services on a fee-for-service basis.

Development of a modern system of primary health care was a major priority of health reform. One feature of the reform in primary health care was the replacement of the former internist, pediatrician and gynecologist with a new figure – the 'general practitioner'. The GP is to provide a much broader package of primary care services comprising preventive, diagnostic-therapeutic, rehabilitation and medical-social health care activities. Although general practice was to be cornerstone of the reform, at the start of the reform there were no medical professionals specializing in general medicine and the GPs were not prepared to do the new job. The Law on Health Care Establishments gave the right to all doctors with a basic medical specialty or in the process of acquiring specialty, to establish an individual or group practice for the purpose of providing primary medical care. The law gave a ten-year gratis period during which to receive training and acquire a specialty in general medicine.

Access to primary care is not constrained. Every Bulgarian citizen is free to choose a general practitioner within the region where he/she resides and to change her/him once every six months if desired. However, the access of low-income groups can be limited by the financial inability to pay the co-payment for the visit.

In 2009, the average number of people registered with a GP in Bulgaria was 1,472, which corresponds to European practice. There is, however, a tendency for GP practices to concentrate in large cities and university centres and a deficit in smaller areas with worse infrastructure, which generates substantial regional disparities in access to primary care services. Solo GP practices represent 82% of all primary care structures. During recent years, the number of group GP practices has been increasing due to organizational and economic advantages of this sort of structure for the delivery of primary care services (Marcheva 2010).

The elements of payment for primary health care include:

- per-capita monthly payments per insured person on a patient list,
- payment for completion of a package of services for priority cases (it is also a per-capita payment combined with periodic balancing),

- monthly sum as a bonus for working in remote places and in difficult conditions,
- fee-for-visit – 1% of the minimum monthly salary in the country.

Primary care practitioners are financed only by the NHIF and private out-of-pocket co-payments; they do not receive any government subsidies. The payment methodology for primary health care has undergone certain changes since the beginning of the reform. The share of preventive activities' payments is increasing with a special emphasis on child and maternal care. It is acknowledged that a system that combines payments for performed activities and per-capita payments is adequate for primary care specificities. This system will be sustained in the future by increasing the weight of preventive care activities by primary care physicians.

GPs act as 'gatekeepers' to the system of specialized care. Visits to outpatient specialists and to hospital care require referrals from the primary care physician. The two groups – patients and specialists – suffer some negative consequences of the GPs' gatekeeper function. Patients have limits on visits to specialists while the income of the specialists is reduced. As a result, the latter are underpaid in comparison with primary care physicians, especially in areas with high coverage by outpatient specialists.

Access to specialized outpatient care is limited due to the restricted financial resources provided by the NHIF. The Fund pays for a defined number of monthly visits to specialists and medical-diagnostic laboratories. Any examinations that exceed this number are put on a waiting list or are paid by the patients themselves. While people with higher incomes can afford to pay for specialized outpatient treatment, this is not possible for patients from low-income groups who represent a significant proportion of the population. Pensioners, pregnant women, children and patients with chronic illnesses need more specialized consultations and medical tests but quite often they have to wait or pay themselves to receive adequate and timely medical treatment. Specialists in outpatient care are paid on the basis of number of visits received. Conditions of payment are negotiated between the NHIF and the professional organizations, and included in the National Frame Contract (NFC).

The elements of payment for specialized outpatient care include:
- payment for initial visit with a payment for follow-up visits at half the fee of the first visit,
- payment for services that require expensive equipment or additional specialization,
- payment for expertise of permanent incapacity and professional diseases,
- payment for diagnostic tests,
- fee-for-visit – 1% of the minimal monthly salary in the country.

A process of horizontal integration of outpatient specialized care into MCs and diagnostic-consultative centres is observed in correspondence with the patients' preferences and for securing higher efficiency.

Regional coverage with specialists per 1,000 insured persons is even more unequal than primary care, and there is a shortage of specialists in remote rural areas. A positive trend is the increasing number of specialized care activities secured within the insurance package and negotiated within the NFC, which indicate improved responsiveness to patients' needs. A gradual increase is also observed in the defined number of referrals by GPs allowed monthly to outpatient specialist care.

With the introduction of compulsory health insurance, access to dental care was the most restricted service covered by the NHIF. Every insured person has the right to choose one of the dentists who have signed contracts with the insurance fund. So far, the number of services paid by the NHIF is very narrow; most people must pay privately or they cannot afford dental care. With the new Framework Contract for 2009, insurance coverage of dental care services for children has been expanded.

3.7 SUMMARY

Health care reform in Bulgaria is an ongoing process that involves all parts of society. Reforms started in 2000 with the introduction of the NHIF, the statute on GPs and clinical paths for hospital treatment, and private choice to supply and demand for health services. Thereafter, Bulgarian political parties reached a consensus about the next steps of health reform and prefer to retain the current health system in order to avoid resistance and unexpected crashes. In 2010, a set of measures has been accepted that will push forward the reform:

- better funding of NHIF through an increase of health contributions from 8% to 10% of the employee's salary,
- introduction of co-payment for specific hospital treatments,
- elaboration of a health map in order to optimize the number and location of hospitals and possible implementation with support of EU funds,
- the shift from clinical paths of hospital care to the diagnostic-related groups (DRGs) with a testing period during 2012-2013 and complete implementation after 2013-2014.

In fact, real changes were postponed until after elections in the autumn of 2011 so they could commence in early 2013. However, some steps have been taken such as closing several small and inefficient municipal hospitals; merging a few multi-profile neighborhood hospitals; increasing the level of generic drugs delivered free of charge by NHIF; and enhancing salaries of medical staff. All these measures are adaptive, so the second wave of comprehensive reforms is ahead of the country. Inevitably the reforms – other than restructuring the hospital system for efficiency – have to find a solution for the rise in medical expenditures through higher premiums for health insurance, higher private payments or direct government budget support. To some extent a delay in reforms can be an advantage because a better shape of measures is important for the success of any changes. Yet despite political consensus, the lack of sufficient budget resources is a barrier to health reforms.

4 Health Reforms in the Czech Republic

Ivan Malý, Marek Pavlík and Zuzana Darmopilová

Situated in central Europe, the Czech Republic is bordered by Poland, Germany, Austria and Slovakia. With an area of 78,864 km^2 and a population of about ten million, its capital and largest city is Prague with 1.3 million inhabitants. In the 20th century, following the collapse of the Austro-Hungarian Empire after World War I, the independent state of Czechoslovakia was established. Between the world wars, Czechoslovakia was a highly industrialized country with a democratic government. After the Munich Agreement and later German occupation, the country was divided into three parts – lands assimilated by Germany, the Czech-Moravian Protectorate, and an independent pro-Nazi Slovak Republic. After World War II, perhaps in gratitude for the liberation of Czechoslovakia by the Red Army and disillusion caused by the Munich Agreement, the Community Party won a majority in the 1946 election. After 1948, Czechoslovakia became a communist-ruled state. By 1968, dissatisfaction with the regime had produced the so-called Prague Spring during which attempts were made to reform communist doctrine into a social-democratic state. This attempt ended with another Soviet invasion.

However, in 1989 the Velvet Revolution returned the country to democratic principles, and in 1993 the Czech Republic was established after a peaceful dissolution of the Czech-Slovak Federative Republic. Although both countries are independent, their relations are amicable and their languages are very similar. The Czech Republic is a member of the European Union, NATO, OECD, OSCE, the Council of Europe and the Visegrád Group.

Table 4.1 indicates that as life expectancy and infant mortality have positive trends – upward and downward, respectively – the Czech Republic is among countries with very good social indicators, especially among post-communist states. Female life expectancy crossed 80 years in 2006. The total number of inhabitants is growing and the share of net migration as well as natural increase is proportional.

During 1990-2000, the Czech economy grew by 150% and by 167% during the next decade (Table 4.2). With some fluctuations, the inflation rate had declined to 1% in 2009 but then rose to 2.3% in 2010.

Although health expenditures as a percentage of Gross Domestic Product (GDP) were quite stable during 1990-2010, the structure of those expenditures changed. Like other post-communist states, the Czech health system faced the problems of induced and

Table 4.1 Demographic Characteristics

	1990	1995	2000	2005	2010
Population	10 362 740	10 330 759	10 272 503	10 234 092	10 517 147
Population density	131.4	131.0	130.3	129.8	133.4
Urban population (%)	78.9	74.7	74.5	74.5	74
Life expectancy (male)	NA	70.0	71.7	72.9	73.9
Life expectancy (female)	NA	76.6	78.4	79.1	80.11
Infant mortality rate	NA	7.7	4.1	3.4	2.7

Source: Czech Statistical Office; European Health for All Data Base.

Table 4.2 Economic Data (US$)

	1990	1995	2000	2005	2010
Total GDP (billions)	626	1 534	2 270	3 116	3 775
GDP per capita	60 428	148 457	220 949	304 478	358 957
Inflation rate	9.7	7.9	4.0	2.2	2.3

Source: International Monetary Fund; Czech Statistical Office.

never-ending demand. Problems with effectiveness together with limited resources have generated to an ever-larger portion of private out-of-pocket payments. The key reason was to involve the patient in the 'price' of health care; in other words, patients had to learn to value the cost of health services. The first phase was cost-participation on pharmaceutical drugs; the second phase (2007) was the implementation of regulatory fees.

The introduction of regulatory fees in the Czech Republic provides an example of the two-way interaction between politics and health policy. Between 1998 and 2006, despite rhetoric about government intentions for health reforms, no appreciable progress occurred. Every government found it difficult to construct a majority in the House of Representatives so weak and unstable government mandates inhibited systematic reform. In 2006, a new centre-right cabinet introduced a radical health reform plan, part of which included regulatory fees. The introduction of regulatory fees was necessitated by the need to rationalize over-usage of health services, especially contacts with physicians and prescription drugs. The government sought to increase the out-of-pocket share in financing Czech

Table 4.3 Health Expenditures (US$ Millions, Current Prices)

	1990	1995[b]	2000[a]	2005[a]	2010[a]
Central government outlays	NA	294	216	515	698
Regional & local government outlays	NA	274	229	373	583
Total Outlays	1.031	568	445	888	1 281
Percentage of total intergovernmental budgets[d]	**NA**	**11.7**	**14.1**	**14.1**	**13.3** (2009)
Public insurance	NA	2 916	3 001	7 103	11 193
Public expenditures	1.031[b]	3 484	3 446	7 991	12 474
Private out-of-pocket outlays	NA	277[c]	359	965	2 191
Total health expenditures (public + private)	1 031	3 793[c]	3 805	9 136	17 868
Total health expenditures as percentage of GDP	**4.7[d]**	**7.0[d]**	**6.5**	**7.2**	**7.5**

Sources: a) Czech Statistical Office.
b) Zdravotnická Ročenka ČR 1995 (Health Care Yearbook 1995).
c) Zdravotnictví České Republiky 2001 ve Statistických Údajích. ÚZIS, Praha 2002.
d) Health For All Database WHO, Copenhagen. January 2012.
e) Czech Statistical Office <http://czso.cz/csu/2012edicniplan.nsf/t/CD003F998E/$File/330612k2.pdf>.

health care, which at that time was the lowest of any OECD country. Figure 4.1 compares the Czech Republic with selected countries in the incidence of outpatient contacts.

After January 2008, a series of basic regulatory fees came into force:
- CZK 30 (approximately €1.20) for each visit to a physician,
- CZK 30 for every pharmaceutical paid fully or partially by health insurance and prescribed regardless of the number of packages,
- CZK 60 for each day of institutional care,
- CZK 90 for emergency service by a health facility providing first aid medical service

There was also an upper limit (CZK 5 000; approximately €200) for those who suffer chronic diseases.

As Figure 4.2 reveals, the political situation of the cabinet in 2007 was extraordinarily strong compared with previous periods. Between 1998 and 2006, the cabinet had always

Figure 4.1 Outpatients Contacts

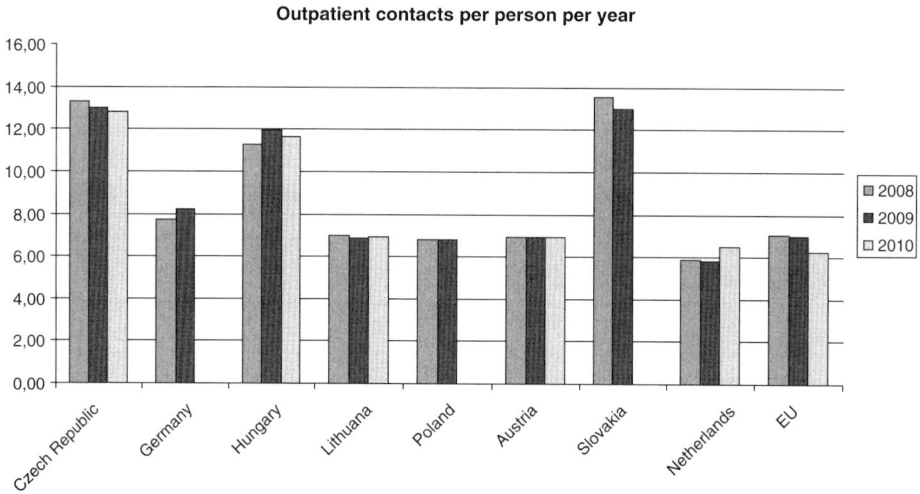

Source: <http://data.euro.who.int/hfadb/tables/tableA.php?w=1600&h=900> (modified by authors).

had a majority in the Chamber of Deputies but a minority position in the Senate and in the regions. Only during 2006-2007 did the cabinet achieve a majority in all regions as well as in the Senate and Chamber of Deputies. Based on the criterion of majority control, no cabinet had ever achieved a better position; hence the space for reform seemed sufficiently large.

However, the implementation of regulatory fees became controversial and generated public frustration. The government failed to explain the change as a part of a broader, sophisticated, and beneficial reform supported by major interest groups. Instead, unity inside the coalition weakened. Opposition parties used regulatory fees in their campaign arguments during the 2008 regional elections and obtained overwhelming success. Consequently coalition deputies did not pass other reform bills in the House of Representatives.

At the beginning of 2009, the cabinet lost its majority, so Premier Topolánek resigned and a 'nonpolitical' caretaker cabinet was formed without authority to introduce for any changes other than its duty to lead the country to early elections. The opposition's victory in regional elections strongly affected the impact of regulatory fees policy. Other than in Prague, all regional governments boycotted the policy in different ways. Most decided to repay the regulatory fees incurred by patients but only in regional hospitals.[1] There were differences in the methods of repayment as well as in the spectrum of regulatory fees covered. Table 4.4 shows the key differences by region.

1 The Czech Republic has four types of hospital: national and university (19+5), regional (24), local (17), and private (124).

Figure 4.2 Strength of the Coalition in Key Representative Bodies

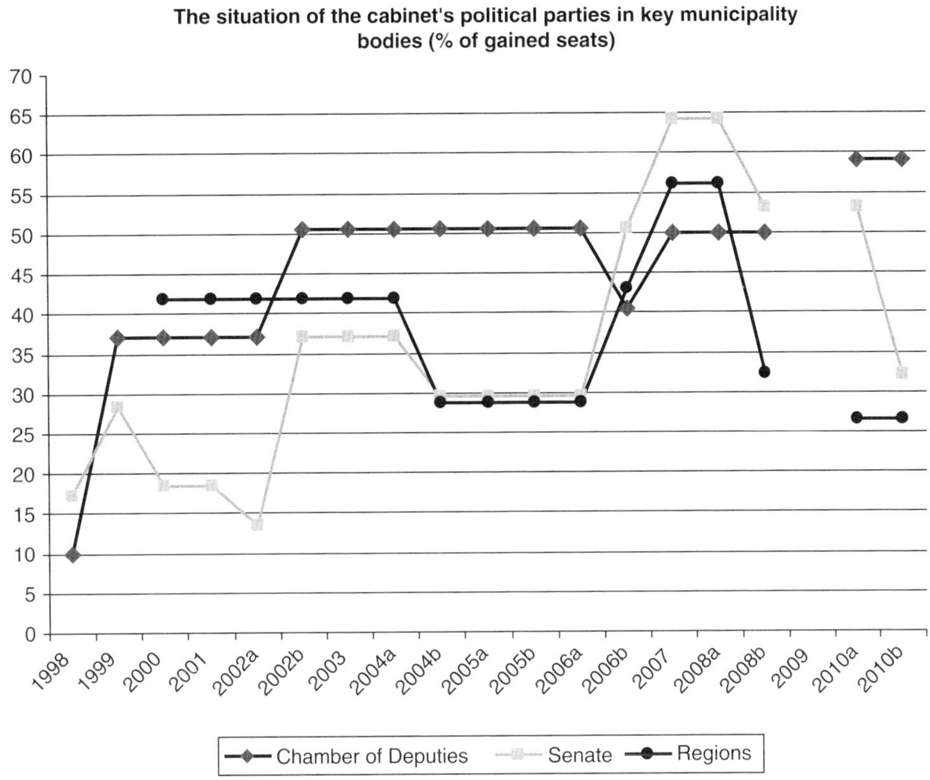

Source: Pavlík 2010 (translated); years marked as "a" or "b" display the situation before or after an election; interrupted lines indicate the period of a non-political caretaker cabinet.

As the regions began to repay the regulatory fees, the following problems became evident:

- discontinuity between the cabinet's policy and policy in the regions,
- discrimination against patients outside the regional hospitals,
- fragmentation of repayment methods and confusing information for patients.

The central government 'fought back' when the Ministry of Internal Affairs declared that the regions had acted beyond their authority. The only approved way to pay the fees would be retrospectively through a written deed of gift. Hence patients had to pay the fee, then request a refund. Consequently, one by one, the regions stopped paying the regulatory fees during 2010. Only one region – central Bohemian – insisted on refunds. In the end, regulatory fees became a regular part of the Czech health system. In 2008, they generated CZK 10 million (Pražáková and Dušek 2011), reduced the demand slightly, and allowed the Ministry and the health insurance companies to reallocate money to more urgent purposes like oncological care.

Table 4.4 Regional Attitudes to Regulatory Fees

Region	Review of Regions' Attitudes to Regulatory Fees					
	30 CZK Physician Visit	60 CZK Per day in Hospital	90 CZK Emergency Visit	Fees for Drug Prescription	Method of Repayment	Percentage of Involved Persons
South Bohemian	Yes	Yes	Yes	Yes	Written deed of gift	70
South Moravian	Yes	Yes	Yes	Yes	Written deed of gift	65
Karlovy Vary	Yes	Yes	Yes excluding dental care	Yes	Written or oral deed of gift	63
Hradec Králové	Yes	Yes	Yes	Yes	Written or oral deed of gift	65
Liberec	Yes	Yes	Yes	Yes	Written affirmation	51
Moravian-Silesian	Yes	No	No	Yes	Written deed of gift	45
Olomouc	Yes	Yes	Yes	Yes	Written deed of gift	65
Pardubice	Yes	Yes	Yes	Yes	Written deed of gift	46
Central Bohemian	Yes	Yes	Yes	Yes	Possibility to ask the region for gift	25
Central Bohemian	Yes	Yes	Yes	Yes	Oral deed of gift	95
Ústí	Yes	Yes	Yes	Yes	Written affirmation	40
Vysočina	Yes	Yes	Yes	Yes	Written deed of gift	60
Zlín	Yes	Yes (only youth and pensioners)	No	No	The patient has to ask the Region for gift	25
Prague	No	No	No	No		

Source: Malý, Pavlík and Krůtilová 2012.

This case provides several lessons. First, it is important to reach a consensus within all relevant levels of the government. Regions can strongly affect a policy, and sometimes they can completely abolish it. Second, successful health policy requires strong political support. On the other hand, it can both generate and take away a considerable political power. And third, the ability to communicate complex social issues with the public and other stakeholders is one of the most important prerequisites of a successful reform.

Table 4.5 shows information about the resources for Czech health care such as an increasing number of physicians and a decreasing number of hospital beds. Debates about optimization of providers are linked with problems of optimal structure and the number of hospital beds. The decline is affected by two factors: economic limits of hospitals and changing trends in hospital care. Although the total number of hospital beds declined by 27%, actors in the system argue about the optimal number of hospital beds, especially in acute care. Efforts to optimize the network of providers are strongly affected by changing 'beliefs' about which key principle is better – market forces or state intervention. Hence the state had a period of state intervention as well as privatization and strengthening of 'market forces'.

Overall, the number of physicians increased by about one-third and seems to cover the needs of the system. Although sometimes the number of physicians in a given specialization or region has been deemed to be insufficient, this problem was never considered to be important. But a special factor affecting the number of physicians is the wage problem. Popular opinion feels that physicians as well as other health professionals are not sufficiently rewarded. The low salaries for nurses are inducing increasing numbers of foreign nurses – mostly from Slovakia because there is no language barrier.

Table 4.5 Health Resources

	1990	1995	2000	2005	2009
Physicians	28 036	30 942	34 604	36 381	37 351
Physicians/100,000 population	271	300	337	355	357
Other health professionals (nurses, pharmacists, midwives)	99 267	100 967	104 268	97 234	97 096
Other health professionals/100,000	958	977	1015	950	941
Hospital beds	113 204	95 217	87 820	85 723	83 667
Hospital beds /100,000 population	1092	922	855	838	811

Source: European Health for All Database.

4.1 CONTEXTUAL ISSUES

The Czech health system is based on the solidarity principle with its roots in the era of centralized economic plans during 1948-1990. After the 1989 Velvet Revolution, structural changes occurred in the health system that were market-oriented but retained the principle of a public insurance system. Left-oriented as well as right-oriented political parties accept the principle of solidarity. Despite attempts since 1990 to reform the health system, none has been fully implemented and most of the changes were nonsystematic. Nonetheless, the aims of the reforms were usually the same: to ensure sufficient financial resources, to improve effectiveness of financial resources allocation, and to improve the quality of care.

Cultural orientations can be described through public opinion polls (Figure 4.3). Questions were posed about the financing system and the behavior of health insurance companies; the quality of care was considered as well.

The system of public insurance theoretically guarantees each necessary service for each insured person. The Czech health system lacks strict gatekeepers so citizens have free choice of physician or health facility. Except for dental services, medication and health aids, direct co-payments were not implemented until 2008. After the most recent reform attempt (by a right-oriented coalitional cabinet), direct co-payment was included in the

Figure 4.3 Problems in the Czech Health System

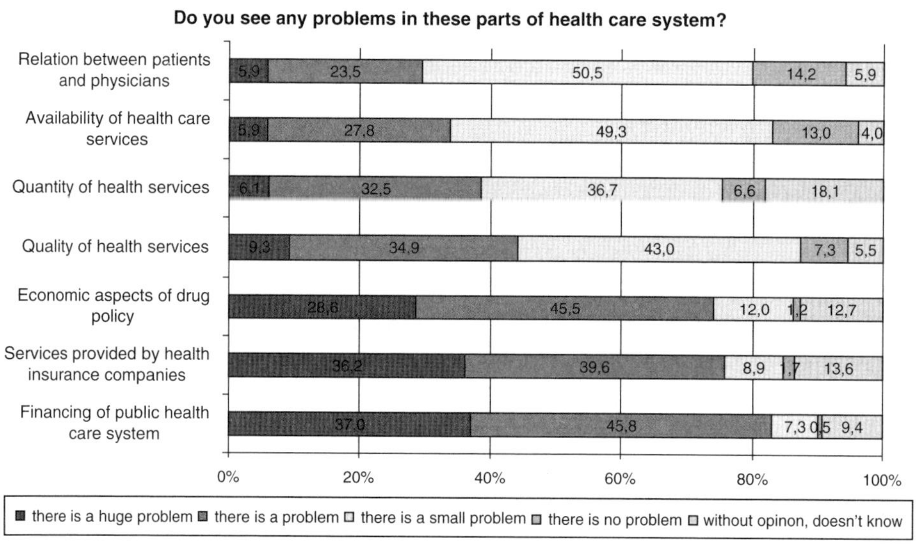

Source: Sociologický ústav AV ČR 2006 (translated).

health system as patients pay a fee for physician visits, prescriptions and hospital stays. The solidarity principle is retained due to the limit of CZK 2,500 (approximately €100) on total expenditures for direct co-payments per year.

Health insurance premiums (more precisely, a health payroll tax) are based on income. Every citizen is formally eligible to obtain care according his or her needs. However, because there is a lack of 'care standards', the extent or quality of care to which a person has a right is not clear.

The state (particularly its cabinet) is traditionally considered to be a strong player in the health sector at both national and regional levels. State authority is based on legislative powers and the state is traditionally perceived as an important policy-maker, especially the Ministry of Health. However, the Czech state consists of two strong players – the cabinet (specifically the Ministry of Health) and self-governments. Both have legislative powers and although regional and local self-governments must formally conform to the cabinet they have power to oppose cabinet policy. For example, in 2007 the cabinet decided to impose fees on patients – *i.e.*, fees for a visit to a physician visit and fees for prescriptive drugs. As part of the intended health reform, fees were considered to be a tool to teach patients about the 'value' of services for health care. However, some regions (mostly with a left-oriented majority in their representative bodies) began to refund money to patients in their regional hospitals. Each region had its own method of repayment but overall the regions sought to boycott the cabinet's decision. Eventually the constitutional court ruled that this situation is unconstitutional and that the regions had to stop such refunds. The prevailing situation is that right-oriented cabinets face opposition in the regions because a majority of the latter have left-oriented representative bodies, and vice versa.

4.2 Role of Government

The government is not directly involved in relations among patients, providers and health insurance companies. However, the legislature determines all the basic variables of the health care system. Laws determine the levels of insurance premiums, the duties and discretion of the insured, the extent of services to be covered fully by providers and those to be covered partly, and the reimbursement to be paid by health insurance companies to providers for their services.

The government determines the level of insurance premiums. For employees and self-employed persons the law determines the percentage of wages to be deducted; for those who are 'state insured' – *i.e.*, persons who lack income like students, pensioners, prisoners – the cabinet decides on the amount to be contributed for each. At present, the 'state insured' are 58% of all those insured in the system. The amount paid by the government for the 'state insured' is always lower than the minimum amount that employees or self-employed persons must pay. Hence any decision about the amount for state insured has an impact on health care resources.

The cabinet's role is very important during the annual negotiations with health insurance companies (HICs) and providers about the level of reimbursement for services. The cabinet also influences the level of reimbursement for pharmaceutical drugs. Finally, the cabinet is able to influence the HICs through appointing members of their executive councils or board councils. Although disputed, this practice is typical not only for health care but for all sectors.

Hence the government influences the methods of providing health care. The state influences the extent of basic care by defining which services are to be provided free (from the patient's point of view). It also specifies the duties and discretion of providers and HICs; the education of health staff and conditions of their work; and the production, distribution and consumption of drugs and medical aids.

4.3 Dominant Values in Health Policy

The first official reform document issued in 1990 (SKUPR 1990) announced a new system of health care in order to ensure transparency, economy, democratization, humaneness and a higher standard of care. During the past 20 years, three values have been evident in Czech health policy – solidarity, equity and plurality. Codified by the Constitution, *solidarity* is the dominant value but it has never been seriously tackled. Despite controversies about the scope of solidarity, the principle itself is generally accepted across all political parties and other health policy actors. There have been few attempts to introduce or to strengthen elements representing principles of equivalence such as clear definitions of a 'standard' or slightly higher regulation fees.

With the exception of a brief period during the early 1990s, Czech society has understood *equity* as *equality*. By comparing data from 1991 and 1999, Řeháková (2001) measured public attitudes about income inequalities and concluded that inequalities are considered to be higher and less fair; there was large support for the view that the government should reduce it. There is a strong proclivity towards egalitarianism within the general public, which is even truer with respect to health services.

The demand for *plurality* was a reaction to the long-term state monopoly on health services. It is reflected in many elements of the Czech health system such as freedom of choice for patients, a public-private mix of providers, multi-source financing, and health insurance through several HICs competing for enrollees. The belief in 'automatic' benefits stemming from plurality (like cost control, quality, and efficiency) has weakened due to misuse of services by 'shopping' patients, virtually no real competition among HICs, and other factors.

4.4 Governance of the Health Sector

The Czech Republic has a multi-source system of financing health care. The sources include health insurance (76.9%), state and municipal (8.3%) and out-of-pocket payments (14.8%). The system is financed mainly by contributions from individuals, employers and the state. Contributions are defined by law as a percentage of wages (before tax). Employees pay 4.5% and employers pay 9% (13.5% combined); the self-employed pay the same total percentage (13.5%); and the Ministry of Finance contributes approximately €30 per month per person on behalf of certain categories of the population – the unemployed, pensioners, children and dependents up to 26 years of age, students, women on maternity leave, men serving in the military, prisoners, and people receiving social welfare. Health insurance contributions have been redistributed in order to lower the potential for risk selection and to ease the financial difficulties of health insurance funds (HIFs) with adverse risk structures. All collected contributions are liable to redistribution; they are reallocated according to two criteria – age and the extent of resource utilization (*e.g.*, treating chronic disease or morbidity). The General Health Insurance Fund (GHIF) administers these funds.

Taxes cover expenditure at both national and regional levels. At national level, the Ministry of Health finances the capital investments of facilities that it directly manages, such as regional hospitals, university hospitals and specialized institutions for research and postgraduate education. Public health services are also financed directly by the Ministry of Health. Direct funding by the Ministry of Health covers part of the cost of training medical personnel and of running specialized health programs such as AIDS prevention, drug control, the operating costs of long-term care institutes, research and postgraduate education. Social care is paid partly by the Ministry of Social Affairs and partly by users of the services. Cost sharing is required for selected drugs, dental services and some medical aids. Since January 2008, with a maximum annual limit, Czechs pay regulatory fees for medical prescriptions, hospitalization days, emergency visits, and visits by medical specialists.

HIFs are relatively independent bodies responsible for entering into contracts with health care providers. Contracts are generally for a two-year period. In accordance with health insurance legislation, there are regular negotiations – usually every six months – among the HIFs, providers (hospital associations, hospitals and private physicians) and professional chambers. These bodies negotiate the range of services to be covered under the compulsory health insurance system as well as the number of reimbursement points per service in the fee schedule; the monetary value of points used to determine actual reimbursement; and conditions for delivering services in the major sectors of health care. The ministry evaluates the results of such negotiations for their compliance with legal norms and public interests. The government is entitled to make the necessary decisions if no agreement can be reached.

As for reimbursement methods, hospital inpatient care is reimbursed according to a budget based on the relevant period of the previous calendar year and taking the inflation rate into account. Since 2001, in addition to the budgets, a flat fee is paid on the basis of the number of cases treated in each hospital. General practitioners (GPs) are paid through capitation fees per patient but the number of patients per physician is limited because exceeding that limit means smaller per capita payments. In addition, some GP services like preventive examinations and visits to patients' homes are paid through fee-for-service (approximately 30% of their income). Services by ambulatory specialists are reimbursed through fee-for-service. There are, however, limits on the volume of services and reimbursement depends on the number of hours worked. Dental services are reimbursed according to a special price list, the individual items of which are calculated directly in monetary terms.

About 95% of primary health care was privatized in 2002. Most primary health physicians work alone but a group of them may work together in health centres or in the few polyclinics that provide primary health care in addition to specialist care. The municipality or local community owns these centres. Currently the Czech network of health care facilities for secondary and tertiary care consists of the offices of specialized outpatient physicians, hospitals, and specialized bed facilities. While approximately three-quarters of outpatient physicians have become private in recent years, most bed facilities remain public. However, their status is undergoing changes in relation to reforms in public administration. Hospitals are owned both by the state and by private for-profit and not-for-profit organizations. Nineteen hospitals are managed directly by the Ministry of Health (9.5% of all hospitals, with 26.9% of the total number of beds); other hospitals are regional, municipal and town. There are also private hospitals and church hospitals. Faculty hospitals have a special status.

The Ministry of Health is responsible for procuring the uniform professional management of public health care. Regional offices and the Ministry of Health are responsible for the network of health facilities. The regional offices cooperate in the creation of the health care institutions and perform tasks related to the establishment and management of health care facilities in their respective territories, with the exception of large hospitals. They execute those tasks as part of their regional powers. As part of the powers transferred to them, regions decide on the issuing, changing or withholding the registration of non-state health care facilities; they keep records on the capacities of health care facilities and enter into contractual relationships for the provision of necessary health care services with respect to first-aid medical services and rescue services.

4.5 Political, Contextual and Historical Features

From a political viewpoint, the Czech Republic has three strong parties: the Civic Democratic Party (ODS), the Czech Social Democratic Party (ČSSD) and the Communist Party of Czech and Moravia (KSČM). At the beginning of the 1990s, KSČM was a one of the weaker parties but has since established itself as the third strongest party. Despite its power, the KSČM was never invited into a government coalition. This decision was made by the right-oriented party ODS as well as the left-oriented party ČSSD for the same reasons – fear of reactions by non-KSČM voters and the past history of the party because during 1948-1990 KSČM had been the lead party. Table 4.6 presents the results of elections from 1996 to 2010. During elections in 2010 two new parties entered the Chamber

Table 4.6 Election Results (Percentage Gained Seats in the Chamber of Deputies) 1996-2010

	1996	1998	2002	2006	2010
ČSSD	30.5	37.0	35.0	37.0	28.00
ODS	34.0	31.5	29.0	40.5	26.5
ODA	6.5	0.0	0.0	0.0	0.0
KDU-ČSL	9.0	10.0	15.5*	6.5	0.0
KSČM	11.0	12.0	20.5	13.0	13.0
SPR_RSČ	9.0	0.0	0.0	0.0	0.0
US-DEU	0.0	9.5	*	0.0	0.0
SZ	0.0	0.0	0.0	3.0	0.0
VV					12.0
TOP09					20.5

Source: <www.volby.cz> (*coalition partners in the 2002 election).

of Deputies. The first is TOP09 (same abbreviation as the name of the party); the second party is called *Public Affairs (VV)*.

Before the 2006 parliamentary election, the right-oriented *Civic Democratic Party (ODS)* introduced a complex health reform vision based on principles of managed competition. Its proposal sought to increase competition among health insurance companies; to define the rules and right for all health actors; and to involve patients in the cost of health care. The Minister of Health (an ODS member) began the reform process but failed. The Cabinet appointed in 2006 (a coalition of ODS, KDU-ČSL and SZ) lost the support of the Chambers of Deputies. Since 2009 a temporary cabinet has existed according an agreement between the two strongest parties in the Chamber of Deputies – ODS and ČSSD. After the elections in 2010, the party entered the cabinet together with fragile coalition with TOP09 and Political Affairs (VV). Although the *TOP09* defines itself as right-oriented party, the second party (VV) is hard to categorize on a right-left continuum. *Public Affairs (VV)* has political program based on populist slogans without a clear program of action.

The left-oriented *Czech Social Democratic Party (ČSSD)* supports solidarity and some of its members strongly support the idea of only one health insurance company. In general, the party supports more regulation in the health system. During 1998-2006, representatives of the party held the post of Health Minister but frequent turnover of occupants caused a lack of systematic health policy. The ČSSD has disagreed with additional out-of-pocket payments by patients and boycotted implementation of co-payments by patients through using regional budgets to cover fees for visits. This position enabled victory by ČSSD in most regions during the 2008 election. ČSSD has made coalitions with left-oriented parties or with ODS.

The 2010 election to the Chamber of Deputies brought a 'pyrrhic' victory for ČSSD. While the party gained the most votes and received 28% of seats in the Chamber of Deputies, it was unable to form a majority coalition. Instead ODS formed the cabinet together with TOP09 and VV. In 2012, there are signs that ČSSD is backing away from its fundamental rejection of regulatory fees.

The *Christian Democrats (KDU-ČSL)* is a right-oriented party – usually one of the two weakest political parties in the Chamber of Deputies – without a vision on health policy. The party generally declares support for the solidarity principle and the improvement of quality of health services. The *KDU-ČSL* has been in each cabinet during last three governments whether the ČSSD (1998-2006) or the ODS (2006-2009) led the coalition.

In 2004, the *Communist Party of Czech and Moravia (KSČM)* introduced a vision of health reform based on the principle of solidarity and a strong role for the state. Although usually the third largest party in the Czech Republic, the KSČM has never entered a cabinet. The *Green Party (SZ)* has no health program but supports the solidarity principle. It accepts the necessity to involve patients in paying the costs of care through fees paid by patients. However, in the 2010 election SZ was unsuccessful; instead, two new parties entered the Chamber of Deputies.

Table 4.7 compares the pre-election programs of the three strongest parties. Although this analysis was done for the year 2006, those three parties retain the same principles.

Table 4.7 Comparison of Party Political Programs in the 2006 Election

	ODS	ČSSD	KSČM
Health Insurance System	More HICs and managed competition	Merge HICs (long-term vision of one payer in the system)	Only one HIC
Determination of Patients' Rights	Yes, by the law	Not mentioned	Not mentioned
Increasing salaries of health staff	Yes, for nurses	Yes	Yes
Legal form of 'public' hospitals	Non-profit (directed by the state or university)	Non-profit hospitals	Network of state and non-profit hospitals
Creation of skilled centers of care	Yes	No	Not mentioned
Financing system	Co-payments for services above defined standards	Increase GDP portion to 8%	Cancellation of patients' fee
	Possibility of private insurance in addition to public insurance	Increasing insurance premium for 'state insured'	Increase GDP portion to 8%
	Limits to co-payments for basic care (equity)	Decrease patients' fee; fixed limits for co-payments	Higher insurance premium for 'state employees'
Pricing drugs	Decrease price of drugs and reimbursement tariffs	Centralized drug policy	Standardize drug co-payments
	Transparent pricing system		

Source: compiled by the author.

Health policy seems to be irrelevant in 2012 compared to the political issues of corruption, growing distrust by a large part of public in the whole official political structure, and the social consequences of governments, restrictive fiscal policy. On reflection, there are two competing postures similar to other countries – health services as a non-for-profit public undertaking and health services as a well-organized business, efficient but not necessarily not-for-profit.

4.6 History of Health Reforms

After World War II, the socialist model of a health system – centralized and hierarchic – was established in Czechoslovakia. Regional and municipal districts of national health hired all medical staff. The state had a monopoly in providing health care. The system was fully financed from the state budget and had large capacities (more physicians and greater number of hospital beds in international comparison), but was relatively cheap (approximately 5% of GDP). The system was characterized by low effectiveness; it did not react flexibly to citizen needs and there was a lack of modern management, economic stimuli and quality control. Thus, the Czechoslovak health system lost the ability to make rational decisions about the resources allocation so a great deal of money, human potential and confidence of the citizens was squandered. The social prestige of health workers was low. The system was said to be equal for all citizens, but in reality, privileges existed for certain social and political groups while others experienced discrimination. The possibility of choosing a physician or health facility was limited. In summary, health services in Czechoslovakia at that time could be described as undemocratic, uneconomical and often lacking a human approach.

Initially, of course, the system had functioned well. Some diseases disappeared and the rate of infant mortality indicators declined. Between 1960 and 1964, the Czechoslovak health system held the tenth position among 27 European countries. However, health indices then stagnated or declined. These indices indicated that citizens were sicker and died sooner than nationals of other European as well as some non-European countries. From 22nd place in 1970, Czechoslovakia dropped to the 27th place in 1980. This situation revealed a chronic crisis of health and health care. Political, economic and social changes after November 1989 brought new impulses for the health system and for the whole economy.

4.7 Transformation (1989-1991)

In the early 1990s, initiatives by citizens began to appear and to cooperate with the Ministry of Health. Together they formulated the first principles for changes in the health system. It was evident that modifications of the system would not suffice because a completely new system of health care was required. The target was to create a flexible system capable of adjusting to the changing needs of society while ensuring a balance of professional, economic and human aspects. In other words, a complete transformation from the centralized model into the more democratic and liberal system would provide better health services to all citizens and have a better control of its efficiency and economy.

Even if the monopolistic position of the state in providing and managing the health care services was to be abolished, the state continued to play an important role in the health system by guaranteeing adequate health care for all citizens. The creation, implementation and control of health policy were de-monopolized when it was agreed that the community would implement the principles of public health within its own territory. It was decided that the health services would be financed from different sources (state budget, resources of communities, enterprises, citizens) and that obligatory health insurance would be an indispensable part of the new system of health care. There was an intention to introduce competition into the delivery of health services. The principle of free choice of provider and health care facility was agreed to be introduced.

Important changes were adopted in financing the health system, in providing institutions for services, and in public administration. Regional and municipal health districts were abolished as health care facilities became independent with their own legal and economical liability. The centralized system of health care financed from state budget was replaced by a system financed by different sources although still based on the principle of solidarity. Obligatory health insurance was chosen to be the most important source of finance while patients would have the right to choose their physicians and their health care facilities.

The transformations between 1990 and 1993 occurred quickly and were oriented mostly to financial topics. Physicians greatly influenced the approach to these initial changes – even within the citizen initiatives mentioned above in which physicians sought to increase their social prestige and income. Because legal and economical details were not discussed during the creation and implementation of this transformation, there has been a long period of instability in the health system. The importance of control while using public funds was underestimated, a situation that remains in the current Czech health system.

4.8 Privatization (1992-1996)

The year 1992 was characterized by introduction of privatization into the health system. The first idea was to privatize everything except large hospital complexes. Because the legal system had no rules for nonprofit organizations, most health facilities took the form of business enterprises. In 1993, a law introducing obligatory health insurance came in force, which stressed competition. Initially, 27 health insurance companies were established that subsequently merged or collapsed. By 1996, two-thirds of them had become bankrupt and their liquidation was a problem for the state budget. Today, nine health insurance companies remain in the Czech Republic.

Among the effects of privation were an increase in the quality of services, better technical equipment and the introduction of economical principles in the health care system. Health care management began to be divided among public administration, professional chambers and insurance companies. Unfortunately, the rationalization of the health care facility network, expected as one of the outcomes of the privatization, did not occur.

4.9 Rationalization of the Hospital Network (1997-1999)

In the mid-1990s, the health system was in financial crisis. Many hospitals fell into serious debt and financial imbalances occurred in the insurance companies. Consequently, government health policy began to regulate the supply side of the economy. The goals were to reduce the number of acute hospital beds, to reinforce specialized acute hospital beds, to reduce the number of physicians and to control drugs and investment policy. These goals are still discussed in the Czech Republic. The problem is not the number of hospital beds per se but their geographic mix.

4.10 Public Administration Reform (2000-2003)

Within the framework of public administration reform, 82 state hospitals among the 203 hospitals in the Czech Republic became the property of regions. These hospitals were in debt with total indebtedness of about €20 million. Because the state commitment subsidy to regions represented approximately 60% of the debts, some regions changed the legal form of these hospitals to joint-stock companies. According to regional representatives, this change stabilized the economy of hospitals due to higher motivation and personal responsibility of boards of management and higher transparency of asset and commitment status. Nevertheless, this measure was controversial. Even though a region owns hospitals, they should be managed as any other private company. Some politicians presented this situation as defiance of the principles of equity and solidarity. This problematic continues in the Czech Republic.

4.11 2005 and 2006 Developments

The necessity of change was amplified by the accumulated debt of the GHIF (the biggest insurer in the Czech Republic) and of several large hospitals. Lawmakers sought to centralize decision-making of all financial flows in the sector as much as possible in order to influence the development and management of the debt. Another government target was to increase the price of work by doctors and other medical workers (whose pay is very low compared to other EU members) and to exert pressure on quality.

Changes in the reimbursement procedure meant an increase in prices of services by doctors and other medical workers (expressed by higher numbers of 'points' for some concrete activities) and setting the maximal limit on income for single providers. The result was not only discontent among providers, ending in protests and walkouts, but also a real threat to the accessibility of health care by patients. Therefore another regulation was issued that softened the original limits on reimbursements.

In a proclaimed apprehension of 'tunneling' the regional hospitals, the social-democratic government blocked further 'privatization' of hospitals and enforced the law on the establishment of non-profit hospitals network according to the key 'one hospital in every district'.[2]

This law obliged the health insurance companies to conclude a contract with every non-profit hospital. In conformity to this law, several issues started to be ordained by the Ministry of Health – for instance, the scope and structure of health care provided, equipment, number of beds, personnel capacities, salaries and the remuneration of doctors.

4.12 Julínek Reform Proposal (2006-2009)

Parliamentary elections in 2006 generated high expectations among specialists in the health sector. After 15 years of inactivity and inability to enforce reforms, a certain change seemed to occur in the Czech Republic. Although the government coalition was fragile (102 to 98 seats), Health Minister Julínek (the 14th minister since 1990) did not lack the will to enforce radical changes in the system (carefully prepared long before he entered the position). As early as autumn 2006, the minister presented the objectives of the Ministry of Health for the 2006-2010 period.

2 A district is a municipality smaller than the region; a region is comprised of several self-governing districts.

Reform measures were divided into two phases. The first phase sought to stabilize the system and reform institutions; the second phase included the reform of finances and thus securing long-term sustainability of the solidarity principle. The first phase of the reform ('Institution Reform' from 2006) consisted of four goals: (1) enhance citizens' choices and responsibility, (2) increase the responsibility of health insurance companies, (3) modernize the network of health care facilities, and (4) reimburse drugs according to their asset. This stage of the reform was a preliminary phase that brought partial changes to the existing system and should have been followed by a system change that would transform the financial system of Czech health care. The concept of this new system as well as its framework are relatively clearly defined; nevertheless, in order to finalize its detailed form, a team of specialists at the Ministry of Health began working on the so-called 'Round Table' project. In August 2007 amendments to laws on health care were adopted. The changes sought to stabilize the system and prepare it for subsequent reforms. Within the scope of these amendments, regulatory fees for medical prescription, hospitalization days, emergency visits, and visits of a medical specialist (with maximum yearly limit) were introduced.

The process of determining reimbursement for drugs was changed in compliance with EU requirements, and likewise, the relationship between the state and the General Health Insurance Company. Following these changes, at the end of 2007 the Ministry proposed seven reform laws that were supposed to begin in 2009 and can be divided into three mutually linked sets of legislative and non-legislative measures: public health insurance; provision of health care services; and education, science and research. However, the reform strategy was not enforced and Minister Julínek left office in early 2009. Pursuit of the reform was influenced by three factors: the weak mandate of the government; the weak will of the Ministry to seek consensus within the government coalition; and poor communication strategy with other actors in the health policy. As a result, the Ministry became isolated; this isolation reached a peak after the introduction of regulatory fees. Table 4.8 summarizes the history of health reforms in the Czech Republic.

4.13 Short and Medium-Term Reform Outcomes

No long-term reform has been implemented in the Czech Republic. While there were health reforms at the beginning of examined period, later attempts failed. Some changes occurred but not as an outcome of reforms. Causality between health policy aims and implemented changes is questionable. Most changes were incremental like changes in the legal form of hospitals. Initially competition among health insurance companies was enabled and supported by 60% redistribution of insurance contributions. Later the level of insurance contributions increased and all collected contributions were redistributed. During the period, there have been contradictory opinions about the effects of having

Table 4.8 Health Reforms in the Czech Republic

1990-1991
– Preparation of basic changes – Starting these basic changes – Regional and municipal districts of national health abolishment – Creation of Czech Medical Chamber, Dental Chamber and Pharmaceutical Chamber
1992
– Preparation of the health insurance system – Preparation of privatization
1993
– Introduction of the health insurance system (payers plurality) – Some branch health insurance companies founded – Start of the privatization process (mostly ambulatory care)
1994-1995
– First serious problems in financing the health system – Majority of branch health insurance companies founded – Legal limitation of competition among health insurance companies – Need of fundamental reform begins to be generally recognized
1997-1998
– Leftwing government seeks purely non-profit orientation of health policy – Escalation of expenditures kept down (lump sum payment) – Attempt to re-structure the hospital network
1999-2001
– Stagnation
2002-2009
– Continued escalation of health expenditures – Several reform proposals but only on paper – Transfer of hospitals to regions – Controversial transformation of some regional hospitals to joint-stock companies – Partial amendments in the system – Julínek reform proposal (2006) – Stagnation (since 2009)

Source: Vepřek *et al.* 2002.

more than one health insurance company. Currently, there are nine insurance companies with no real competition; the general agreement is that the current situation is not optimal. However, previous changes provide no clue about the future form of health insurance companies. There are two possibilities: shift to a system of managed competition that enables competition among HICs, or shift to a noncompetitive system by establishing a single health insurance company.

Between 1990 and 2010, there were many changes. First, all the health status indicators were improving due to both better quality of care (based on improved technical equipment) and changing life-style. During this period, reimbursement principles repeatedly changed but only incrementally. Many HICs were established and subsequently liquidated. The number of HICs stabilized at about 9 (+/− one) and has remained stable during the past decade, but the debate about system principles remains open. The question whether only one HIC would be better than a system of managed completion among HICs is still discussed. One important argument is 'effectiveness' – *i.e.,* whether one HIC would be more effective than nine HICs; however, comparison of operating costs (Figure 4.4) indicates that this topic is not 'hot' in the Czech Republic. During the period, health expenditures grew constantly and consuming an increasing proportion of private resources.

Figure 4.4 Comparison of Operating Costs of Health Insurance Companies (% Total Revenues)

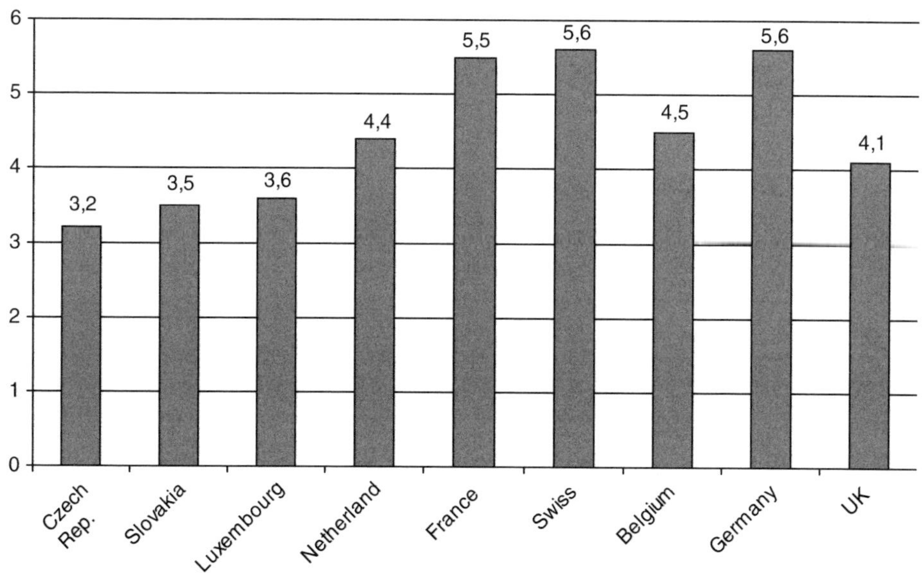

Source: AIM Brussels (<http://szpcr.cz/reforma/100204_strategie_SZPCR.pdf>).

The weakest point during this period is the absence of a comprehensive health policy. All changes were *ad hoc* and incremental within the never-ending debate about reforms. Consensus among strong actors seems to be unreachable. On average, the Minister of Health changed every 14 months so he had little time to defend his position or follow through on proposals. Since 2007, regulatory fees have been implemented, but other fundamental bills to change the health care system have not been passed.

After the 2010, election the current Government has agreed to apply four principles: to open the legal way for patient's co-payments by introducing an explicit "basic benefit package" (so-called "covered standard"); to apply mechanisms in order to regulate new technologies and to reduce their impact upon costs; to enforce changes in HIC´s behavior, mainly to make them accountable for costs, access, and quality of care; and to allow the money to follow the patient. After roughly two years of quite chaotic development, the Ministry has prepared a number of reform bills and successfully presented them in Parliament. A set of reforms comes into effect in 2012 in which the position of patients has been strengthened, insurance claims have been defined explicitly, and procedural requirements have been established.

4.14 Remaining Problems

The system is based on the solidarity principle in terms of access but not in cost participation.[3] The position of actors (regions, state institutions, HICs) remains ambiguous. One major problem – low salaries of health staff – led to a strike by physicians during 2011. From the physicians' point of view, this strike was successful because they were promised increased salaries. The debate about optimizing the network of providers and the extent of guaranteed care (compulsory and optional health insurance) is now resolved in the new legal proposals. The remaining problem of the Czech health care system is evident in Figure 4.5 although the latest data are unfortunately only from 2006.

4.15 Summary

The recent history of Czech health reform reveals ups and downs. A fundamental and possibly too fast transformation in the early 1990s changed the old Semashko system without harming a universal and quite generous access for the public to health care. Several

3 The Czech Republic has the different levels of insurance premiums: an employee together with employer pays 13.5% of wages (average wage CZK 2,000 or €66); self-employed pay 13.5% or at least CZK 1,500 per month (€50); for the 'state insured' the state pays CZK 723 per month (€25).

Figure 4.5 Possible Solutions of Problems in the Health System

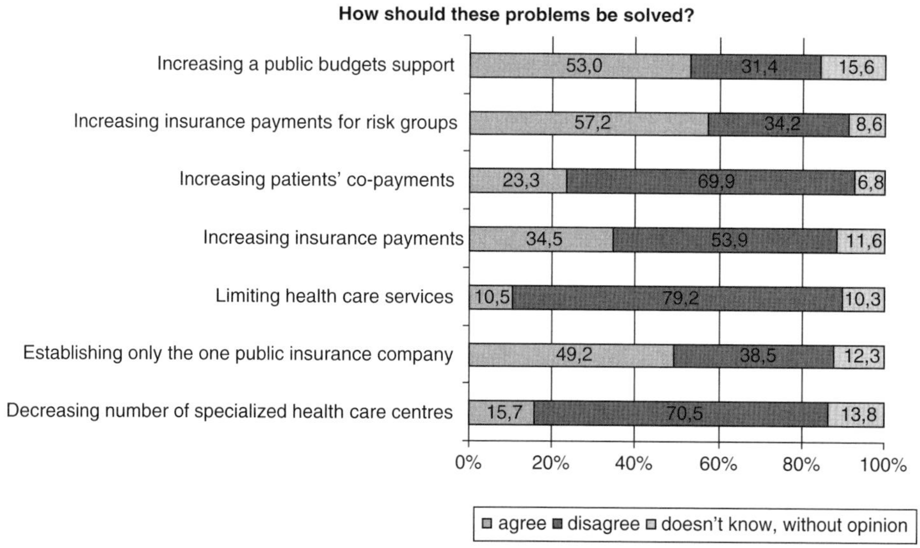

Source: Compiled by authors from poll results published by *Sociologický ústav AV ČR, 2006.*

fundamental pieces of reform were omitted as a price for that speed, such as clear identification of responsibilities and a guaranteed package of benefits. Rising deficits and growing frustration among health professionals have had consequences. After 1995, voices for a fundamental reform began to be recognized. The following fifteen years had many proposals but almost zero implementation.

Apart from excessive and unrealistic expectations of all actors – a major problem of reforms everywhere – other factors influenced the failures of policy. Due to the electoral system, every government has found it difficult to construct a majority in the House of Representatives. Weak and unstable government mandates slowed attempts at systematic reform. Additionally, the post of Health Minister seemed to be the shakiest in the Cabinet. Since 1990, 16 persons have held that post. Ministers have been characterized by a lack of will or capacity to obtain consensus within government coalitions or to communicate strategies with other actors in health policy. While reform is a primarily political process that requires widespread support among different stakeholders, such efforts have been weak and partial. The role of some stakeholders such as health professionals was sometimes completely misunderstood. Most of documents on 'reform strategies' presented their aspirations, goals and preferences poorly without a proper idea about how to implement them.

The Czech health system demonstrates troubles, inefficiencies and a need for reform, but it is far from failing or even from collapse. During the past twenty years, several 'factors of success' indicate some hope for future developments. The most influential actors (providers and HICs) show considerable flexibility as well as an ability to learn quickly. And the system has proved its ability to bear crises and to solve conflicts of interest in a civilized way. Recently, *e.g.*, a large protest action by physicians that said 'Thank you, we're leaving' produced a compromise solution.

Are any lessons to be learned from the case of health reforms in the Czech Republic? Its experiences support theoretical as well as empirically tested prerequisites for the successful reform of public (health) policy (Saltman 1998; Mazmanian 1989; Hill 2002). It is apparent that reform is primarily a political process that requires widespread support among different stakeholders. A strong political position of the government and its ability to communicate complex social issues with the public and other stakeholders are among the most important prerequisites.

5 Health Policy in Hungary

Sándor Gallai

This chapter[1] describes the context and the contents of health policy-making in post-communist Hungary. After an overview of the country's transformation and new political framework, it presents basic indicators, economic data and health-related statistics. Its main section outlines the main steps of reforms before discussing their outcomes and assessing their results. Although the health sector witnessed considerable changes, the legacy of the communist era continues to prevail in some areas because party politics and electoral considerations reduced the policy options of successive governments.

5.1 Legacy and Political Context

In the 1960s, following the suppression of the 1956 revolution, the Hungarian communist system became less rigid and less oppressive than other regimes in the region (Tőkés 1998). In return for recognizing the ruling position of the Hungarian Socialist Workers' Party (MSZMP) and its party secretary, János Kádár, the citizens obtained a certain level of individual freedom (without political liberties) and enjoyed the benefits of steadily increasing standards of living. To offset the negative impacts of the oil crises of the 1970s, Hungary took international loans. The country became heavily indebted and by the early 1980s debt services impeded the policy of improving standards of living. Compensation was provided in the form of economic liberalization (such as legalizing the second economy) and popular measures like reducing official working hours and easing restrictions on travelling abroad. Many people supplemented their salaries at a price of overtime in new types of public and some forms of private enterprises.

The beginning of Hungary's economic transition preceded its political transformation. During the second half of the 1980's a two-tier banking system was established while corporate tax, personal income tax and value-added tax were introduced. Market-oriented enterprises were permitted that led to an early phase of ('spontaneous') privatization. Managers of state-owned companies and other people in the nomenclatura set up private businesses and took over the assets, products, production chains and/or markets of the most profitable branches of state enterprises at almost no cost.

1 This study was written as part of the TÁMOP-4.1.1.A-10/2/KMR-2010-0011 research project. Parts of the description of health management in Hungary are rewritten text of a separate article that was published in the (Chinese) *Journal of Public Administration*.

Political transition in Hungary was elite-driven, negotiated, and peaceful (Gallai 2003a). Pluralization started early, and a multiparty system emerged – quite exceptionally – *before* the first free elections (Bozóki 2003). In 1989 the ruling MSZMP declared its dissolution, and the Hungarian Socialist Party (MSZP) was formed as its replacement (Bihari 2005). At the same time several new (opposition) parties were founded, but only six political parties managed to enter the unicameral parliament at the first free election in 1990. Extensive modifications to the Constitution – both before and after the election – resulted in the declaration of the Third Republic of Hungary and the introduction of a complex system of checks and balances that included many new institutions, a rather fragmented structure of local governments,[2] and the requirement of a qualified (two-thirds) majority in several legislative areas (Körösényi *et al.* 2003). The initially weak position of the government was considerably strengthened by the introduction of the institution of a constructive vote of no confidence, which increased the role of the prime minister and shifted Hungary's form of government from the classical parliamentary to a (German) chancellor-type (Gallai 2003b).

After the elections of 1998, the increasing centralization within government, stronger coordination and leadership in governance, and a more resolute personnel policy changed both the environment and the ways of policy-making. The executive branch in general and the prime minister in particular considerably strengthened their power vis-à-vis other political institutions. That development was reinforced in 2006 by changes to the legal and political environment of the cabinet (Gallai and Lánczi 2006). As a result, the Hungarian institutional arrangement has moved away from a mixed system towards a majority model (see Lijphart 1992) that paralleled developments in party politics. Compared with other countries in the region, the Hungarian party system demonstrated a relatively high degree of stability (International IDEA 2007). Between 1998 and 2009, the party system underwent a considerable degree of concentration, and, although the pattern of consolidation ended with the 2010 election (when two new parties entered parliament), the position of the government was strengthened by subsequent institutional changes.

5.2 Basic Data and Health Resources

Within its 93,030 km^2 the Hungarian population has declined from approximately 10,375,000 in 1990 to 9,986,000 in 2011. In two decades Hungary has lost nearly 400,000 inhabitants and its current population is below 10 million. The proportion of urban population has increased (61% in 1990 and 69% in 2010), while population

2 Nearly 3,200 local governments were established at municipal level (Temesi 2000). They obtained broad competences but remained financially dependent on transfers from the central budget. County governments continued, but their influence was considerably curtailed.

density has decreased (112 persons per km^2 in 1990 and 108 in 2010). Life expectancy has improved (female: 73.7 years in 1990 and 77.9 in 2010; male: 69.2 and 77.3, respectively) and likewise the infant mortality rate (IMR) (14.8 per 1,000 births in 1990 and 5.9 in 2010).[3]

Both before and during the transformation Hungary managed to avoid hyperinflation (Table 5.1). By regional standards economic growth remained low even in the best years of transition, and during the early stage of transition, Hungary experienced an economic crisis. Data from the Hungarian Statistical Office demonstrate that both industrial and agricultural production fell by more than 30%, one-third of export markets and 30% of jobs were lost, and unemployment rocketed from 0.44% in 1990 to 13.20% in 1993. Economic recovery began in 1992-1993 but serious imbalances demanded major readjustment that took the form of an austerity package in 1995. Subsequent economic expansion was steady but relatively low, and it ended abruptly in the global crisis of 2008-2009 (Figures 5.1 and 5.2).

The low growth rate has been particularly deficient in the light of Hungary's foreign debt service. The country began to become indebted in the 1970s. The level of state debt (Figure 5.3) peaked in 1993 at 90.7% of Gross Domestic Product (GDP) and declined to 52% of GDP in 2001. Following another period of steadily rising foreign debt (65.9% of GDP in 2007), the level rapidly increased to 80.1% of GDP in 2010. When hovering at its highest level, the country's annual debt service accounted for 4%–5% of its GDP.

General tax revenues initially covered social expenditures. With the establishment of the Social Insurance Fund, contribution-based financing was introduced. In 1992 the Social Insurance Fund was divided into two separate funds: a Pension Fund and a Health

Table 5.1 Changes of GDP and Inflation, 1980-2010 (%)

	1980-1990	1990-2000	2000-2010	1980-2010
Average change of GDP, constant prices (1990 = 100)	1.14	0.70	1.88	1.24
Average change of inflation, constant prices (1990 = 100)	10.71	20.03	5.62	11.96

Source: Hungarian Central Statistical Office and Hungarian National Bank; calculation by the Department of Economic Analysis, Institute for Public Policy Research.

3 Hungarian Central Statistical Office (<http://portal.ksh.hu/portal/page?_pageid=37,592228&_dad=portal&_schema=PORTAL>).

Figure 5.1-5.2 GDP Growth, 1990-2010

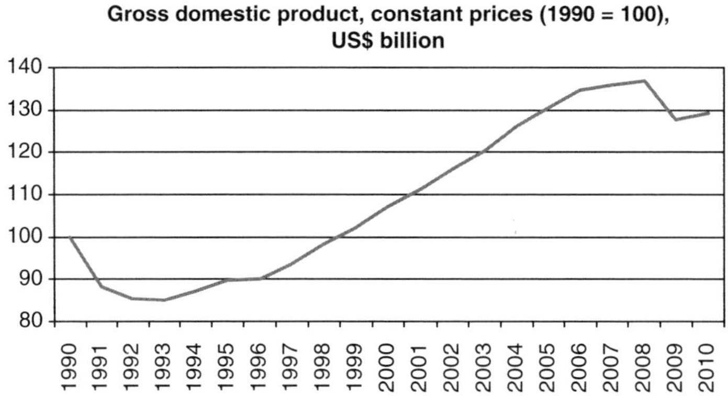

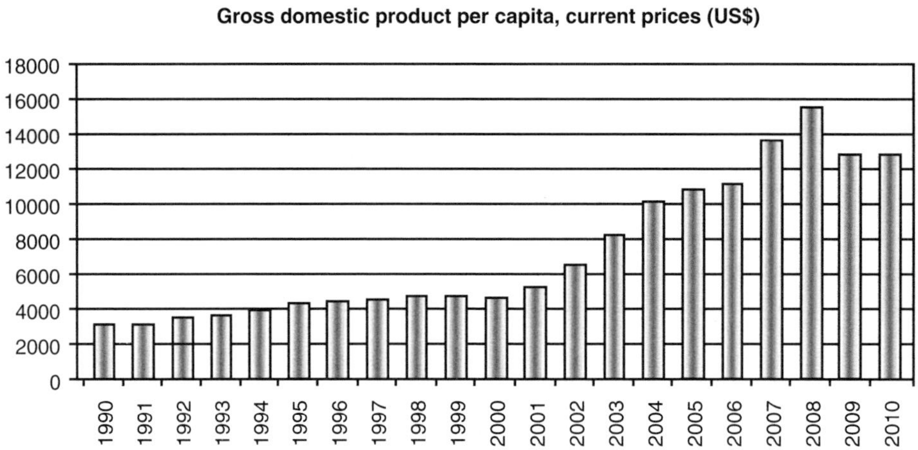

Source: Hungarian Central Statistical Office; data processed by the Department of Economic Analysis, Institute for Public Policy Research.

Figure 5.3 General Government Gross Debt (% of GDP)

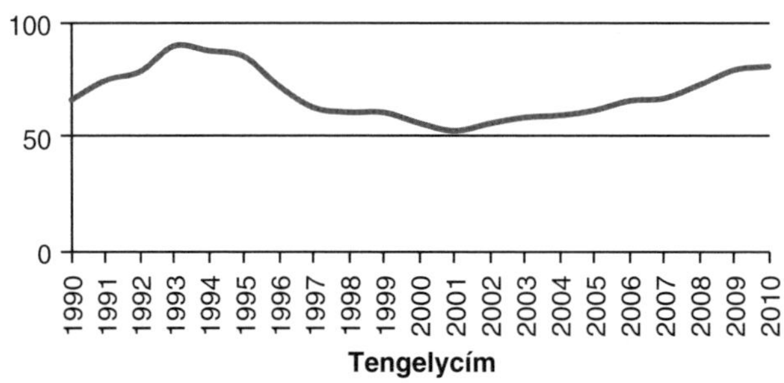

Source: Ministry of Finance (1990-1994); Eurostat (1995-2010).

Table 5.2 Health Insurance Contributions by Employers and Employees (%)

	1992	1995	1996	1998	2000	2005	2006	2007	2008	2010
Employers	19.5	19.5	18.0	15.0	11.0	11.0	11.0	8.0	5.0	2.0
Employees	4.0	4.0	4.0	3.0	3.0	4.0	6.0	7.0	6.0	6.0

Source: Respective Acts, own collection.

Insurance Fund. Thereafter health insurance contributions (Table 5.2) have provided the main source of revenue to the health budget. However, as not all incomes were subject to payment of contributions, such exemptions violated the insurance principle. Therefore, in 1998 such incomes were subjected to a 'health contribution' formula. As opposed to health insurance contribution, the new contribution was introduced as a tax that originally existed in two forms: one payable as a lump-sum contribution[4] and the other one defined as a percentage of income. Health contributions partly 'bought' their payers the eligibility for health services and partly supplemented health revenues.

Potential revenues have been considerably curtailed by two problems: the relatively small proportion of economically active population (of nearly 10 million inhabitants only 3.7 million pay contributions) and relatively widespread tax evasion (nearly half of employees reportedly earn the minimum wage, and the black and grey economies remained significant). In order to reduce the incentives for and the possibilities of evasion, the contribution base was broadened in the mid-1990s, a new lump-sum (hypothecated) tax was introduced, and the rate of health insurance contributions paid by employers was actually decreased. A few years later the government further lowered the rate of health insurance contributions while the health tax was extended and increased. After 2006, greater emphasis was laid on the eligibility of accessing services. Although the number of contribution payers increased, macroeconomic imbalances and increasing health expenditures did not allow major cuts in the health budget.

Health expenditure per capita in Hungary has been far lower than the average of OECD countries. Among the Visegrád countries,[5] health spending per capita in 2007 was highest in the Czech Republic and lowest in Poland, while the respective figures for Hungary and Slovakia were in-between (Figure 5.4). In 2009, nearly 80% of all HIF expenditures were devoted to service providers and approximately 17% were spent on cash benefits. The remaining 3% paid the pension contributions of mothers on maternity leave. Of the cash benefits

4 In its first year the contribution was HUF 60 per day. It increased annually and reached its peak (HUF 150) in 2002. During the last four years it has been HUF 65 per day; it was then eliminated in 2010 (Acts 88/1996, 66/1998, 42/2002 and 78/2009).

5 Visegrád (or V4) countries include the Czech Republic, Slovakia, Poland (V3) and Hungary.

Figure 5.4 Health Expenditure per Capita (Insured Population, US$, PPP), 2009

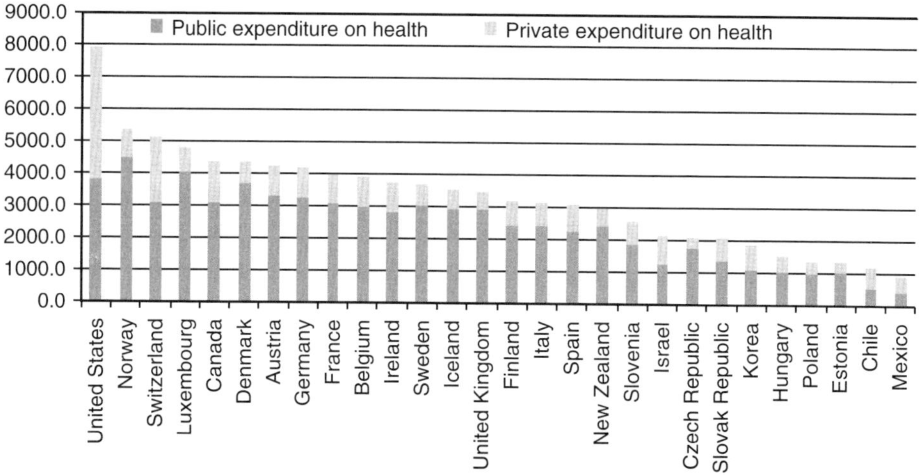

Source: OECD Health Data 2009 <www.oecd.org/health/healthdata>.

more than three-quarters were allocated to finance the costs of maternity leave (36%) and sick leave (40%). In terms of in-kind benefits, the Fund spent more than 30% on subsidizing medicines, 30% on buying services for inpatient care, close to 10% on outpatient care, and about 9% on primary care (of which one-quarter financed dental services and three-quarters went to general practitioners). The remaining 20% purchased other medical services (like chronic care, diagnostics, dialysis, ambulance) and medical equipment.[6]

In Hungary, the three years 2007-2009 (Table 5.3) demonstrated a considerable decline of central and local government expenditures, a significant expansion of private insurance schemes, and a small increase in the financial role of the non-profit sector. The expenditures of both the National Health Fund and the households first grew moderately, and then declined slightly.

Table 5.4 provides an overview of changes in the numbers of physicians, dentists, pharmacists and nurses. As compared with the first year of the transformation, the size of each professional group has expanded. However, some professions still exhibit a shortage of health professionals. In underdeveloped and remote areas the hiring of general practitioners causes difficulties and requires assistance from the national government. The shortage of nurses and certain specialists (*e.g.*, anaesthesiologists, pathologists) is increasing

6 Author's calculations from data of the 2009 balance of the Fund (<www.oep.hu/pls/portal/docs/PAGE/LAKOSSAG/OEPHULAK_UVEGZSEB/KOLTSEGVETESEK/P%C3%89NZFORGALMI_2010_J%C3%9ALIUS.PDF>).

Table 5.3 Health Expenditures (HUF billions)

Year	Public Sector			Private Sector				
	Government (central/ local)	Health Fund	Total Public	Private insurance	Out-of-pocket	Non-profit	Total Private	Grand Total
2007	232.92	1 095.79	1 328.71	39.26	458.62	36.13	534.01	1 862.72
2008	228.01	1 143.81	1 371.82	42.22	460.84	36.21	539.27	1 911.09
2009	212.28	1 140.72	1 353.00	52.23	460.53	42.01	554.78	1 907.78

Source: OECD STAT.

Table 5.4 Human Resources in Health Care (professionals per 100,000)

Year	Physicians	Dentists	Pharmacists	Nurses
1990	454	N.A.	339	N.A.
1995	501	N.A.	342	4 948
2000	516	N.A.	451	4 972
2005	502	451	484	5 206
2010	493	526	540	5 273

Source: Hungarian Central Statistical Office.

because the number of emigrating doctors is growing. The replacement of ageing general practitioners is particularly troublesome as their average age is nearly 60 and GPs in one-third of the 6,800 districts are over retirement age.[7] Every year, from among the approximately 100 new resident doctors, fewer than 60 continue as GPs.

In Table 5.5 the high initial figures for hospital beds reflect two facts: a strong emphasis on inpatient care and the use of hospital capacities for social care. In addition to the gradual decline in the numbers of both licensed and active beds, there were two major cuts. First, although the Constitutional Court rejected the way that the 1995 austerity package reduced hospital capacity,[8] indirect intervention by the government (through a

7 <www.hirado.hu/Hirek/2011/08/27/19/Csabitjak_a_kezdoket_aggasztoan_magas_a_haziorvosok_eletkora.aspx>.

8 The minister for welfare had instructed the National Health Insurance Administration about how much capacity to contract with individual service providers.

Table 5.5 Changes in Hospital Bed Capacities (Numbers of Beds)

	Licensed		In Acute Wards		Inactive	Beds in Use	
Year	*N*	*per 10,000*	*N*	*per 10,000*	*N*	*N*	*per 10,000*
1990	104 686	100.9	73 902	71.3	2 732	101 954	98.3
1995	93 147	90.2	64 847	62.8	544	92 603	89.7
2000	84 277	82.6	57 632	56.5	847	83 430	81.8
2005	80 185	79.6	60 243	59.8	580	79 605	79.0
2009	71 489	71.4	44 406	44.3	425	71 064	71.0

Source: Hungarian Central Statistical Office.

need-based formula of hospital beds per county) caused a significant reduction in capacity of approximately 9,000 beds. Second, in 2006-2007 the government decided to close five hospitals, transform eleven into chronic care rehabilitation centers and to merge six hospitals into one with reduced capacities. The overall outcome was a reduction of about 15.5 thousand beds for inpatient care (of which about 7,000 were transferred to chronic care). Despite the reductions, OECD data suggested that the per capita figures of 2009 were still among the highest in Europe (with Germany and Austria being the only two ahead of Hungary).

5.3 NORMATIVE ISSUES

Communist regimes were characterized by centralized power structures and extensive state activities. In the 1960s, however, the Kádár regime became less rigid and less oppressive than other dictatorships in the region. In the so-called 'happiest barrack' politics remained under strict control, but individual freedom in other areas was extended and the standard of living steadily increased. The oil crises during the 1970s ended the period of steady economic growth, but the policy of increasing living standards continued as it was financed by international loans. Deteriorating financial conditions and economically irrational use of loans caused debt servicing to increase, which seriously burdened the entire economy.

The Communist Party tried to offset the successive cycles of financial crises by additional economic liberalization. Liberalization had started in 1968 when the so-called New Economic Mechanism was introduced. Post-1968 economic management included financial incentives and eased rigidities of the planning system. The new system was characterized as 'neither plan nor market' (Bauer 1982). The parallel economy was legalized along with the establishment of new forms of public and private enterprises that offered additional jobs to many people who – at the price of extensive overtime – could maintain their standard of living. Major economic reforms were introduced before the regime change: a two-tier banking system was instituted, personal income tax and value-added tax were imposed, and market-oriented forms of enterprises were permitted. An early phase of uncontrolled privatization began in which members of the nomenclatura acquired valuable assets and profitable branches of state enterprises at almost no cost. At the same time, popular measures were launched such as reduction in official working hours and lifting some restrictions on traveling abroad.

Despite relative individual freedom and the early emergence of market elements, support for the regime was no stronger than in the other communist countries. As economic difficulties mounted, the legitimacy of both the political system and its leadership began to evaporate. The political culture of the declining Kádár era (see Kurtán 2003; Körösényi *et al.* 2003) was marked by the following characteristics:

- 'Restrained toleration' of the regime: moral-emotional support for and affiliation with the political leadership was less and less expected. People approached politics as 'consumers'; political loyalty was awarded by increasing affluence, and the latter made political acts – including illegal and undemocratic practices – acceptable.
- Distrust of political institutions: respect for political institutions and representatives remained low, and their reputation was tainted by widespread corruption. A dual set of political values developed. While 'official' political values were formally accepted, individual acts were rather driven by unrecognized 'unofficial' values. In the lack of shared political values and public interest, individualization reached a high level and citizens emphasized private (family) life over public affairs. The political environment was regarded unchangeable so individual accommodation strategies were pursued.
- Political 'infantilism' and cynicism: general knowledge on politics was limited and few people believed that they were able to influence decision-making or protect their interests. Since fundamental moral values were ignored, collective political immorality and the extensive violation of rules and laws were widely accepted.

These characteristics have, to a great extent, continued to dominate political culture after the change of regime. Even in the post-communist era, 'consumer politics' prevails as a strong element of Hungarian political culture that often overrules fundamental political and moral considerations. Material expectations were key motivations behind public support for democratization. At the beginning of the transformation, more than four-fifths of the population agreed to the statement that one of the most important attributes of capitalism was welfare, and half a year after the first free elections three out of four respondents believed that the concept of democracy included a better economic situation (Sándor and Vass 2007).

Figures 5.5 and 5.6 reflect the strong correlation between the perception of family affluence and the judgment of Hungary's development. In both respects the perception of election years was generally positive. The highest and lowest values mark two major governmental interventions of opposite nature: in 1995 an austerity package was introduced; in 2002 a 'welfare' package was implemented that included a 50% salary increase for public employees.

At the start of the transition, support for a market economy hovered at a relatively high level, but data from the first three years demonstrate rapid disillusionment. Steadily growing dissatisfaction with market economy was temporarily broken in the election year of 1994, and reached its peak in 1995 at the time of the austerity package. Thereafter both satisfaction and dissatisfaction with market economy remained relatively stable.

Figure 5.5 The Financial Situation of Your Household Compared to Last Year (%)

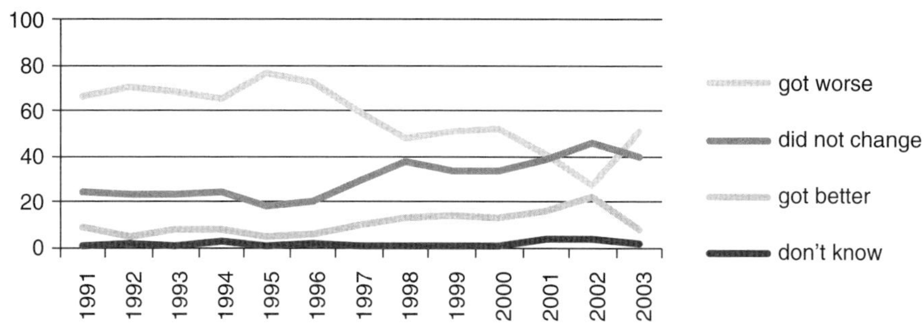

Source: TNS Hungary.

Figure 5.6 Is Hungary Going in a Good or Wrong Direction? (%)

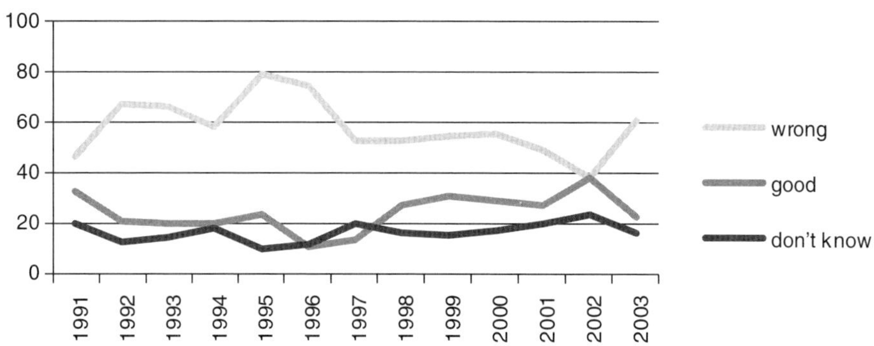

Source: TNS Modus.

Figure 5.7 Is the Creation of a Market Economy Good or Bad for Hungary? (%)

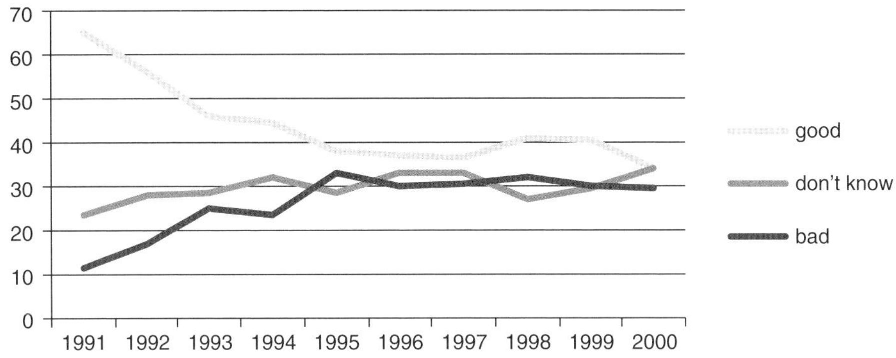

Source: TNS Modus

Political cynicism has prevailed in the new system: apparently accepted rules have been repeatedly violated and loopholes have been actively sought. The new political system could not gain strong moral foundations[9] due to the elitist nature of the regime change, the looting of valuable state property and the lack of sufficient justice[10] to the victims of communism. Low confidence in the system and its institutions demonstrates the lack of moral support. Moreover, the majority of the population has had an ambivalent attitude towards the state: polls suggest that a large proportion of citizens like the state as such (*i.e.* in principle) but do not like the state as it is.

Although many people expect the state to be active, pay for and guarantee a great variety of social benefits, respect for the state and its institutions is rather limited (Sándor and Vass 2007). Obedience to the law remains problematic; corruption, tax evasion, and weak law enforcement continue to present serious impediments to the rule of law. Respect for laws has also been undermined by numerous legal cases where appeal courts – without apparent new evidence – turn down initial verdicts, or where obvious crimes remain unpunished, or where convicted persons turned out to be innocent, or where punishments are perceived by the public as disproportionate to the seriousness of crimes committed. The same applies in cases where political institutions and other representatives of the state have openly violated laws – without facing the consequences. Such attitudes have bred anti-state and anti-politics feelings and encouraged citizens to disobedience.

9 For the importance of the moral foundations of democracy, see Lánczi 2007.

10 Lustration was narrowed to people who collaborated with the communist secret services (that is, it did not affect the agents themselves or their former superiors). Compensation was limited, and its level remained far below the value of the original property.

5.4 Health Governance and Reforms

Prior to the change of regime the exclusive role of the state was evident in the health sector. Being responsible for health services, the state owned all health institutions and facilities as well as managed, provided and financed their services. Coverage was universal and services were provided free at the point of use. Nevertheless, the actual quality of services available to citizens depended on the latter's residence, informal connections, willingness and capacity to offer under-the-table payments and gratuities. The laws of the time did not recognize the concept of patient rights and failed to address ethical issues in health care.

Structural problems (inefficiencies and redundant capacities) in the health sector became apparent by the 1980s when the emergence of private arrangements was officially accepted. While policy management remained centralized and while professional interest groups were tightly controlled, part-time private practices for specialists (dentists, dermatologists, urologists and gynecologists) were permitted. A dual structure emerged in which public services continued to dominate the sector but private services began to gain a share. In 1988, when restrictions on private provisions were completely eliminated, previously existing private practitioners were recognized and full-time private entrepreneurship was legalized. In the same year the financing of the health system switched from taxation to compulsory social insurance contributions. The Social Insurance Fund was detached from the central budget and became the main source for financing health institutions. Also in the late 1980s, university clinics followed international developments and began to address ethical questions as well as the rights of patients.

After the change of political regime, the roles of regulator, owner, purchaser and service provider in the health sector were separated from one another, and the institutional landscape of the sector transformed (Gaál 2004). Parliament became the supreme law-making body; responsibility for public welfare was assigned to the national government while the organization of services and the operation of institutions were regulated in a decentralized manner. In 1990, the privileges of public institutions were eliminated: both natural persons and legal entities obtained the right to pursue medical activities and to set up and maintain health institutions on condition that they meet the appropriate personnel and professional requirements. Parliament determined the size and structure of the annual health budget as well as the annual contribution rate to the HIF. Those issues are decided by simple majority (plurality), while decisions affecting the competences of municipal governments must be adopted by qualified (two-thirds) majority in parliament.

The central government is the main driving force in the formulation of health policy. Given stable backing in parliament, governments were usually able to maintain control over the size and operations of the HIF. This became more apparent after 1998 when the Self-government for Health Insurance – a supervisory body of employer and employee representatives – was abolished, and control over the HIF was transferred to the government. First, a political state secretary in the Prime Minister's Office controlled the area and proposed to replace the state-run HIF with competing private funds, but his proposal failed to obtain cabinet support. Control over the Fund was soon transferred to the Ministry of Finance. In 2001, the Ministry of Health obtained the right to supervise the HIF, and it has remained with the portfolio ever since.

Despite the important role and responsibility of municipal governments, it is the responsibility of the central government to cover deficits of the HIF that finances public health services, ambulance, blood supply, health education, research, and the health insurance scheme of social groups exempted from contributions. It also contributes to the health expenditures of citizens with low income; transfers earmarked and targeted subsidies to local governments; negotiates with pharmaceutical retailers on the subsidies of (certain) medicines; and supports the members of voluntary health funds with tax rebates. Within the government the health portfolio has always been at the centre of making health policy. Between 1990 and 1998, the portfolio belonged to the Ministry of Public Welfare, then to the Ministry of Health that was incorporated into the Ministry of National Resources after the 2010 elections. It has been in charge of the management of the entire sector; however, in financial and capacity issues the ministry shares responsibility with the Ministry of Finance, while in health education and training it collaborates with the Ministry of Education. For specific medical issues, the minister/state secretary for health can rely on several professional advisory bodies.

Since the deficit of the National Health Insurance Office must be covered by the central government budget, the Ministry of Finance (now part of the Ministry for National Economy) carries an important weight in determining resource allocation. The Ministry of Education (now part of the Ministry for National Resources) was made responsible for medical higher education, while control over clinics together with the coordination and supervision of health R&D and professional training have rested with the Ministry of Health. Some administrative functions and powers of the Ministry – the registration and licensing of pharmaceuticals, the licenses of medical equipment, or the assessment of the performance of service providers – were assigned to non-departmental public bodies of national competence. The supervision and coordination of public health services were transferred to the National Public Health and Medical Officer Service, whose competences include the licensing of health care service-providers, disease prevention and disease control, health promotion and public hygiene. The Service registers and monitors the facilities and the professional quality of health service providers. The National Emergency Ambulance Service also operates as a non-departmental body of the Ministry, but it has no monopolistic role; on the contrary, a great number of ambulance cars and units are run by private companies, charity and non-profit organizations.

The services of both public and private operators are equally funded from the HIF. Guarantee of blood supply was originally the task of the respective hospital units, but in 1998, those were reorganized under the umbrella of the National Blood Supply Service. Highly specialized methodology centres operate as national health institutes. They issue clinical guidelines and medical protocols as well as support clinical work, education, research and patient care. While the HIF funds their clinical services, their other costs are typically financed by the central government budget.

The HIF has been the primary institution of financing health services and sickness allowances. Established in 1992, it is managed by the National Health Insurance Administration that through its county offices registers contracts with and coordinates financial transfers to local health providers. The Health Insurance Supervisory Authority was officially established to monitor the operation of health institutions, assess the quality of health services, and protect patient rights. In fact, it had been set up as part of an aborted plan that had anticipated the replacement of the state-run health insurance system by compulsory private funds. After the failure of the multi-insurance initiative and the election of 2010, the new government decided to abolish the Authority only three years after its establishment.

In 1990, local governments obtained broad competences including responsibility for local health services. In order to meet that task, they became owners of most primary care facilities, hospitals and polyclinics – more than 90% of all health facilities. Nevertheless their freedom in capacity planning remained restricted; they could only reduce capacities if their decision had been approved by the respective (local or county) chief medical officer while the expansion of capacities had to be jointly approved by the ministers in charge of health and finances. On the other hand, municipal governments could decide on how to organize and guarantee health provisions at local level so they had the freedom to choose between providing services through their public institutions and employees or to contract services to private providers. Responsibility for secondary care was shared between municipal and county governments. While the HIF covered the operational costs of both municipal and county institutions, the owners were put in charge of raising capital/stock costs of investments and development. Local governments also received earmarked financial support from the central governmental budget to cover the wage costs of public health employees. This system prevailed until as late as 2011.

In 1993, access by citizens to services was – in principle – conditioned by contributions to the public health insurance system. In practice, however, eligibility was universal due to broadly defined exemptions and to services provided on social grounds. The insurance principle was taken seriously only from 2007 when an IT-based registration system was used to check the eligibility of patients. That move brought approximately 100,000 new contributors into the system. Nonetheless, the estimated number of free riders remained four times higher (about 400,000), and the package of basic services has not been drawn properly.

In addition to being covered by the state-run health insurance system, citizens may join voluntary insurance funds. Adopted in 1993, the Act on Voluntary Insurance Funds permits the foundation of private health funds where membership is voluntary and supplementary to the compulsory national scheme. These funds offer both complementary services (which are not covered in the state-run system) and services of better quality. In order to encourage membership in the private schemes, tax rebates were introduced for contributions paid to the voluntary funds. Although membership in voluntary private funds has expanded, their impact on the financing and the operation of the health system remained limited.[11]

In 1992, 'family physicians' replaced the former system of district physicians. Family physicians serve as general practitioners (GPs) who are the main providers of general primary care services. They help patients preserve their health and prevent illnesses by regular consultations, screening tests and check-up examinations. In fact, however, most family doctors put little emphasis on preventive testing, and doctor-patient meetings mainly occur in case of illnesses. Ill patients are treated by their GPs and – if necessary – they are referred to outpatient specialists or inpatient services. Unnecessary reference of patients to diagnostic laboratories or outpatient specialists is a widespread practice to avoid risk-taking and to transfer responsibility to a higher level. General practitioners have regularly been criticized for prescribing too much and too expensive medicines. Most GPs are specialized in either child care or adult care; very few have mixed practices. In a few municipalities, the local government employs doctors so they are public employees, but the bulk of the family physicians operate as private service providers; thus they are registered 'entrepreneurs'. In the latter case the services are contracted out, *i.e.*, the responsibility for organizing primary care lies with the municipal government, while actual services are delivered

11 There are 37 private health funds with approximately 932,000 members. While they only pay HUF 1.3 billion to the funds, contributions from their employers exceed HUF 8.5 billion (<www.pszaf.hu/bal_menu/jelentesek_statisztikak/statisztikak/pszaf_idosorok/idosorok>).

by the entrepreneurial GPs. Such physicians usually rent their offices and medical equipment from the municipal government with which they have a contract.

Insured persons are allowed to register with a service provider whom they choose freely. However, in smaller places, particularly where there is a shortage of operating GPs, free choice remains a mere declaration that cannot be translated into practice. Most physicians operate within one of the country's 6,800 districts, the boundaries of which are determined by the municipal governments. General practitioners affiliated with districts are obliged to provide care for all local residents who had not registered with other GPs. Given guarantees of primary care for patients with high risks of disease and for the elderly, 'cherry picking' is impossible. Some general practitioners, particularly in bigger towns, lack district affiliations, so they are free to attract patients from anywhere regardless of their residence. Above a given number of registered patients, GPs may run their practices as well as receive state funding for their services.

GPs become eligible for state funding after they have contracted the respective county (regional) office of the National Health Insurance Administration. Regardless of district affiliation, GPs in primary care receive per capita payment from the HIF. In principle, their state funding is paid according to the number of their registered patients, but the final sum is corrected by age-group points (given for older patients) and qualification multipliers. Per capita funding accounts for 75%-80% of an average GP's total funding. The rest comes from complementary territorial allowances (that serve to compensate GPs working in disadvantageous areas), traffic payment, money earmarked for office maintenance, and payments for urgent (*ad hoc*) cases of patients registered with other GPs. In 2005, an increased monthly price was introduced for doctors filling in permanently vacant medical districts. While the operational costs are financed from the HIF, development costs should be covered by the municipal governments. However, due to the shortage of sufficient resources, the GPs in many districts could not obtain enough funding. Therefore, from the early 2000s the government made it possible for the GPs to apply for extra support from the HIF to buy new equipment, furniture or real estate. At the same time the government provides subsidized loans for purchasing the facilities from the municipal government.

Outpatient services are provided in outpatient centres, clinics and outpatient departments of hospitals. After the regime change the owners of those facilities employed doctors working in outpatient services so they were public employees of local and county governments. While this pattern prevailed as the main form of employment, in some cases the owners decided to contract out the operation of outpatient facilities. In such cases, services were organized by private companies who employed doctors and other staff members through private contracts, the conditions of which are regulated by the Labor Code. The foundations of outpatient financing were laid down in 1992-1993 when a fee-for-service point system was introduced. It adopted the principles of the German system that nationally fixes (*ex-ante*) the weight ('share') of the values of every service and pays for the delivered services accordingly. In order to control expenditures, the system applies a monthly ceiling on outpatient funding. Should the overall value of delivered services exceed the ceiling, the value of the points in each service category will be reduced proportionally. Service providers must document their activities daily and report to the Fund once a month.

After 1990, patient choice became so respected that patients were allowed to choose and visit their outpatient service provider so freely that no referral was required. In the lack of effective gatekeepers, outpatient service providers became unreasonably overburdened. Following the introduction of some restrictions, the government restored the requirement of territorial affiliation, according to which the GPs must send their patients to the outpatient institution nearest to the patient's residence. Patient choice is therefore limited to the doctors of a given institution. Choice becomes a real possibility only in places (typically bigger municipalities) where more than one specialist works in the same field.

Most hospitals and clinics are publicly owned. The few exceptions are comprised of privately owned institutions and church-sponsored hospitals. In inpatient services most doctors are public employees; only those who work in private institutions are employed under the Labor Code. Patient choice in both inpatient and outpatient care is similarly regulated: apart from emergency cases, patients are obliged to go to the nearest hospital in their district so real choice is limited. The main exemption from the rule applies to patients who have a recorded history with another institution; they may choose between returning to the previous institution and going to the nearest one.

The financing of hospitals was redesigned in the early 1990s and remained basically intact until 2012. Owners of institutions were responsible for maintenance and development expenditures while the HIF reimbursed the costs of services. In that system acute and rehabilitation cases were financed along a modified version of the Diagnosis Related Groups (DRGs) scheme. As in the American version, the Homogenous Disease Groups (HDG) system was performance-based; funding was based on the type and number of cases reported. Patients treated in inpatient care were categorized into diagnosis groups. The weight ('share') of each diagnosis group was fixed annually (*ex-ante*). The sub-budget of acute inpatient care was also capped and as in outpatient care – discretion was applied. Part of the sub-budget was reserved for compensation and seasonal variations. High-cost interventions were not part of the scheme; they were decided on a case-to-case basis. Chronic cases were paid on the basis of patient days that were adjusted according to the complexity of the case.

In the United States diagnostic weights carry the same monetary value nationwide; in Hungary a different value was set for each individual hospital. Oddly enough, that system favored the least efficient hospitals, the average operation costs of which were higher than usual (*e.g.*, hospitals that had had fewer patients than other institutions with similar capacities). As a result, treating patients with identical diseases in two different hospitals could bring more money (sometimes twice as much) to one hospital than to another. Differences in the financing of identical services in various institutions were widely publicized, which generated serious tension and dissatisfaction within the health sector. In response, the government ended the unequal funding of identical services and by 1998 all hospitals received equal payments for identical cases. Retrospective payments to individual hospitals were replaced by prospective base-fees for each diagnosis group in a system where fees were valid nationwide and fixed in advance. Since some HDG categories were underfinanced while others were over-financed, providers were financially inspired to (mis)report their cases; whenever possible, they classified under-financed cases into better paying categories. It was general practice to report unnecessary (or even unperformed) medical examinations as well as more hospital days than actually spent in bed.

The administration of the HIF is obliged to scrutinize the activities of service providers and to fine those that had breached the rules. Although successful investigations did occur,[12] due to the limited administrative capacities, it has been impossible to monitor the operation of all hospitals fully. Soft budgetary constraint forms an even more serious obstacle to disciplined financial management (Kornai 2009). Capping the sub-budget, allocating less to hospitals or cutting back their capacities could only have been effective if the indebted institutions had been closed down. However, closures rarely occurred. On the contrary, the government has always found resources for the financial consolidation of hospitals. Repeated consolidations have demonstrated a political fear of reducing the number of hospitals. In addition, financial consolidation did not help to restructure the sector because the distribution of additional funds was not conditioned to the rationalizing of the institutions.

Therefore, in 2004, when the deficit of the HIF rocketed to new heights, the government imposed a new limit to hospital funding. The performance volume limit presents a financial cap on the activities of hospitals as their services are reimbursed by the HIF up to a

12 In such cases providers were compelled to repay their unjustifiable reimbursement (<www.nol.hu/belfold/mutet_papiron__milliardos_csalasokat__tulszamlazasokat_tart_fel_az_oep>).

certain limit. Above that threshold no intervention or treatment is paid by the state. From a fiscal point of view, the system of administrative control over active inpatient care has proved to be effective, but from the patients' point of view, it caused considerably longer waiting lists and serious delays in treatments. Hospitals reducing the number of interventions have had to face embarrassed patients who are disappointed (or literally sickened) by the postponement of examinations and surgeries. On the other hand, carrying out all interventions generates serious debts, and usually results in a cry for fiscal consolidation. There are examples for both options and also for a strategy that falls in between: some hospitals intervene in certain areas while producing endless waiting lists in others. The system of reimbursement was modified in 2009; the HIF reimbursed hospitals up to 70% of the value of their previous year's performance while the value of additional services was determined by a formula that calculated both the remaining balance of the sub-budget and the performance of other service providers. That policy had deepened the under-financing of services and increased the indebtedness of hospitals to such an extent that yet another round of hospital consolidation was required.

Changes to the pharmaceutical sector were even more drastic and rapid because the liberalization of the pharmaceutical market was accompanied by large-scale privatization. National drug producers, together with the pharmaceutical wholesale and retail industries, were by and large privatized. The Act on Pharmacies set the conditions for the privatization of pharmacies and nearly all pharmacies were privatized. State control over drug prices eased, and the high consumption level of medicines with considerably increasing prices put a serious pressure on the HIF. In certain years the expenditures on subsidized medicines surpassed even the costs of inpatient care. In 2009, the respective figures were HUF 343 billion and HUF 325 billion, making the sub-budget of subsidized medicines the largest of all. Therefore, control over drug expenditures has always been crucial for the balance of the Fund.

The issue of keeping price increases under control has been on the political agenda under nearly all governments. In 2000, during the first Fidesz-led government, drug prices came under control by the establishment of the Social Insurance Price and Subsidies Committee that negotiated and concluded a three-year agreement with stakeholders in the pharmaceutical industry. The agreement kept price increases below the level of inflation and – in cases of expensive medicines – it stipulated decreasing margins between wholesale and retail prices. Following a change in government, the new cabinet renegotiated the agreement with the pharmaceutical companies and a more differentiated price increase was permitted. Nevertheless, the companies agreed to pay the costs of subsidies on their products if their medicine was sold in a quantity above the level of originally agreed. In 2006, when the senior governing Socialists left the position of the health minister to the junior governing liberal Free Democrats, a new law made it easier to open pharmacies and legalized the sale of medicines in stores and petrol stations. At the same time the expenditures of the pharmaceutical sub-budget were cut at the expense of producers and suppliers, and a minimal fee for medicines was introduced for chronic patients, who had not previously paid for their drugs.

Although health reforms in the first years of transition resulted in a more decentralized and deconcentrated institutional arrangement, responsibility for and decisions on the financing of health policies remained highly centralized (Füzesi *et al.* 2005). The HIF has operated with a deficit for most of the years and the central budget had to pay HUF 30-80 billion annually to cover the deficit (Figure 5.8). Despite upper ceilings on the sub-budgets and the mechanisms protecting the expenditure caps, from 2002 the balance of the Fund started to deteriorate dramatically, and by 2006 the deficit exceeded HUF 300 billion. Government policies introduced in 2006-2007 reduced the deficit so successfully that – for the first time in its history – the balance of the Fund turned into a slight surplus.

The successful elimination of the deficit of the Fund was the outcome of two developments. First, the government applied all existing administrative and financial brakes on expenditures on health care – with no respect to medical and political consequences. The second element of financial consolidation was the introduction of a policy mix that incorporated four components: the size of the health budget was reduced (*i.e.*, the fund available for health spending was cut back); the introduction of a comprehensive co-payment scheme to reduce unnecessary use of services while bringing in additional revenues; the privatization of health institutions and/or services in hope of raising (investment) capital and improving efficiency; and the introduction and expansion of managed care to save

Figure 5.8 The Balance of the Health Insurance Fund (HUF, billion)

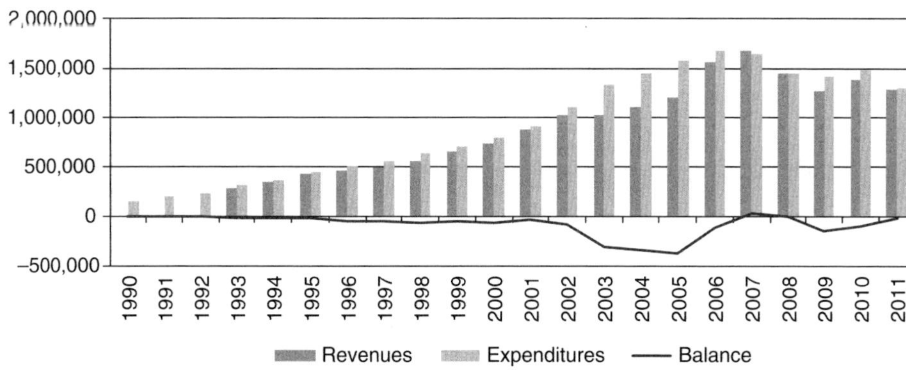

Source: Data collected from the Health Insurance Fund (<www.oep.hu>).

money by way of better resource allocation. The overall result of changes was financially positive; although the sector had lost substantial resources to the central budget, the balance of the HIF turned into a surplus.

For the past three decades (except 1997-2003), the Hungarian economy was characterized by fiscal imbalances, external debt and slow economic growth. Due to persistent economic difficulties, Hungarian macroeconomic management has cyclically been forced to introduce austerity programs. Economic needs and electoral considerations usually translated into circles of stop-and-go policies. After the regime change, the most serious fiscal adjustments programs were implemented in 1991, 1995, 2006 and 2009. Although all four programs included considerable cuts in public spending, the health sector was affected with particular severity in two cases: in 1995 and 2006. With the cut in 1995, the health budget hit the bottom in its post-1990 history. The number of hospital beds was reduced while the HIF stopped the financing of dental services[13] and the subsidizing of spa treatments. Patients had already been expected to pay either a reduced or the full price of their medicines, but in 1995 co-payment was extended to the transportation of patients. At the same time, the state shifted responsibility for providing health services at workplaces to the employers. The austerity package provoked serious legal (and political) criticism, and the Constitutional Court ruled that several measures were in conflict with the Constitution and other standing laws. At the end, nevertheless, the health sector suffered a considerably reduction of both capacities and financial resources.

In 2006-2007, the government introduced further cost-saving measures that made waiting lists even longer. The minister for health readjusted the cap on financing by setting it at the level of 95% of the formerly reported activities (Sinkó 2008). At the same time the government decided to reduce hospital capacities. Hospitals were classified by range of services: the highest category was reserved for clinics and hospitals of regional importance while the lowest category applied to small local hospitals with limited capacity, resources and activities (Mihályi and Molnár 2006). In the original plan redundant (unused) capacities, shortage of professionals and loss making were the key characteristics of institutions that were marked for closing down. However, political lobbying distorted the plans, and the list of affected institutions was modified. Although it weakened the legitimacy of the decision, the outcome was nonetheless a considerable cut in hospital capacities.

The most symbolic element of the 2006 package was the introduction of a comprehensive co-payment scheme. After 2007, the government introduced the so-called visiting fee and hospital fee. The former had to be paid by the patients after each visit to their doctor. The

13 A year later tooth-preserving treatments were returned to the list of publicly funded services.

latter was paid by patients for each day they stayed in hospital. The fees were set at HUF 300 (€1.10 at the exchange rate of the time) per visit and per day. Although the fees were relatively modest, they became the target of a bitter political conflict between the governing MSZP and the senior opposition Fidesz. The opposition wanted to block government policies and create tension within the coalition so they put the issues of visiting and hospital fees – and that of the tuition fee – on the agenda of a referendum initiative. The so-called 'social referendum' in March 2008 turned into a strong protest vote against the government, and all fees were voted down with a convincing majority. The turnout was 50.5%; the proportion of votes rejecting the hospital fee exceeded 84% while it was more than 82% in the cases of both the visiting fee and the tuition fee.[14]

In terms of the role of private capital, two opposing health care models emerged by the mid-1990s. On the one hand, liberal economists and politicians, financial circles (particularly insurance companies), and certain private entrepreneurs operating in health care tended to advocate a much bigger role for both private insurance schemes and out-of-pocket payments as well as limit public financing in the sector to the very poor and to a relatively narrow circle of basic services. On the other hand, social policy experts, health economists and politicians rejecting liberal economics envisaged a publicly financed health system in which the citizens could enjoy free services provided by various enterprises (private, non-profit, municipal and state-owned). In their views, co-payment or full payment could only be extended to a limited and well-defined package of (extra) services with private funds reserved for voluntary supplementary schemes.

In the past two decades the role of private actors and capital in the health sector increased considerably. In fact, private participation now involves private practitioners, family physicians, private clinics and specialists, factory physicians, diagnostic laboratories, mostly foreign capital-based enterprises of artificial kidney centres and other high-tech-based services, supplementary service providers (*e.g.*, washing, cleaning and maintenance), pharmacies, some emergency ambulance operators, and insurance companies. All in all, private service providers deliver some 10% of the health care services. The once state-owned pharmacies have all been privatized. Some 90% of artificial kidney centres and around one-third of CTs and MRIs are run by private companies. Nearly 90% of family physicians and almost 70% of dentists operate as private entrepreneurs (Gaál 2004). Many specialists run private practices, often as a supplement to their full-time (sic!) job in the public sector.

Privatization in its classic meaning (*i.e.* the transfer of ownership rights from public to private owners) remained a rare phenomenon in the Hungarian health sector with

14 <www.valasztas.hu/hu/ovb/42/42_0.html>.

pharmacies and a few hospitals returned to the churches as the only marked exceptions. Functional privatization (outsourcing), on the other hand, has become a general practice in primary care; it has also gained ground in secondary care services. Nevertheless, private capital in secondary care went mostly for cherry-picking and took over the operation of certain units and (profitable) services (Herczeg 2002). Outsourcing the operation of complete secondary care institutions remained rare in inpatient services: by 2008 the operation of less than ten public hospitals were taken over by private enterprises (out of approximately 150).

The first 'spontaneous' privatization of hospitals took place after the 1995 austerity package. The cutbacks affected the public institutions quite painfully and left them with no reserves in their budget. Since the owners of the health institutions have been responsible for providing capital for investments, equipment and renovation, the lack of sufficient resources led some municipal governments to seek the possibilities of incorporating private capital by contracting out both supplementary and medical services. In response to spontaneous privatization, two attempts were made to regulate the conditions of the process. The first, enacted by the Fidesz-led majority in 2001, was repealed and replaced by a new one after the change in government. However, that second, Socialist-Liberal-sponsored Act did not come into effect because the Constitutional Court declared it null and void. When the law was passed, the President of the Republic used his veto power and sent it back to parliament for reconsideration. Parliament decided to overrule the presidential veto without discussing his reservations. The Constitutional Court declared that parliament had not fulfilled its constitutional obligation of 'reconsidering' the bill. Although the ground for the ruling was a formal mistake in the decision-making, the government did not resubmit the bill to parliament and once again left the possibility of privatization unregulated. Despite the failure of the two legislative attempts, the privatization of health institutions and health services did not stop. Although legally nothing hampered the process, its scope and scale remained limited. In inpatient care there were two main groups that – in hope of future benefits – invested in the sector, and one of them became bankrupt in 2009. The bankruptcy, along with unfavorable prospects for financial returns and the lack of stable and transparent legislative environment, did not help to attract private capital. Moreover public sentiment remained skeptical about the role of and the need for private enterprises in the health sector; the medical staff was also alienated by infamous labor conflicts with private managements.

Under such conditions it was unsurprising that the most ambitious privatization plan – the privatization of the health insurance system itself – had failed. Between 2006 and 2008 the junior governing Liberal party, which controlled the Ministry of Health, wanted to replace the state-run system with a multi-insurance system in which compulsory health insurance would have been provided by competing private funds. The senior governing Socialists, on the other hand, preferred the decentralization (regionalization) of the state-run fund to its privatization. The compromise was presented as a bill on the establishment of regional health funds. According to the agreement between the governing parties, the state would have kept a majority stake in the funds while the management of the funds would have been controlled by private (financial) investors. Although the respective Act was adopted, following the defeat over the issue of co-payment in the March 2008 referendum, the government initiated the repeal of the Act on Health Insurance Funds, and parliament voted for the motion.

In 1999, the government approved the introduction of the so-called managed care experiment that combined elements of the American-managed care system and the British GP fund-holding model. The experiment started with nine pilot projects and covered 160,000 people from different territories. Three years later nearly 500,000 people were involved; participation peaked at more than 950,000 (nearly 10% of the population) in 2004. The objective of the experiment was to see if better coordination, monitored cases, and reallocation of resources between sub-budgets could reduce service costs and improve higher efficiency and better quality. Therefore, care coordinators received per capita payment from the HIF after the number of the insured inhabitants; they also received a fee for their organizing activities and some support for prevention. They were in the position to sign contracts with service providers freely. Their costs had to match their revenues because those coordinators who had produced a deficit for more than three consecutive months had to be deprived of their permit of operation. The first assessments of the pilot projects were positive[15] so the government decided to extend the project to two million people. However, the State Audit Office negatively assessed the project (ÁSZ 2006) and more critical voices started to gain ground. Criticism focused on three main points: the time-scale was too short to measure changes in the health condition of the patients; the best performing projects were able to raise extraordinary revenues (through political channels), so the actual balance of managed care was not necessarily positive; and there was a segregation of patients because care coordinators often excluded the old and the sick whose treatment would have cost them dearly. So although all parliamentary parties supported the initiative in 1999, the projects were stopped. In recognition of the political defeat in 2008 of government-sponsored health reforms, the parliamentary majority voted for the silent termination of the managed care (Baraczka and Mihályi 2009).

15 Participating doctors earned more than their colleagues; patients reported that they received more attention and better care; prevention got more emphasis; the consumption of medicines decreased significantly; and the budget of care coordinators was kept in balance.

As the government has primarily shaped Hungarian health policy, the influence of social and professional groups has depended on the will of the governing forces; therefore interest-representation has been over-politicized. Despite their low impact on policy formulation, organized interests and institutionalized forms of interest representation do exist in the health sector. Health professionals are organized into three chambers: the Hungarian Medical Chamber (established in 1988), the Hungarian Chamber of Pharmacists (1994) and the Chamber of Professional Health Workers (2003). The chambers play an important role in professional training and further education, issue codes of ethics for medical practices, and have the right to impose sanctions on those who do not comply. They also have the right for being consulted on medical issues. The Hungarian Medical Chamber has veto power over the conditions of contracts between medical doctors and the National Health Insurance Administration.

Membership in the chambers was made compulsory in 1994 when the chambers were also assigned some regulatory competences. In 2007, however, compulsory membership was eliminated and their competences were curtailed. Since the change came after the Medical Chamber had expressed strong opposition to the policies of the minister for health, the move looked like political retaliation. Three years later the change in government resulted in the restoration of compulsory membership; nevertheless the rights and competences of the chambers remained limited. Two other important professional organizations, the Alliance of Hospitals and the Association of Health Financial Managers, tend to express similar views especially when it comes to the issue of hospital financing. On the employee side, the Democratic Trade Union of Health Workers has become the largest union. Union representatives participate in various interest reconciliation forums, but – despite their often loud voice, occasional demonstrations and strikes – their impact on policies remained limited.

After the change of regime, more than 100 patient associations were founded and registered. Many of them are organized along disease groups to represent specific patient interests; other organizations focus on patient rights with the aim of providing legal protection. Representation as a collective right of patients appeared gradually and its scope remained limited (Heuer 2002, Molnár 2001). Nevertheless, patient organizations have gained representation in advisory and coordinating bodies such as the National Health Council, the regional health councils,[16] hospital supervisory councils,[17] county ethics committees,[18] and

16 Regional health councils were founded in 2005 to monitor and assess regional health programs, give advice on the allocation of regional capacities, and reconcile the interests of regional stakeholders.

17 In 1999, supervisory councils were set up in hospitals to monitor their operation, and to give opinion and make proposals to institution managements.

18 In 1999, local ethics committees were set up in the health institution to issue protocols on ethical questions and make general recommendations. Individual cases, on the other hand, had originally been investigated in the respective committees of the Hungarian Medical Chamber, but in 2007 that competence was transferred to the then established county ethics committees.

waiting list committees. They also participated in negotiations over pharmaceutical prices. Moreover, they are free to register with parliament and the Ministry of Health in order to join the system of compulsory consultations. Ministries are obliged to consult the interest organizations on all health-related draft proposals. If registered with parliament, they can receive draft bills for comments, but they may only attend the meetings of the respective standing committees on invitation. In fact, however, their opinion is usually requested at short notice and rarely taken into account. The lack of significant policy influence is partly explained by financial and organizational shortcomings because their organization is usually weak and their capacity of expertise is often limited (interview, ministry official, 15 November 2007).

In contrast with the general situation, there were two relatively successful exceptions in the area of patient interests: the Chain Alliance (founded in 1989) and the Advocate Foundation for Patient Rights (1994). The former was established as an umbrella organization of 27 associations of chronic and disabled patient groups. It was particularly active in the drafting of a new law on health care in 1997. Later, however, internal conflicts (of personal nature) weakened the organization considerably (interview, co-founder, 22 May 2008). The Advocate Foundation for Patient Rights was inspired by the Anglo-Saxon school of legal theory that not only expressed rights but also offered effective protection through legislation (Exter and Sándor 2002). The main objectives of the Foundation were to monitor relevant laws and practices, formulate policy recommendations, and invent new solutions and mechanisms. The Foundation set up a Consultation Centre for Patient Rights to give legal assistance to ill-treated, humiliated and vulnerable patients (Blasszauer, year not available). When the drafting of the new law on health care began in the Ministry of Welfare, the chapter on patient rights, patient involvement and representation was mostly built on contributions from experts connected with the Advocate Foundation for Patient Rights (interview, ministry official, 15 November 2007).

After two years of preparation and deliberation, the Act on health care was approved in parliament. In parliament several modifications to the bill had watered down the chapter on patient rights. Nevertheless, a relatively wide-ranging catalogue of patient rights and a new institution to advocate the rights of patients were enacted. Although the Act came into force in mid-1998, the first full-time advocates started their job only in January 2000. The number of advocates has never exceeded 60, yet they deal with about 8,000 cases per

19 Due to low salaries, specialists who do not receive under-the-table payments are forced to work extra hours or seek a job abroad. The number of doctors and nurses working in foreign countries has significantly increased after Hungary's accession to the European Union. The Chamber claims that 3,000 specialists have left the country since 2004.

year. By law they are obliged to cover every single service providers in the country. Since their total numbers nearly 40,000, the advocates are practically limited to hospitals.

5.5 Policy Outcomes and Deficiencies

On the positive side, the separation of roles in health policy has been achieved. Purchaser, provider and financing roles were separated from one another. At the same time regulatory, monitoring and supervisory bodies are in place and respective mechanisms were introduced, albeit not always functioning effectively. In terms of financing, incentives of various types exist although they have often proved to be ineffective, sometimes even counter-productive. Keeping the financing of hospitals and pharmaceuticals under control has always been crucial for the balance of the HIF. When it failed, bureaucratic control was imposed to deliver the anticipated financial success but it also led to a serious setback in services. Notwithstanding the gap between laws and reality, the institutionalization of patient rights and their protection are among the important outcomes of policy changes.

Despite the long list of institutional changes and policy reforms, however, the health sector remains poisoned with several problems. Health insurance is still based on national risk-taking; the HIF is run by the state; and most health institutions are publicly owned. Nevertheless, the expansion of private practices and private facilities has reinforced the dual structure of public and private patterns while the conflict of interest for double-hatted doctors has not been properly regulated nor have existing rules been respected. Thus, free riding on public facilities prevails; it continues to be a typical misuse of dual roles in which publicly employed doctors see their patients for (expensive) medical tests and examinations in public institutions (where the costs of services are covered by the HIF); then they give the diagnosis and provide care in their private practice where the patients are requested to pay out-of-pocket fees for their visits. Various forms of corruption and cheating also impede the efficient functioning of the sector. Underfinanced health institutions often try to generate revenues by making unnecessarily interventions, misclassifying the reported cases, reporting undone activities, and misreporting the number of days spent in hospital. Many publicly employed doctors offset their low salaries by multiple employment, under-the-table payments and gratuities.[19] In principle, under-the-table payments are pursued by law while gratuities are subject to taxation. In fact, however, gratuities are rarely reported to the tax authority, and in several areas (surgical operation and child delivery are the most notable ones) the majority of the patients fear uncertainty and mistreatment so they retain the system of under-the-table payments. In primary care, some doctors are allegedly sponsored by pharmaceutical companies in return for favoring their products when prescribing medicines to the patients.

The health sector has not only been tainted by financial inefficiencies but also marked by professional ineffectiveness. In comparison with other countries of the region, Hungary has been characterized by serious public health problems and produced very poor health indicators in most areas. Although life expectancy has increased, Hungary remains a laggard within the Visegrád group of countries (Figure 5.9). The difference between the Hungarian figure and the average of the other three Visegrád countries (V3) has not changed over the past 20 years (Egészségjelentés 2010).

In health-related mortality cases, Hungarian indicators are 20%-100% above the corresponding figures of V3, while indicators for serious illnesses show 20%-70% higher numbers. The only exception is depression, where Hungary stands exactly at the level of V3 (Egészségjelentés 2010). The male population over 50 produces the worst indicators of all, and their mortality rate is worryingly high. The poor indicators reflect partly an unhealthy way of life[20] and partly the limited emphasis on prevention. The prevention budget in 2008

Figure 5.9 Health Expenditures and Life Expectancy

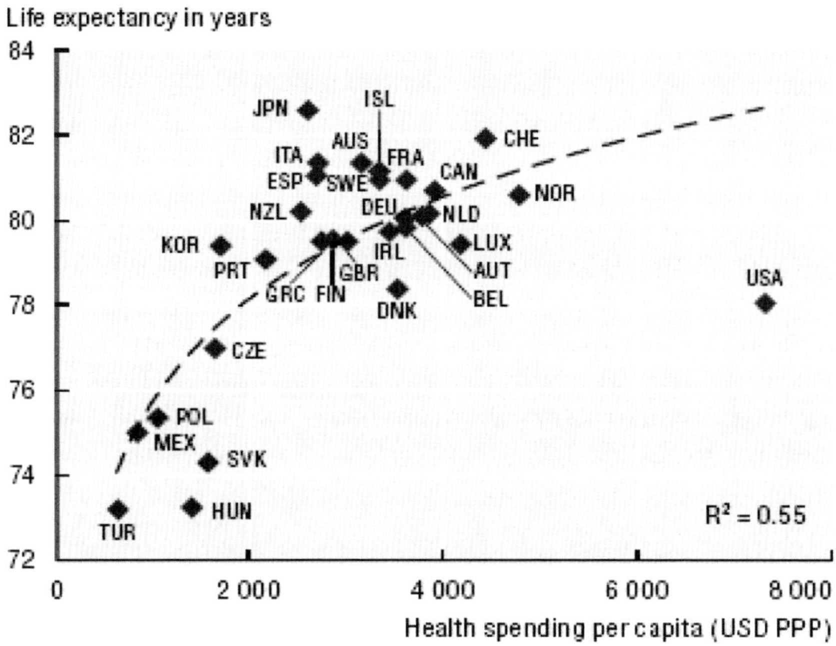

Source: OECD 2009 (<www.oecd.org/health/healthdata>).

20 For example, eating unhealthy (fat, salty, spicy) food, drinking too much alcohol, working heavy overtime, and living in a stressful environment.

was only one-third of the fund available in 2001. At the same time, the traditional attitude of doctors changes rather slowly. They tend to prescribe drugs and medicines far too often; many GPs do not act as real gate-keepers but needlessly refer patients to specialists; the number of medical interventions remain very high; hospitalization is unnecessarily common (Figure 5.10), and inpatient services are often used for the purposes of social care. Due to ineffective prevention and to traditional reflexes, Hungary registers a high numbers of surgeries and particularly high numbers of days spent in hospital (twice the EU average).

5.6 Politics of Health Reform

Both stakeholders and party politics have impeded the introduction of structural changes and financial measures in health policy. The main impediments can be identified around four factors: incumbent interests, fiscal constraints, political culture and party politics. Underpaid doctors who earn more – sometimes several times more – from under-the-table payments and gratuities are not interested in changes. Although a minority within the medical profession, they have strong motivations to impede certain reform measures. A survey conducted by Tárki research institute indicated that a majority of respondents regarded payment of a gratuity for home visits by GPs as customary while in surgical operations and obstetrics 80%–90% felt it habitual; therefore, if GPs had no queues and operations were fewer, the income of doctors would be reduced (Bognár *et al.* 1999:12-13).

Structural reforms are generally considered beneficial for both fiscal balance and economic growth in the short run (D'Auria *et al.* 2009), but, due to (politically) necessary compensation of the expected losers, they require additional resources in the short run. Even in social policy areas the long-term gain can exceed short-term pain (van den Noord and Cournède 2006). In the health sector, both cutting subsidies and introducing or increasing co-payment will save money for the budget; however, a shift from cure to prevention,

Figure 5.10 Hospitalizations per 100 Inhabitants

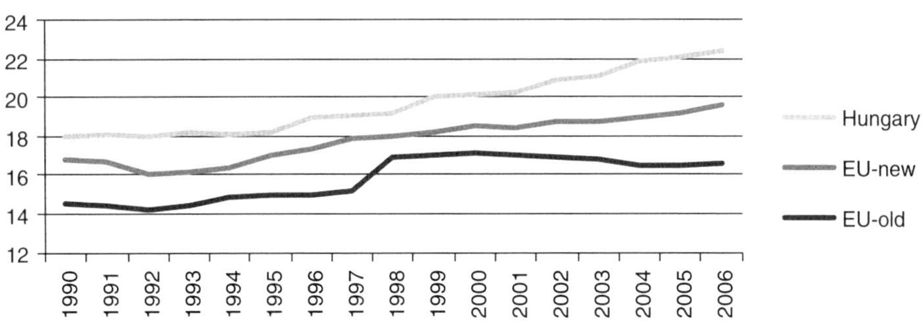

Source: Egészségjelentés 2010.

from hospitalization to one-day surgery, or from a fragmented infrastructure to a more efficient one – each shift requires the allocation of extra funds to the sector. Therefore, fiscal constraints do not create favorable conditions for comprehensive transformation; the lack of sufficient funding and recurring cuts to the health budget have limited the scope of reforms.

The third and fourth impediments are of a political nature. As discussed above, political culture is tainted by its communist legacy; neither anti-market sentiments and dependence on state benefits nor corruption and free riding favor the establishment of a transparent, effective and fiscally balanced health sector. Nevertheless, the Socialist-Liberal government of 2006-2008 had chosen health care to be the flagship of its reform policies. Most changes were driven by the need to reduce the expenditures of the Health Fund while some policies were designed to weaken incumbent interests by shaking the existing structures in the health sector. But the ultimate goal of the government was to privatize the health insurance system and to create an environment in which citizens could have chosen among competing private funds of compulsory membership. But the plan collapsed; the flagship of health reform was wrecked on the sea of party politics. In order to understand the importance of party politics, four characteristics of the Hungarian political system are relevant: the strength and stability of cabinets; the extraordinary role of the prime minister; the concentration of the party system; and the bipartisan (two-block) nature of electoral contests.

The Hungarian election system (Gallai 2000) has effectively filtered the contesting political forces: the nomination process – together with the high (implicit) threshold – has kept the number of effective parties low. At each election only four to six political parties were able to enter parliament; and the overrepresentation of the winner of the individual constituencies (when there was a definite winner) also helped the formation of majority governments. The institution of constructive vote of no confidence further strengthens the position of the cabinet. Since the regime change – quite exceptionally in the region – there has been no need for early elections, and the rare (3) replacements of prime ministers before the end of their term took place without major reshuffles. Therefore, the strength of the cabinets depends primarily on their internal cohesion; their power is limited mainly by undisciplined governing MPs and coalition partner(s) while external barriers exist in the form of the need for qualified majority votes in parliament for certain decisions,[21] and legal review exercised by the Constitutional Court.

21 For the election of high-ranking public officials the support of at least two-thirds of all MPs is usually required. In a few areas, the adoption of laws is only possible with the support of two-thirds of the MPs present. This requirement affects health policy primarily through the Act on Local Governments that is also subject to qualified majority.

Under such conditions, when the government enjoys stable support in parliament, the opposition has no legal means to get rid of the ministers or the cabinet. It can only try to put pressure on the cabinet by blocking policy initiatives and/or by winning the public discourse and turning public opinion against the government. Policy initiatives can be stopped by using legal or political procedures. In cases of legal incoherence or unconstitutionality the opposition may request legal review by the Constitutional Court. The most powerful political means of blocking government initiatives is the referendum: if backed by at least 200,000 voters, the opposition could initiate a referendum which only succeeded if at least one-quarter of all eligible voters cast their ballot in support of the initiative and they win a majority over their opponents.[22]

Starting with the June 1990 modifications to the Constitution, the position of the executive and its leader have considerably strengthened vis-à-vis the parliament (Gallai 2003b). The prime minister plays an extraordinary role: (s)he selects and replaces ministers who are formally appointed and dismissed by the president of the republic, but the head of state does not make decisions. Ministers have limited responsibility to parliament because neither the motion of vote of confidence in, nor the vote of no confidence against individual ministers exists in the Hungarian legislature. Therefore, the loyalty of the ministers is primarily expressed towards the prime minister, who is not simply the first among the equals but definitely the leader of the cabinet.

This has been expressed by three important developments. First, the Prime Minister's Office (MeH) was considerably strengthened in 1998 when it was transformed into a centre for stronger coordination and leadership in governance (Körösényi *et al.* 2003) and – for the first time – a minister was appointed to lead the unit. Its central political role was reinforced two terms later. Second, in 2006 the right to select and appoint ministry leaders together with the right to approve the organizational structure and operational rules of the ministries were assigned to the prime minister. And third, in 2006 the prime minister was also officially given the right to command the ministers. The other side of these developments was the weakening of the ministerial positions, the detachment of key political decisions from the formal decision-making structure, and the emergence of an informal power centre (Gallai and Lánczi 2006). After 1998, not only the position but also the political style of the prime minister began to show similarities with the executives of presidential systems (Körösényi 2001). The new government structure of 2006 amplified this change and shifted the Hungarian political system further from a mixed towards a

22 In the first half of the 1990s validity was conditioned to a turnout higher than 50%. After 2010 the new governmental majority decided to reinstall the same requirement.

majority system (see Lijphart 1992). In fact, after 1998 the political party system began to move from 'moderate pluralism' (Sartori 1976) towards a quasi-two-party system.

Compared with other countries in the region, the Hungarian party system has demonstrated a relatively high level of stability. By 1998, the Hungarian Socialist Party (MSZP) was able to consolidate its position in the left while Fidesz emerged as main contender from the right.[23] The filtering effect of the election system has also helped the main parties absorb more and more votes. The small parties either had to run together with a senior partner or they struggled to pass the electoral threshold. In 2002 and 2006 MSZP and Fidesz each obtained more than 40% of the votes. Such a high concentration of votes demonstrated the consolidation of two main parties (to be precise: two party blocks). In the first two terms after the change of regime, there were examples of collaboration of left wing and right wing policy experts in the standing committees. By the turn of the 21st century the deepening post-communist versus anti-communist political cleavage had excluded the possibility of cooperation between the two sides, and the relationship between the main parties has deteriorated further after the 2002 parliamentary elections.

The outcome of the 2002 election came as a real surprise because it contradicted the forecasts of all polling agencies. For the first time in the history of democratic elections in Hungary, the losing side challenged the fairness of the contest. The change in government was followed by political retaliation. Many civil servants were fired (Szilvásy 2003) and a state secretary, who was appointed to investigate the suspected corruption scandals of the previous government, made dozens of accusations. Unsurprisingly, when the Socialists were ousted from power in 2010, a government commissioner was appointed to reveal the illegal and unethical cases of the outgoing cabinet; once again several accusations were submitted to the police. Since then conflict-seeking has become the standard pattern of party strategies. Especially after 2004, the year of EU accession, there were few issues in which the opposition did not reject entire government proposals out of hand. The chance of collaboration has definitely gone when Prime Minister Péter Medgyessy was replaced by Ferenc Gyurcsány of the ruling Socialist Party, when strong leadership and personalized politics became equally important on both sides. The invalid referendum of December 2004 erected a strong wall between MSZP and Fidesz because the Socialist prime minister campaigned against the idea of giving citizenship to those Hungarians who live in the neighboring countries. The other question in the referendum intended

23 It is important to note the use of left and right is correct in cultural respect, but in some policy areas, most notably in economic policy, the left is on the right, and the right is on the left: Fidesz represents a more étatist economic policy and rejects further privatization, while MSZP advocates privatization and market competition.

to impose a ban on the privatization of public health institutions and hospitals. Due to low turnout, the referendum was invalid but compared with the other question a large proportion of Socialist supporters rejected the official party line: on dual citizenship only 52% voted in favor of the initiative, whereas 65% voted for the ban on privatization. Deep conflicts and distrust between the main political parties made co-operation impossible.

In such a situation, the 2006 election and the subsequent political scandal produced serious frustration among rightwing politicians and voters. A few months after the election a tape was made public in which the re-elected prime minister – talking to the Socialist MPs in a closed meeting – admitted that his first cabinet had lied about the state of the economy, avoided crisis by 'hundreds of tricks' and won re-election with campaign strategies built around deliberate lies. The speech drove masses of people to the streets demanding the resignation of Prime Minister Gyurcsány. Despite the protests, the subsequent riots and the lost municipal elections, the prime minister was confirmed in his position by a vote of confidence. Police brutality during the 50th commemoration of the 1956 revolution poisoned the government-opposition relations. Since the opposition had no means to force a politically discredited prime minister to step down, they declared him *persona non grata* and rejected every government initiative.

In the health sector this standoff has meant the rejection of cuts, capacity reductions, privatization and co-payment. Since most decisions of 2006 and 2007 were imposed on the sector (Dózsa 2008), the government was unable to win the support of the affected interest organizations. In addition, the majority of the population opposed the changes because the withdrawal of funds had resulted in cancelled surgeries, expanding waiting lists, and more expensive medicines. The government could have offset the severe cuts on health expenditure and the reduction of hospital capacities by generating higher revenues to the sector, but already high taxes and social contributions did not allow a significant increase of health contributions. Privatization and the introduction of co-payment schemes into new areas could have offered further possibilities to bring in additional revenues, but both options were politically executed. Although private actors are important service providers and in some areas they have played a vital role, public sentiment has never been in favor of privatizing entire health institutions (not even in the form of contracting out their operation). Yet, to a great extent the really profitable services in the sector have already been privatized while the operation of most institutions is financially not promising. This left the privatization of the public health insurance scheme as the only possibility of generating considerable private capital for the sector. Public attitudes towards co-payment have also been rather ambiguous. Co-payment for medicines has had a long tradition, and out-of-pocket payments at private service providers, such as dentists and gynecologists, are also broadly accepted. These examples and surveys (Baji *et al.* 2011) suggest that many patients are willing to pay user fees for easier access and services of better quality. Therefore, in the 2008 referendum the rejection of the relatively low visiting fee and hospital fee was primarily politically motivated. In the fierce bipartisan contest of a strongly polarized party system the referendum was used by the opposition to express a strong protest against the government and Prime Minister Gyurcsány.

The referendum demonstrated that politics in general and electoral contests in particular could lead to U-turns in policies. The situation converted Fidesz, a centre-right party, into a bitter opponent of privatization in the health sector while the outcome of the election drove the government to not only give up the introduction of co-payment but also to drop the idea of privatizing the HIF. After the referendum, the halting of health reform and the firing of the minister for health, a member of the junior governing party, broke the coalition. A year later, amidst the international financial crisis, Prime Minister Gyurcsány decided to step down. The new cabinet devoted its incomplete one-year term to crisis management and introduced further cuts without implementing any significant change to the health sector.

In the 2010 election, dissatisfaction with the performance of the Socialist governments, mounting corruption scandals, increasing distrust in politics and politicians, and growing disappointment with the outcomes of transition (Pew Research 2009) have shaken the Hungarian party system. The two main opposition parties of the regime change have disappeared, the Socialist party has lost more than half of its supporters, and Fidesz won a major victory by obtaining qualified (two-thirds) majority in parliament. Therefore, the second Fidesz-led government enjoys nearly unlimited legal freedom in the formulation of health policy.

5.7 Recent Developments

In 2010, the new government received unexceptionally high political (electoral) support, but it also inherited a country in its worst financial trouble during the past two decades. The extremely strong budgetary constraints as well as the fierce opposition from Fidesz to both privatization and co-payment during the previous term reduced the possible elements of the government's policy mix. Thus, the strongest post-1990 government could only choose from a limited range of policies of which the introduction of powerful central management and imposing serious cuts dominated the agenda. Brussels did not allow the government to leave the convergence path and loosen its fiscal policy. Therefore the government was forced to reduce state expenditures. The health sector was seriously affected as government financing in this sector was reduced by HUF 76 billion in 2011, and an additional cut by more than HUF 110 billion can be expected for 2012. At the same time revenues to the health fund were increased by an additional taxation of a broad range of unhealthy drinks and foods. This extra tax has been levied on products with high fat, salt, sugar and caffeine content.[24] Nevertheless, the expected revenues (HUF 20 billion in 2012) are considerably lower than the losses of the sector, and they will be most absorbed by the salary increase of doctors and other health professionals.[25]

Cost containment in subsidizing medicines and financing inpatient care traditionally presents a challenge to every cabinet. The new government decided to transform the support of the pharmaceutical sector. On the one hand, the tax burden of the pharmaceutical companies was raised. Subsidies on medicines, on the other hand, were considerably lowered by the introduction of a very strict (negative) bidding system. Bidding takes place twice a year. In cases of generic products (of the same agent) the medicine of the lowest bidder wins the title of 'reference product', and receives full subsidy. Other bidders have the option to modify their previous bid and make a choice: they may adjust their price to stay within a 5% range of the reference product that would make them eligible for full compensation; or they may stick to a higher price level but then they lose either 15% of their subsidy (if they stay within the 30% range) or the entire sum (outside the 30% range). The financial benefits of the new system were apparent: blindfold bidding saved the fund for medicines approximately HUF 20 billion in 2011.[26] However, the first side effects soon became noticeable; in order to squeeze out incumbent producers, foreign and smaller pharmaceuticals bid below the actual cost level and caused supply problems for some products. In addition, there is a high probability of losing jobs and tax revenues in the sector.

In the case of hospitals the decision on the future status was primarily driven by fiscal and political considerations. During 2002-2010 the general government debt had rocketed from 52% to 82% of GDP. Consequently, the new cabinet put the debt reduction on the top of its economic priority list. This decision seriously affected local and county governments, which owned most of the hospitals. In 2010 many institutions for inpatient care were at the brink of bankruptcy[27] while their owners were not in the position to bail them out because they too had generated considerable debts.[28] In response, the new cabinet introduced a constitutional limit on general debt (temporarily suspended) and applied an

24 Despite an early correction of the regulation, the range of heavily taxed products is still not consistent.

25 The salary increase was agreed between the government and the Hungarian Residents' Association when more than 2,700 residents threatened to quit. The wages of other doctors and health professionals also had to be increased for two reasons: higher wages of residents could have compressed (unfairly) the scale of salaries in the sector; and OECD found Hungarian salaries in the sector to be the lowest in East and Central Europe.

26 By 2013 the government intends to reduce public expenditures on medicines by one-third compared to 2010.

27 Their overall debt in December 2011 hovered around HUF 123 billion.

28 Many local governments and nearly all county governments are heavily indebted. Their share in the general government debt increased steadily and by 2010 accounted for about 5%.

administrative brake on debt generation by local governments.[29] Moreover, instead of the usual pattern of a consolidation without restructuring, the new cabinet took over the ownership of the hospitals, which will be reorganized and supervised by the National Institute for Quality and Organizational Development in Healthcare and Medicines. The Institute, which will even have the authority to instruct the hospitals in management related issues, is a government agency that operates under the Ministry of Human Resources.

In order to improve the scale of the economy and the management of the hospitals, the government decided to divide the country into eight territorially integrated units. Each unit has about 1-1.2 million inhabitants, and their boundaries differ from the units of local public administration. The reason for not following the division of (NUTS-2) regions was to leave the natural patient routes intact. The new division takes hospital capacities into account and aims to restructure capacities by strengthening central hospitals, promoting the specialization of other inpatient institutions, and transforming hospitals with low capacities into institutions of social care. With the introduction of the coordinated management the government also expects to reduce the supply costs of medicines and medical instruments, and to increase efficiency by the reinstallation of managed care.

5.8 CONCLUSIONS

In general, political considerations and the logic of electoral politics limit the policy options of governments. In Hungary the strongly polarized two-bloc system reduced the policy choices of the cabinets during the past decade and often made policy rationale the victim of a fierce party contest. Taking the strength of incumbent interests and the weakness of the civil society into account, it is not surprising that successive governments have been unable to implement their policies despite having properly diagnosed the problems of health care management.

Persistent financial difficulties are the result of significant informal payments, free riding, inefficiency, and revenue-generating (misreported and unnecessary) interventions. Multiple employments of doctors cause conflicts of interests and examples of state capture; this issue remains legally unresolved. An increasing shortage of labor in certain areas, limited emphasis on prevention, high number of surgeries, too many days spent in hospital, and high consumption of drugs and medicines are both symptoms and causes of inefficient resource allocation. The quality of services remains uneven and likewise access to services.

29 Local councils may only take government generating loans or issue bonds if their decision also receives approval by the minister for national economy.

The package of basic services has not been defined. Waiting lists are expanding, while the population is characterized by indicators that – even by regional standards – are generally poor. The male population over fifty years of age produces particularly worrying health indicators.

The strong electoral mandate and legal freedom of the new government facilitate the introduction of policy innovations. In contrast, uncertain external conditions and tough fiscal constraints limit the cabinet's policy options. While the initial costs of restructuring generally cry for additional resources, the current government is obliged to reduce public spending. Under such conditions it is impossible to optimize policy goals and electoral considerations.

6 Health System Reforms in the Republic of Macedonia, 1991-2010

Vladimir Lazarevik, Blasko Kasapinov, Dance Gudeva-Nikovska and Branko Dimeski

In order to investigate and evaluate health system reforms in the Republic of Macedonia since 1991, desk research was conducted on literature in English and Macedonian about health sector reforms as well as on laws relevant documents available at the Ministry of Health and the Health Insurance Fund (HIF). Official data on demographic and health status indicators were collected from the Institute of Public Health and the State Statistical Office, which were cross-checked against international data sets. In addition, interviews were conducted with stakeholders working in the health care system to assess their perceptions about the impact of health system reforms.

The Republic of Macedonia inherited the former Yugoslavian health system with its widespread and easily accessible health infrastructure, large hospitals and a regional network of institutes of public health responsible for preventive activities as well as the notion of social ownership of health facilities. After independence in 1991, the health system was re-established to protect and promote the values of solidarity, equity and participation. The health system is predominantly financed by compulsory social health contributions by employees (7.2% of gross salary). For two decades, the monopoly position of the HIF as the single purchaser of health care services constrained the fragmentation of scarce health resources. Recently, however, financial stability of the HIF has been jeopardized by an increased number of insurees, smaller transfers of funds from the central budget and a generous package of basic benefits.

Three periods of health system reforms are evident in Macedonia: post-socialist, pro-market and manifesto-driven. These periods are based on reforms developed and implemented during political developments in the country. Over the years, poor maintenance, low efficiency and high operational costs have increased out-of-pocket expenditures for health and reflect the deterioration of public hospital infrastructure. This has reduced quality in the provision of health services in public facilities. Parallel to these processes, liberal health care market regulation produced a trend in the commercialization of health care services and investment in new private for-profit hospital services. Long transitions and ineffective reforms in the public health sector impelled many health personnel to move to the private sector, but to remain in Macedonia. Disappointed in the quality of services provided in the public health sector, many citizens now opt for services in private health care facilities where they pay out of pocket.

Despite many reforms and initiatives, political promises and actions, health sector reforms in the Republic of Macedonia are fragmented. Key problems are poor quality and low efficiency of the services provided in public health facilities, distortion of the social health insurance system and politicization of the health sector. The success of future health reforms depends on many factors but crucially on the diminished influence of politics over health institutions. A promising step in such a direction would be to adopt new legislation for the autonomy of selected health providers that would transform public hospitals into corporate entities. Such legislation would open opportunities to rationalize hospitals, to initiate mergers and to stimulate entrepreneurial behavior among the managers of public health care institutions. These reforms require political wiliness and courage that unfortunately in the current political setting cannot be envisaged.

6.1 Background

With an area of 25,713 km^2, the Republic of Macedonia is located in the middle of the Balkan Peninsula. Macedonia's neighbors are Bulgaria to the east, Albania to the west, Kosovo to the northwest, Serbia to the northeast and Greece to the south. In mid-2008, the total population was estimated to be 2,046,898 inhabitants comprising 1,026,022 males and 1,020,876 females (State Statistical Office 2009a). Their multiethnic composition is an important characteristic of the country. According to the 2002 census almost two-thirds of the population is ethnic Macedonian (65%); minorities include Albanians (25%), Turks (4%), Roma (3%), Serbs (2%) and Vlachs (1%). Although there was a slight decline in population after independence due to emigration of ethnic non-Macedonians to the new countries that emerged from former Yugoslavia (Croatia, Slovenia, Bosnia and Serbia), the number of inhabitants has been relatively stable throughout the last 20 years. In 2008, population density was 80 people per square kilometre.

Despite relative stability in numbers, there have been significant changes in demographic structure. The ageing index (the ratio between older and younger populations) has climbed from 0.18 in 1948 to 0.62 in 2008. Since independence the proportion of urban population has been steady at 60%. In 2008 life expectancy at birth was 71.95 for males and 76.14 for females (average 74.0), which represents a slight increase compared to previous years; gender differences have remained the same, in favor of females. According to the World Bank, average life expectancy at birth for 2010 is estimated at 74.6 years and the trend is increasing. Life span in the Republic of Macedonia is five years lower than the EU average (World Health Organization 2010). Child health indicators are valid indicators of development achieved as a result of investment in health professionals, a network of health institutions for maternal and child health, programs for maternal and child health, programs for immunization, developed patronage service and quality of health services.

The infant mortality rate (IMR) in the Republic of Macedonia has steadily decreased from 88 per 1,000 births in 1970 to 31.6 in 1990 and 9.7 in 2008. In 2009 the IMR unexpectedly rose to 11.7/1,000 (WHO 2010) that triggered an alert among health policy makers. During the last two years the IMR again fell below ten per thousand live births; in 2011 the rate was 7.6/1,000 live births (State Statistical Office 2012).

Since independence, the Republic of Macedonia has undergone several administrative reorganizations. Under the federal structure of Yugoslavia, the Republic of Macedonia was divided into 30 municipalities. A territorial reorganization after independence in 1991 produced 124 municipalities. With the latest administrative revision in 2004, the number decreased to 84 municipalities, including 10 new municipalities within the capital Skopje. In total there are 1,762 populated localities, 34 of which are cities and the rest are villages (State Statistical Office 2009b).

Since independence, the Republic of Macedonia's domestic economy has had radical reforms in order to establish market economy structures. In the early 1990s the country experienced hyperinflation. Since 2001, the Central Bank has employed a strict monetary policy to avoid inflation, which has produced macro-economic stabilization as well as price stability in goods and services (Gjorgjev *et al.* 2006). World Bank data indicate that total Gross Domestic Product (GDP) in 1990 (US$4.5 billion) had doubled by 2010 (US$9.2 billion) (World Bank 2010). In the early 1990s, the rate of inflation was 1,690%; since 2001 the economy has been stable with inflation no higher than 10%. In 2012 the State Statistical Office reported an unemployment rate of 31.6% while poverty is estimated to be 30.4%. The most significant determinants of poverty are the size of the household and the number of employed persons within a family (World Bank 2003). However, because Macedonia has a large informal economy, the figures (especially those related to unemployment rates) should be considered with caution.

As a percentage of total government expenditures, public sector expenditure on health has ranged from 14.7% in 1995 to 15.8% in both 2000 and 2005. According to the latest available data, the percentage decreased to 12.1% in 2009 (WHO 2012). The estimates for private expenditure on health as a percentage of total expenditure on health are 27.6% in 1995, 29.1% in 2000 and 33.3% in 2009. According to these data, public sector expenditure as a percentage of total health expenditure is around 66.4% for 2009. As a percentage of GDP expenditure on health was 7.6% in 1995 and 2000, 8.1% in 2005 and 6.9% in 2009 – the lowest recorded rate among countries in the region (WHO 2012).

Curative health care in Macedonia is organized at three levels – primary, secondary and tertiary – while preventive health care is organized through a network of one national institute and ten regional centres of public health. Official data show that the total number of physicians and other health professionals (dentists, pharmacists, nurses, midwives, laboratory technicians and others) has been relatively stable throughout the past twenty years. There were 4,396 physicians in 1990 and 5,052 in 2007. In 2008, the ratio of physicians in the general population was 262.95/100,000, well below the EU average (330). In total there were 12,838 health professionals in 1990 compared to 14,082 in 2007 (Institute for Public Health 2010). Prior to 2006, the exact numbers of health personnel might be underestimated, especially for private physicians and other health professionals, because the Institute of Public Health did not collect complete reports on the staff employed in private health organizations. However, given the process of privatization of primary health care as well as the emergence of new private hospitals, data for health staff and procedures conducted in private organizations are now routinely recorded. During the past two decades, the massive hospital capacity has been reduced, although not sufficiently. Rationalization of hospital capacity is evident in the reduction in the number of hospital beds from 11,119 in 1990 to 9,434 in 2010. In 2009 the ratio of hospital beds was 449/100,000 population, and the trend shows a steady decline over the years. The average length of stay in hospitals decreased in favor of home treatment and patient care. Day-care hospitals, day-care treatment centres (community mental health centres, addiction disease treatment centres) and patronage services have been developed.

At the beginning of the 1990s, Macedonia's health system was organized within so-called 'self-governing communities'; it was governed and owned by 30 municipalities and the city of Skopje. Health care was financed on the municipality level with a solidarity fund at central level to finance those municipalities that contributed less revenue for health and thus were unable to provide appropriate health care. In August 1991, a Health Care Law (HCL) was adopted to reestablish the health care system. Based on the values of equity, solidarity, reciprocity and universal coverage of the population, the HCL defines the organizational structure of the health system. It envisaged the formation of the HIF and the mechanisms for financing and delivering health care services. Adopted in 2000 the Health Insurance Law (HIL) provides rights, obligations and responsibilities to plan and collect the revenues for compulsory health insurance and to determine the rights of insurees. Its responsibilities are to purchase health services following efficient, effective and economic use of funds, to protect financial risk of the citizens in case of health service need, and to follow other rights and obligations as specified in the compulsory health insurance legislation (HIL 2000; HIF 2008).

6.2 HEALTH SYSTEM FINANCING

The health system in the Republic of Macedonia is funded by social contributions deducted from the gross salary of all employees. The rate of health contributions in 2010 was set at 7.3% of the gross salary. This percentage is rather low compared to other countries with similar organization of the social health system financing (Saltman *et al.* 2004). The trend to reduce social contributions started in 2007 with changes in the law consistent with the newly elected government's policy to reduce the costs of labor and to stimulate new employment. By 2010, health and pension contributions, together with contributions for the unemployed, were subsequently reduced to 7.3%, 18% and 1.2%, respectively (OG 2008a). Before these tax reforms, the rate for health contributions was 9.2%, adjusted by a complex formula to consider the education status of the employees (Donev 1999, 2009; Misovski 2004). Contributions by pensioners were 21% and 10.5% for the unemployed. At 55%-58%

Table 6.1 Republic of Macedonia, Categories of Data (1980-2010)

Demographic Characteristics	**1990**	**1995**	**2000**	**2005**	**2010**
Population	2 028 000	1 965 984	2 031 541	2 036 855	2 055 004
Population density (per km^2)	78.9	76.5	79.0	79.2	79.9
Urban (%)		59.76	59.44	59.66	57.8
Life expectancy at birth (male)	69.98 (1991)	70.04	71.18	71.44	72.5
Life expectancy at birth (female)	74.53 (1991)	74.48	75.74	75.88	76.14
Infant mortality rate per 1 000 live births	31.6	22.67	11.81	12.8	7.6 (2011)
Economic data	**1990**	**1995**	**2000**	**2005**	**2010**
Total GDP (US$ million)*		2 377	3 588	4 534	9 189
Total GDP (US$ million)&#	4 471	4 449	3 586	5 814	9 189
GDP per capita (US$)*		1 209	1 771	2 226	2 980 (2008)
GDP per capita (US$)&#	2 205	2 263	1 765	2 854	4 570
Inflation rate*	1 690.7 (1992)	15.9	10.6	0.5	1.6
Inflation rate (GDP deflator)#	93.7 (1991)	17.1	8.2	3.8	2.2
GDP growth rate (real)	−6	−1	5	−5	1.8

Table 6.1 Republic of Macedonia, Categories of Data (1980-2010)

Health Expenditures	**1990**	**1995**	**2000**	**2005**	**2008**
Public outlays as percentage of total intergovernmental budgets	n/a	n/a	15.8	15.8	n/a
Private out-of-pocket outlays (estimates)	n/a	n/a	29.1	29.6	33.26
Total health expenditure (PPP$ per capita)	n/a	368	452	601	702
Total health expenditures (% of GDP) @	n/a	7.6	7.6	7.8	6.88
Health Resources	**1990**	**1995**	**2000**	**2005**	**2010**
Physicians (public)	4 396	4 516	4 455	4 392	3 636
Physicians (private)	n/a	n/a	n/a	n/a	1 905
Physicians (total)	4 396	4 516	4 455	4 392	5 541
Physicians per 100,000 population (total)	217	230	219	216	261
Other health professionals (public)	12 838	13 071	12 838	11 511	9 994
Other health professionals (private)	n/a	n/a	n/a	n/a	5 475
Other health professionals (total)	12 838	13 071	12 838	11 511	15 469
Other health professionals per 100,000	633	665	632	565	753
Hospital beds (public)	11 119	10 645	10 248	9 569	8 848
Hospital beds (private)	n/a	n/a	n/a	n/a	335
Hospital beds (total)	11 119	10 645	10 248	9 569	9 434
Hospital beds per 100,000	548	542	504	470	447

Sources: *= State Statistical Office; &=Ministry of Finance; #=World Bank; @=WHO).

of the total HIF budget, health contributions constitute its largest portion (HIF 2008). An additional 21%-23% of the HIF budget comes from the Pensions Fund that covers health services for retired citizens. The health and pension contributions constitute the most stable finances of the HIF budget. Until 2008, the State Employment Agency (SEA) contributed 8%-10% to the HIF budget on behalf of unemployed people in the country.

Recent changes in the HIL to insure all the unemployed have transferred the funding from SEA to the central budget. While sustainability of health financing was jeopardized by smaller than expected transfers from the central budget to HIF, combined with the need to purchase higher volume of services (HIF 2010), during the last three years the percentage of funds transferred from the ministry of finance to HIF increased to around 20% of the total HIF budget. This money compensates for the deficit due to lower contribution rates and the generous basic benefit package. The negative aspect of such increased transfer of money from the central budget reflects the limited autonomy in decision making by the HIF, which does not have total control and is therefore politically influenced by the government. A small portion of the health budget (4%) comes from copayments and additional sources (HIF 2009). Since 2002 the HIF budget has increased from 14 billion MKD to a projected 22 billion MKD in 2012 or approximately €357 million (€1 = 61.5 MKD). However, this budget is probably overestimated and may be rebalanced due to poor economic performance of the country during 2012. The annual growth of the budget peaked in 2008 when it increased by 12.4% compared to 2007. Since then annual growth has been around 5%. Finally, preventive programs are funded by the central budget and administered through the Ministry of Health (MoH) and a network comprising an institute and ten centres of public health.

Apart from public financing of the health system, a significant percentage of total health expenditure comes from private expenditures for health. According to a household expenditure survey, out-of-pocket expenditure (OPE) constitutes 25% of total health expenditures in the Republic of Macedonia (State Statistical Office 2009c). The latest estimate of private expenditure for health in Macedonia is around one-third of total health expenditure (WHO 2010). Due to poor data, however, these figures are probably underestimated so OPE may be as high as 40%-50% of total health care spending. A large percentage of OPE is devoted to pay private providers for health care services, medical devices and pharmaceuticals. A smaller percentage is for official copayment for services delivered in public health facilities, including informal under-the-table payments (MoH 2007).

The rise in costs of access to health care has direct implications for inequities in the country (Lazarevik *et al.* 2009). Given the lack of complementary private health insurance, a portion of private spending is devoted to financing the health services provided in private hospitals. A few insurance companies offer supplementary private health insurance packages, but the health insurance market in Macedonia is small and market opportunities for complementary health insurance are limited due to existence of generous basic benefit package provided by the HIF. There have been many discussions and debates to introduce private health insurance, or to implement competition in the social health insurance in Macedonia (Centre for Research and Policy Making 2005). Some of these initiatives have been announced by the government, but not yet implemented in practice.

The position of the HIF as single purchaser of health care services has so far prevented fragmentation of scarce health care resources and maintained relative financial sustainability of the system. Since 2006, the HIF has been building its profile as a strategic purchaser of health care services. However, in practice the HIF acts more like a simple payer rather than a strategic purchaser. According to the HCL, the HIF is obliged to sign contracts with all providers licensed by the Ministry of Health, whatever the status of their ownership. Since 2007, all interested providers are obliged to apply at the HIF for contracts.[1] As of 2010 contracts are agreed and signed in April each calendar year in order to deal with the fiscal problems experienced by the providers during the previous calendar year.

The HIF purchases services from public health care providers at all levels of the health care system. These providers include primary and specialist clinics, hospitals, public health institutes, laboratories, pharmacies and dentistry. Primary health services are purchased through capitation formulas and contracts with individual doctors. Specialist services in both health centres[2] (HC) and hospitals are paid as part of the global budget of the health institution. Each HC signs a contract with the HIF. Public hospitals also sign contracts with HIF and their budget is estimated according to historical averages from previous years. The contracts include type and volume of the services to be delivered over the year by each provider.

It is important to note that the contracting process is founded on negotiations between the HIF and the providers, but the latter have limited power and autonomy. Thus contracting is based on HIF pressure over providers following the "take it or leave it" principle. In 2007, the government initiated a process to change the financing system in hospitals. In 2009, a Diagnostic Related Group system was introduced in all inpatient facilities, so in future it is expected that hospital budgets will be tailored according to their performance. Diagnostic Related Groups (DRGs) have proved to be an important tool to model health providers' budgets, but its real implications are yet to be analyzed. In addition to the public providers,

1 Prior to 2007 health care providers did not have contracts with the HIF; budgets were allocated according to historical performance and traditions.

2 HCs are organized as traditional polyclinics with primary care and specialist doctors.

the HIF signs selective contracts to purchase certain services from private hospitals. While all public hospitals have permanent contracts with the HIF, there are few active contracts between the HIF and private hospitals but demand is increasing which causes an additional threat to the financial stability of the HIF.

There are three levels in ownership and provision of health care services in Macedonia: primary, secondary and tertiary. The primary level has two types of ownership: primary health clinics that are an integral part of the HCs owned by the central government, and primary clinics owned by private doctors (Table 6.2). Public primary health clinics are privatized, but ownership of the facilities remains with the central government. Decentralization in the health system occurred only in the primary health care sector, mainly in the governance of the HCs, but it has had little effect in practice. Councils of the municipalities appoint two representatives in the managing boards of the HC but their influence over the decision-making process is limited. The secondary level of health care provision is divided between specialists' clinics in government ownership located within the HCs, and many privately owned specialist clinics throughout the country. In addition, specialists practice secondary care within the hospitals.

The central government owns and the Ministry of Health is responsible for running public hospitals. Private investors own the private hospitals that are regulated by health laws. The

Table 6.2 Ownership, Financing and Government Control of Health Providers

Levels of the Health Care System	Ownership	Financing	Government Control
Primary health clinics	Private	Capitation (free access without copayment)	Small
Health centres	Public	HIF + co-payment	Municipalities, central government
Specialist/ consultative care	Public/private	HIF/OPE (copayment, fee for service)	Municipalities, central government
Public hospitals	Public	HIF/copayment/ private patients	Strong central government
Private hospitals	Private	Out of pocket, contracts	Week regulation, private
Public health institutes	Public	Central budget, HIF, laboratory services	Central government, municipalities

country has eight private hospitals – two general and six specialized – covering general surgery, cardio-surgery, ophthalmology, gynecology, nephrology and dialysis. Most of these private investments were developed without an initial HIF contract or government partnership. An early form of public-private partnership was introduced in the case of a cardio-surgery hospital that opened in 2000 and within the publicly owned facility of the military hospital. The government has credited initial purchasing of the equipment, and the HIF was obliged to purchase cardio-surgery services from this provider. Over the past two years the HIF became more proactive and purchase-oriented and has continued to sign contracts with private hospitals for certain type of services.

There have been many discussions and proposals for additional private-public partnerships in the health sector in Macedonia. In 2008, the parliament adopted a law on public-private partnership (OG 2008b), but the Ministry of Health has not developed by-laws or rules of procedure that would make this law operational in practice. Thus the ambitions of three successive governments to introduce public private partnerships remain only as promising statements by several Ministers of Health without further action. In 2012 a new HCL was adopted that includes a new model for concessions where all providers irrespective of their ownership can apply to deliver requested health care services. However, it is too early to analyze its effects in practice (HCL 2012).

In 2010, following the government call to attract new investors in the health care system, three new private hospitals were opened for gynecology, ophthalmology and dialysis. This government initiative was undertaken without envisioning its financial implications for the HIF and the overall health system. It took several years for the government to understand the implications and to adopt more strict legislation about how new providers enter the health care system (HCL 2012). According to the new legislation, in order to ask for contracts with the HIF, each new provider must have approval from the Ministry of Health and be considered as part of the medical map.

Private hospitals have contracts with the HIF only for those services that are either not provided at public health facilities or where there is higher demand from patients (IVF, ophthalmology, cardio-surgery). The private health sector follows entrepreneurial processes and constantly looks for new opportunities in the health care market. Until the adoption of the new HCL in 2012, government control over the private health sector was limited to setting standards and control over quality of services; it did not include governing principles or setting limits in opening and planning new investments. With the new HCL adopted in March 2012 and the Medical Map, the government is expected to strengthen its control and regulations in the health care system especially in relation to the entry of new providers into the health care market.

6.3 History of Health System Reforms

Macedonia inherited the Yugoslavian health system with its widespread and massive health infrastructure, large and overstaffed hospitals, regional networks of institutes of health responsible for health promotion and prevention activities, and social ownership of facilities. One characteristic of the Yugoslavian model of health system organization that left its mark on the Macedonian health system was the notion of universal and free access of health services for all citizens regardless of their ability to pay (Saric and Rodwin 1993). Since independence in 1991, three main periods are evident in the development of health system reforms: post-socialist (1991-1998), pro-market (1998-2006) and manifesto-driven (2006-continuing). These periods are not sharply divided and some aspects overlap in different periods. Shifts in decision-making power over allocation of resources and political influences were used as orientation to select the phases. Each of these periods carries its own specifics that have left a stamp on the current structure of the system (Table 6.3).

In the period after independence, the Republic of Macedonia faced many challenges as a new country emerging after the collapse of Yugoslavia. The country moved to develop parliamentary democracy and a welfare state based on citizens' participation and the right to private property. The Constitution adopted in 1991 included the right to health care protection plus obligations for citizens to protect their personal health as well as the health of the others (Article 39). The organization and functioning of the health care system was reestablished under the HCL adopted in 1991. This law redefined all subjects operating in the health care system, medical chambers and professional associations and, for the first time, opened the possibility of private medical practice. The law also served as a basis for the development of the social health system by introducing compulsory health insurance and the HIF within and under the auspices of Ministry of Health. The health care system was centralized to provide strong control over the utilization of resources and equitable distribution in times of economic crises (Menon 2006).

The transition from socialism to a market-oriented system caused the collapse of many enterprises. Within a few years many socially owned enterprises were privatized, and a huge proportion of the population (over 200,000) became unemployed (Slaveski 1997). The collapse of the socialist economy caused significant deterioration in the health care sector. Breakdown of the socialist enterprises and increased unemployment resulted in evasion in payment of social contributions. Between 1991 and 1995, health revenues decreased by 40%, which had negative implications on the health status of the population, on the satisfaction of health personnel and patients, and on maintenance of the old infrastructure of the health care system (Ivanovska and Ljuma 1999).

Table 6.3 Three Periods of Health System Reforms, 1991-2010

First Period **Post-Socialist (1991-1998)**	**Second Period** **Pro-Market (1998-2006)**	**Third Period** **Manifesto-Driven (2006-2012)**
• Constitutional right to health protection • Adoption of the Health Care Law 1991 • Development of health insurance system • Transfer of ownership from social to public • Reestablishment of professional associations and medical chambers • Introduction of the system of referrals and choice of doctor • Introduction of co-payment for health services • Promotion of private practice ownership • Humanitarian and development assistance programs • Maintaining features of the old system • 1996 World Bank – Health Sector Transition Project #1	• Adoption of Health Insurance Law • Purchaser/provider split reform • Separate Health Insurance Fund from Ministry of Health • Development of capitation model • Continuous medical education • Purchasing equipment • Strengthening perinatal care • Decentralization and new territorial organization • Privatization (dentistry, pharmacies, primary clinics) • Opening of private hospitals • World Bank- Health Sector Transition Project #2	• Political platform (manifesto) for health sector reforms • Health management – two directors in public health institutions • Reorganization of the University Clinical Centre • Strategic purchasing function of HIF • Decentralized procurement • Advanced rights of patients • Reference and set-pricing of pharmaceuticals • Development of contracting process • Health insurance for all • Purchasing new equipment • Renovating health facilities • Development of DRG system • More private investments in health • Migration of health personnel to private hospitals • Constitutional Court • Medical map • New Health Care Law 2012

Due to lack of funds, low motivation and poor efficiency, all health care providers started acquiring financial debts that by 1997 totaled US$40 million. In the post-socialist phase HIF was an integral part of the Ministry of Health and all decisions for allocation of resources, financing of health care providers, and planning of investments came from the Cabinet with different ministers of health. In order to increase the funding of the system, the government in 1993 introduced co-payment for health care services, with safety nets for children up to 14 years and for the elderly above 65. Citizens had the possibility to select their personal doctor and a new referral system was introduced to access hospital services. This period is also marked with huge humanitarian assistance for the health care sector from international donor agencies and friendly countries in pharmaceuticals, medical devices and equipment (Jovan Tofoski, former minister of health, personal communication).

The main features of the post-socialist phase in health sector reforms in Macedonia were oriented to prevent the collapse of the health care system and to maintain some characteristics of the old system such as strong prevention, free access, and solidarity in financing. In this period the government signed its first Loan Agreement (LA) with the World Bank for health sector reforms (World Bank 1996), but its effects on the health care system were felt in the second pro-market period of reforms.

The pro-market period in health sector reforms coincides with the first official shift in political power from left-oriented former socialists to centre-right conservatives (Szajkowski 1999). This period is marked by intensive health sector reforms, mainly initiated and guided by the World Bank's Health Sector Transition Project (HSTP) (Staff Appraisal Report 1996). The influence and the pressure of the World Bank were key in the design of structural and financial reforms in the health care sector. The most important feature of the reforms within this period was the formal separation of the HIF from direct control by the Ministry of Health. In 2000 a new HIL was adopted and the HIF was established as autonomous health insurance agency governed by a managing board of 13 representatives, including six patients, two employers, three health providers delegated by the medical chambers and a representative of the Ministries of Finance and Health (HIL 2000). The establishment of the HIF as an independent agency was expected to improve transparency and efficiency in financing and delivering health care services. Also, it was important to link the purchase of health care services according to defined volume and scope of services, and to replace previously politically driven internal budget allocations. These reforms represented implementation in practice of the global movement led by the World Bank to create markets for health by separation between the purchaser (HIF) and provision functions in health care services (McPake 2002).

The next important developments were preparations for the privatization of primary health clinics and the implementation of a capitation-based model for payment of physicians. These preparations paralleled the development of centres for Continuing Medical Education (CME). Four training centres were opened in which over 40% of primary physicians in the country completed the program and received certificates as well as individual medical equipment (World Bank 2003). A population-based survey was conducted to assess the workload of various doctors (general practice, pediatrics, gynecology and school medicine) and to determine the likelihood of patients by sex and age to visit doctors' clinics (MoH 2001). This survey as well as supplemental work undertaken under the auspices of the HSTP served as a basis to create the risk-adjusted capitation formula. Development of the capitation model was a prerequisite to initiate the privatization of the clinics within the HCs that took place after changes in legislation.

The second wave of health reforms was marked by active – sometimes painstaking but also enthusiastic – participation by representatives of the MoH, HIF, the medical chamber and professional associations. It was clear that successful implementation of the reforms depended primarily on government willingness but also, more importantly, on local ownership of the reforms. Following the internal armed conflict in 2001 (Hislope 2003), health care reforms were slowed down to resume in the following years in parallel with the process of consolidation and democratization of the country (Daskalovski 2004). Decentralization emerged as one of the tenets of the Ohrid framework agreement. While a new law on local self-government was passed and basic health care was decentralized to municipalities, health insurance remained under central government control (Menon 2006). In 2004, the Ministry of Health introduced changes in the HCL that for the first time opened the possibility for privatization of segments of the public health care system, including dental clinics and pharmacies. In 2005, additional amendments of the law were adopted to initiate the privatization of the primary health doctors (HCL 2005).

The privatization process followed long administrative procedures of preparation and development of plans and by-laws by the Ministry of Health. According to the changes, each HC was obliged to prepare a special program for privatization to be approved by the Minister of Health. By October 2007, less than three years after the adoption of the first changes in the laws, a total of 3,521 health workers (doctors, dentists, pharmacists and nurses) were privatized (Table 6.4). The previous salary-based payment of doctors was replaced by capitation, and income was related to the number of citizens enrolled on doctors' lists. The doctors established private practices premises rented at the HCs (*Zdravstven dom*). The privatized doctors used the same clinics where they had worked prior to privatization.

Table 6.4 Privatization of Primary Health Care in Macedonia, 2004-2007

Primary Sector	**Rented Premises**	**Number of Employees**	
		Doctors	**Nurses/Technicians**
Primary health care	888	944	694
Dentistry	431	616	292
Dental laboratories	72		210
Pharmacies	21 sold	64 Pharmacists	414
	51 rented; State pharmacies sold		91
			196
Total	**1 463**	**3 521**	

Source: Ministry of Health 2008.

Primary health care privatization did not result in transfer of ownership of the clinics but only in privatization of medical practice. Each privatized doctor signed a contract with the HIF and receives payment on a quarterly basis. The Ministry of Health reports that, compared to the previous salary-based system, patients are pleased with the services and most of the doctors with their income (MoH 2007). However, a recent survey among primary health care doctors who are paid through a capitation formula found that they feel overburdened with administrative paperwork that reduces the time they need to spend with patients (Lazarevik 2012b). Another survey of primary health care doctors estimated their additional monthly expenses. Based on these disappointing findings, an international project recommends that doctors introduce a small co-payment for visits to GPs (Healthgrouper.com 2012b). Medical nurses are also disappointed because their income is directly related to and depends on that of the doctors.[3]

While the whole process of privatization in primary care was completed without transfer of ownership in health facilities, the biggest failure was the privatization in 2006 of a state-owned company that consisted of a chain of pharmacies called "City Pharmacies" (*Gradski Apteki*). The company was sold on the market with transfer of ownership to several private owners who formed a new company. In 2009, three years after its privatization, the company went into liquidation following a scandal in the media and street protests by employees who lost their jobs.

3 The privatization of primary health clinics was based on standards developed by the Ministry of Health. These standards required each doctor to be privatized in a package with one nurse. This policy protected the jobs of the medical nurses but made their income dependent on the doctors' willingness and financial ability to pay their salaries. It has also overburdened doctors as new entrepreneurs need decent income.

The pro-market wave of the reforms was also felt in the private health care sector. This period marked the development and opening of large private hospitals for cardio-surgery, genecology and obstetrics, and one general hospital.[4] The private hospital sector began its development in parallel to the state hospital system. HIF initially signed contracts to cover the services provided in the cardio-surgery hospital; in subsequent years contracts were signed with other private hospitals for selected services. Unavailability of insurance requires the patients who choose the private hospital sector to pay out of pocket for most of the services provided there.

The third wave of health sector reforms in Macedonia started at the end of 2006 after parliamentary elections and a change in the government. Prior to this phase, most health sector reforms had been initiated and driven by international organizations. The main engines of reform were two projects financed by World Bank loans.[5] Political parties did not have specific programs and manifestos; even if they had, the governments did not implement their pre-election promises. The elections in 2006 marked a shift in the promotion of political platforms for elections. Promotion of new health system reforms was an integral part of the political platform of the elected party (VMRO-DPMNE 2006). Key features of this manifesto were aimed to decrease out-of-pocket expenditures for health, to improve efficiency and transparency at the level of health care providers, to advance patients' rights in all medical interventions, and to strengthen the position of the HIF as strategic purchaser of health care services. Moreover, the government promised to decrease the price of the pharmaceuticals and to introduce a referent-pricing system by providing more choice to the patients.

As a first step in realizing its objectives, the Ministry of Health developed a Health Management and Leadership Training Program (HMLTP) in the fall of 2006. The HMLTP was developed in collaboration between the Ministry of Health, the Medical Faculty in Skopje and the World Bank. The program consisted of ten teaching modules delivered over the period of six weeks, with participation of world renowned management, economics and health policy experts as well as local experts and professors from the Medical Faculty in Skopje. The announcement of the program provoked huge interest among both medical doctors and economists. The first call published in local media attracted more than 700 applications for the places initially limited to 60 participants.

---

4 In 1996 the first private hospital for plastic surgery – 'Dr. Miskovski' – opened with five hospital beds. In 2000 a cardio-surgery hospital 'Philip the Second' started to work. In 2002, a gynecology hospital 'Sistina Medical' and in 2005 a general hospital 'Re-medica' were added.

5 In 1996, the government of the Republic of Macedonia signed a loan agreement (LA) with the World Bank for a Health Sector Transition Project of about US$16 million. After its completion, another LA was signed in 2004 for a Health Sector Management Project of about US$10 million. Details on these projects are available at <www.moh-hsmp.gov.mk>.

The announcement of the program followed an initiative to change health legislation by adopting amendments to the HCL. The changes introduced a new concept in the governance of the public health providers by replacing the previous system of traditional appointment of medical doctors as directors, with a diarchal system of two directors with shared responsibility but different backgrounds – one a medical doctor, the other an economist (HCL 2007). In the following years, more than 700 doctors and economists participated at this program and were provided with the possibility to learn new concepts in health economics, management, procurement, budgeting and contracting, and policy making (MoH 2007). The changes in health legislation enabled economists for the first time in Macedonia to hold the position of director. These posts had previously been exclusively reserved for medical doctors.

This period of reforms was also characterized by strengthening the position of the HIF as the strategic purchaser of health care services. For the first time the process of contracting was implemented in practice; health care providers at all levels of the system were obliged to sign contracts with the HIF. Changes in the law on pharmaceuticals introduced a system of set-prices[6] determined by the Bureau of Pharmaceuticals at the Ministry of Health. The new system had immediate repercussions in the decline of pharmaceutical prices. Another novelty was the implementation of reference-pricing but this innovation produced an opposite effect and increased out-of-pocket expenditures by patients for pharmaceuticals (Lazarevik 2010). In order to deal with corruption in the health care system that was concentrated at the central level, the government decentralized procurement to the level of individual providers. Although health care providers became responsible for financial management, in practice they lacked autonomy. The budgets of individual providers were still decided on the basis of historical allocations, and small differences were mainly driven by political influences as during previous phases of reforms. Decentralization in procurement included decentralization of the University Clinical Centre into 31 independent clinics (legal entities) and one service provision agency.

The next important reform in the manifesto phase is the work in progress to change payment to hospitals from the previous input-based system to an output-based system. This reform required broad acceptance of the concept of E-health system, but its introduction into Macedonia's health care system entails several preconditions and numerous risks. Preconditions include, first, an already developed IT infrastructure to all health institutions in the republic and, second, an e-health service provider who would be able to prepare the appropriate documentation for undertaking technical and organizational measures as well

6 Under the new law, the Bureau of Pharmaceuticals at the Ministry of Health determines the prices of all drugs. Thus, the price of a drug from same producer is identical regardless of the pharmacy where it would be purchased.

as to protect personal data during the process of e-health personal data processing and during the implementation of the provisions for personal data protection. Full implementation of the e-health concept carries certain risks, too, such as insufficient use by the citizens due to weak training, unavailability of IT infrastructure, and insufficient use by the citizens because of mistrust in the system. Despite the risks and financial constraints, there are examples of successful implementation of e-health in the Macedonian health system. Those are the implementation of e-treasury and DRGs.

An e-treasury of public health institutions is a transparent system of payments for public health institutions. Located in the Health Fund and independent of the treasury held and managed by the Ministry of Finance, the main purpose of the e-treasury is to secure efficient and purposeful use of the financial resources of the public health institutions. The treasury is directly connected with the National Bank for income and expenditures realization. By adopting e-treasury, there is better financial planning and management, purposeful use of the health resources, transparency of payments and improved financial and budget discipline by the public health institutions. The crucial measures for e-treasury implementation depend on the availability of hardware equipment and software solutions in the health fund, training the employees in the fund as well as in public health institutions for preparing and adopting annual financial plans for 2011, training personnel to maintain information technology (IT) equipment, and providing them with IT skills and knowledge in the field of e-data exchange between the health fund and all public health institutions.

The health treasury account is a system of accounts that is managed by the Treasury of Health Fund of the Republic of Macedonia in order to perform efficient, accurate and rigorous control of financial transactions in public health institutions and the annual plans for total revenues and expenditures by the public health institutions. Each public health account differs from the national treasury account held by the Ministry. Each sub-account holds a specific amount of money that can be used independently of other public health institutions. Within the health treasury account are the separate accounts for every public health institution: an account for Health Fund resources, an account for own revenue sources and an account for donations.

The DRG policy measure is a budgetary tool to create savings in the public health sector and to increase the efficiency of hospitals. The Macedonian health system has had rather poor financial performance in the past and accumulated a significant debt to the HIF. At the same time, patients remain dissatisfied with the quality of services provided by health institutions while medical staff are discontented with their salaries that do not match the increasing expenditures. The Macedonian government believes that a DRG payment system will improve efficiency, transparency, the just distribution of health care resources, and payment of medical staff according to the number of cases treated.

In 2007, under the leadership of the Ministry of Health, the process to change the payment system for hospitals was introduced based on DRGs. Australia's DRG model was selected as most appropriate and the Ministry of Health purchased the DRG license from the government of Australia. The period of preparation lasted three years and, since 2009, all inpatient services in 56 selected health care providers started to code hospital cases according to the adapted version of the Macedonian DRG system (HIF 2009). All health care providers that have inpatient services and contracts with the HIF were obliged to code and report each episode of hospital treatment. The providers electronically send collected information to the web application (grouper) available at the web page of the HIF.[7] Although financing is not completely linked to DRG performance by hospitals, this process is advancing each year by adjusting provider budgets by a certain percentage according to results obtained by DRGs.

Currently the type and volume of services provided by individual providers as coded by DRGs serve as an approximation of hospital outputs, then compared to previous historical budgets. First year data reveal large differences and inequities in historical tailoring of hospitals budgets.[8] The second year of implementation has been more successful. Most of the problems were corrected and coding errors are limited. In 2011 the HIF published its second annual DRG report that confirms that most expectations have been met. The implementation of DRG depends on the availability of IT hardware and software as well as on professionally trained IT personnel and medical staff in the field of information technology. DRG is a story of successful implementation of IT in the health system of the Republic of Macedonia.

The whole manifesto phase of health system reforms has been influenced by government promises to improve quality in the delivery of services in public hospitals by purchasing medical equipment and renovating their facilities. In the meantime, early elections were called in 2008 in which the ruling party increased its majority in parliament. This was a new opportunity to update the health manifesto and to add new promises. The updated program divided health reforms in four main components: protect the values of solidarity, equity and participation of the citizens in the decision-making process; advance and preserve the social health insurance system; strengthen public health services; and continue to invest in the health care sector. This period in health system reforms will be

7 <www.fzo.org.mk> DRG grouper.

8 First DRG results indicate that a few hospitals provide more services and receive smaller budgets compared to other hospitals with much smaller production of services and higher budgets.

remembered for its promising start, great enthusiasm, profusion of activities, and political promises aimed to improve health system delivery (MoH 2006). The greatest successes over the last four years have been the purchase of medical equipment, renovation of facilities, and adoption of a new HCL.

6.4 Observations

The three periods analyzed in Macedonia's health system reforms provide a mixed picture of some successes and many failures. The key successes during the post-socialistic phase were the establishment of the social health insurance system and the prevention of fragmentation and collapse of the health sector due to rising unemployment in the country after the collapse of the socialist enterprises. In addition, this period promoted the possibility for private ownership of medical practices.

The second phase of reforms during the pro-market period promoted privatization of the primary health care, adoption of the HIL, purchaser-provider division in organization of the health care system and replacing the centralized command and control system directed by the Ministry of Health. The first big private hospitals were opened in parallel to the state-run hospital system, but they did not become an integral part of the health insurance system. Patients were obliged to pay out of pocket for services in private hospitals.

The third or 'manifesto' phase created great enthusiasm and social atmosphere for change in the public health sector. Many amendments to the health laws were adopted[9] while new legislation and by-laws were drafted. This period is also marked by the official introduction of health management within public health facilities, including a new concept of governance in public health institutions represented by two directors, including one economist; by 2011 this change had been abandoned in almost all institutions except university clinics. Overall prices of the pharmaceuticals were decreased and patient's rights advanced. On the financing side, health contributions declined and the HIF began contracting with public and some private health providers. A DRG system was introduced as a way to pay hospitals for inpatient services. In 2010 the first contracts with suppliers of medical equipment were signed; equipment was installed and put into use during 2011 and 2012.

Despite these achievements, the reforms did not solve all problems in the health sector. Old problems remained and new ones emerged. Over the years little attention has been

9 Between 2006 and 2008, more than forty legal documents were adopted, including changes in the legislation as well as drafting by-laws within the Ministry of Health (personal communication from Angelina Bacanovic, lawyer at the Ministry of Health).

paid to proper maintenance and development of massive health infrastructure. Lack of earlier investments caused deterioration of health facilities and poor quality in provision of health services, which opened the opportunity for private health sector development. Reforms in the primary health system did not continue with the privatization of the specialist doctors who belong to the secondary level of the health care system. The delay and hesitation of the government to continue with reforms produced huge inefficiencies and financial losses of two billion MKD or 15 million EUR per year in the health sector (Janez Jelnikar, personal communication).

In 2008, the government announced the transformation of public hospitals into autonomous corporations by drafting an initial version of the law for autonomy of health providers (MoH 2007). However, political interest not to give away power has prevented adoption of the final version of this law. Such uncertainties in the implementation of reforms forced a huge "migration" of senior health personnel into the private sector. Thus, the private health sector experiences progress in building state-of-the-art facilities, purchasing the latest equipment and technology, and attracting patients by aggressive marketing of their services. In 2008, the HIF budget reached its historically highest level, but in 2009 the health system again experienced serious financial constraints.

The local media are replete with negative coverage of conditions in the public health care system. The causes of these problems are partly due to the impact of the global financial crisis but also to unsustainable government policies to decrease the rate of health contributions, to provide coverage to all unemployed, and to introduce new services in the already generous basic benefit package. It required several years after the policy in order to insure that all citizens were supported with extra funding from the central budget. Although the HIF budget in relation to GDP increased in absolute terms, health care spending is declining. HIF is not able to cover the demands by health care providers. Thus the burden of financing health services shifted from the HIF to the patients. Out-of-pocket expenditure is increasing for all citizens, even for the insured, and new hospital debts are accumulating.

In early 2010, many hospitals began to acquire new debts, followed by scandals in the local media about poor quality in the provision of health care (Boskovska 2010; Jovanovska 2010). These developments were followed by information in the media about poorer provision and lowered quality of health services in many general hospitals.[10] In 2006, in order to improve the situation in the public hospital system, the government initiated a process to purchase new equipment and to renovate the old facilities.

10 In less than three months in 2010, three previously healthy women died after deliveries in three different general hospitals in Macedonia.

It took almost four years to complete the tendering procedure and to sign contracts with suppliers (SEEurope 2010). In addition, despite continuous problems in financing, the government was reluctant to deal with known causes of inefficiencies in the system. Privatization within the HCs was not completed, so specialist doctors and numerous administrative staff remain paid by fixed salaries.[11] Health management was officially introduced as part of the government strategy to improve the performance of public health providers, but direct interference by the political parties blocked all mechanisms for successful reforms. The politicization of the health system in Macedonia became a symbol of the transition and the key decision-making mechanism in financing, planning investments, employment and, most importantly, appointing and dismissing directors in health institutions.

These activities in the health system are performed following previous agreements between coalition partners (political parties) in the government. Instead of choice based on the quality and performance of the candidates, government coalition partners negotiate about which party will be responsible to propose politically suitable candidates for directors in selected hospitals. Once a political agreement is reached, proposals for directors are submitted to the Minister of Health who then formally appoints the directors. Similar political negotiation and agreements take place for the employment of new personnel. Part of this politicization in the administration is due to the requirements of the Ohrid Framework agreement to increase the employment of the Albanian minority in state institutions (Brunnbauer 2002; Daskalovski 2002). However, this politicization mainly benefits the political parties in maintaining their influence in local communities while it has direct negative consequences for the health system by stimulating inefficiency, nepotism and poor management that lead to systematic degradation of the public hospitals (Lazarevik 2012a).

The reform of the University Clinical Centre fragmented the largest tertiary health institution in Macedonia into many smaller subunits. The creation of each clinic as a separate legal entity (hospital) with a managing board and two directors has significantly increased operational costs and increased the number of new administrative staff. This reform has created many political problems for the government as well as problems for management, personnel and patients in the functioning of the clinics. Fear of losing patients and, more importantly, increased share of the private hospital sector has forced the government to be more protective of the state-run system. Despite new private investments in the health sector, the HIF signs only limited contracts with the private hospitals; most of the expenses in

11 Following the privatization of primary health physicians, the last phase of privatization in the Health Centres should have included around 1,500 administrative workers and 1,183 health workers (437 specialist doctors, 720 medical nurses, and 26 other health workers). However, this part of the privatization was not initiated and the reforms stopped.

the private sector are paid out of pocket by patients. Such policy in Macedonia has created a two-tier hospital system: the public hospital system covered by health insurance, limited budgets, poor infrastructure and lowered quality in provision of the health services, and a private "state of the art" hospital system without health insurance where citizens privately finance their own health services.

In the meantime, in January 2010 the Constitutional Court opened the possibility for reimbursement of costs in the provision of health services to all citizens regardless of the ownership or contracts of the providers with the HIF (Constitutional Court 2010). According to this decision, anyone who wishes to obtain services in private hospitals is eligible for reimbursement as a portion of the total costs according to the price-list of services authorized by the HIF (HIF 2010). These developments encouraged hundreds of high quality trained personnel to leave the public sector and to join the private hospital sector.[12]

This decision generated extensive public debate and created intense dispute between the government (especially the Prime Minister) and the Constitutional Court due to governmental concerns about possibly huge financial implications for the HIF budget (MIA 2010). But the public welcomed this decision although it would still require patients to pay the difference in the costs that on average are up to three times higher than the cost of the same services provided in public hospitals. The private health sector became a preferable alternative for health service delivery for those with the ability to pay. The financial implications and consequences of the Constitutional Court's decision for the health insurance system in this liberalization in the provision and reimbursement of health services need to be analyzed but initial expectations were that it would divert a portion of the HIF budget to private hospitals.

In March 2010, the government announced a new set of restrictive measures aimed to deal with inefficiencies in the health system. The most important aspects of the new proposal include reduction in the monetary value of the capitation point, adjustment of doctors' salaries, decrease in the number of hospital directors and managing boards, merging of hospitals and new opportunities for public-private partnership (Balaban 2010). In early 2012, an international project Healthgrouper.com – the biggest provider of information on doctors and health care providers in the Balkans – conducted two regional surveys among doctors and patients in Macedonia, Serbia and Bulgaria. In Macedonia the great

12 In March 2010, a new private general hospital – Sistina Medical – was opened; it employs over 700 staff, including highly qualified doctors and medical nurses. Most of these health personnel had resigned from the state hospitals and the university clinics in Skopje. Attracted by higher salaries, almost all of them went to the private sector (personal communication, Ajanovski 2010).

majority (75%) of the surveyed doctors were unsatisfied with the health care reforms, 45% would change their workplace, and a significant percentage consider moving abroad. Similarly, the great majority of the surveyed patients treated in public health institutions were dissatisfied with the quality of services, hygiene conditions, huge administration and long waiting time to be treated (Healthgrouper.com 2012).

6.5 CONCLUSIONS

The health care system in Macedonia is undergoing almost continuous reforms. As in other countries in the region, most of these reforms are partial, fragmented and without clear vision and long-term sustainability. Most of the reform initiatives are aligned with the interests of politicians to promote quick successes; clear direction and vision for strategic development of the health care system are missing. Initiation of the reforms was influenced by many external and internal factors. On the external side the most influential factors were policy pressures and project activities financed by World Bank loans. These projects produced certain changes in the health system, but the processes were confronted with many internal political changes, various interest group struggles and lack of continuity. The most important internal factor for pursuing or obstructing the reforms is the interest of the political parties. Populist political motives to gain votes and over-politicization of the system caused a near collapse of the public hospital sector. Even after more than twenty years since independence, the country still struggles with poor data management and intelligence in the health care system, which leaves more room for political manipulation.

The future success of health reforms depends on many factors, but crucially on the diminished influence of politics over health institutions. A promising step in such a direction may be to adopt new legislation for the autonomy of selected health providers that would transform selected hospitals into corporate entities. Such legislation would open the possibility to rationalize hospitals, to initiate hospital mergers and to facilitate more entrepreneurial behavior among the managers of public health care institutions. Such reforms require political wiliness and courage that unfortunately in the current political setting cannot be seen.

7 Health Reforms in Romania

Răzvan Chereches

During its recent history, especially after the collapse of the communist regime in December 1989, Romania has struggled to improve the organization of its health care system. Given the scarce resources allocated to the health sector, the results can be considered partly successful. However, widely perceived as corrupt, the health sector and health professionals in Romania have attracted popular opposition and mistrusts, although paradoxically, physicians remain well regarded. After providing information about the Romanian context, this chapter presents the successive steps taken to reform the health system and reports the main outcomes that the reform process has produced.

7.1 Demographic and Economic Characteristics

Situated in southeastern Europe with an area of 238,391 km^2, Romania is a middle-income country with approximately 19 million inhabitants. In 2010, Romania's population was almost two million fewer than in 1990 – a 10% decline due to a dramatic decrease in the crude birth rate from 16.5 per thousand in 1988 to 10.4 per thousand in 2009 as well as due to the high rate of emigration. According to preliminary results of the November 2011 census, the exact number of citizens in Romania is 19,043,767. Due to the reduced number, population density declined from 97.3 inhabitants per square kilometer in 1990 to 89.9 inhabitants/km^2 in 2010. While the urban population also declined, its share of the population increased due to the overall reduction in total population. In 2010, 55% of Romanians lived in urban areas – a 2% increase since 1990.

Table 7.1 Demographic Indicators

Year	1990	1995	2000	2005	2010
Population	23 211 395	22 712 394	22 455 485	21 658 528	21 462 186
Density/km^2	97.3	95.1	94.1	90.7	89.9
Urban	12 352 681	12 469 059	12 297 122	11 901 033	11 818 670
%	53.2	54.9	54.8	54.9	55.1

Source: Romanian National Institute of Statistics, Tempo-online database.

Table 7.2 Life Expectancy at Birth (Years)

Year	1990	1995	2000	2005	2010
Total	69.7	69.4	71.1	71.8	73.4
Male	66.5	65.7	67.7	68.3	69.8
Female	73.0	73.4	74.8	75.5	77.3

Source: World Bank 2012.

Life expectancy at birth decreased immediately after 1989 in Romania and through the 1990s. The pattern, however, differs from other post-communist countries in Eastern Europe. Dolea *et al.* (2002) report a decline of 1.71 years in life expectancy for men and 0.54 years for women between 1990 and 1996 – possibly caused by the low level of economic growth and behavioral factors related to food and drinking patterns. Since 2000, however, life expectancy has improved although a seven-year gap between men and women remains evident, a gap partly explained by changes in causes of morbidity and mortality. For example, chronic non-communicable diseases that lead to disabilities have replaced infectious communicable diseases. Improved lifestyle, better education and advances in health care and medicine also contribute to increased life expectancy (Eurostat 2011).

Romania has a long history of high infant mortality. In 2001, the rate was more than triple the EU average. The indicator has since almost halved from18.6 deaths per 1,000 live births in 2000 to 9.4 in 2011 – a reduction attributed to improved clinical facilities, access to a wider range of pharmaceuticals, a significant fall in the birth rate, and greater effectiveness and efficiency of the national programs addressing maternal and child health (Dolea *et al.* 2002; National Institute of Public Health 2011). However, Romania has the worst infant mortality in the European Union (Eurostat 2011).

Despite the recent years of economic constraints due to the generalized financial crisis, the evolution of selected economic indicators – Gross Domestic Product (GDP), GDP per

Table 7.3 Economic Indicators

	1990	1995	2000	2005	2010
GDP (million in 1990 US$)*	39 789	35 731	35 314	46 631	52 672
GDP per capita (in US$)	1 650	1 563	1 650	4 572	7 539
Percent inflation (consumer price index)	—	32.24%	45.66%	8.98%	6.09%

Source: *Romanian National Institute of Statistics, Tempo online database; World Bank 2012.

Table 7.4 Health Expenditures (Percentages of GDP)

Year	1995	2000	2005	2010
Total health expenditures	—	5.20	5.49	5.57
Public health expenditure	—	3.52	4.41	—
Private health expenditure	—	1.83	1.05	—
Public health expenditure as % of total health expenditure	70.3	67.7	80.2	78.1

Source: World Bank 2012.

capita, inflation (consumer price index) – has been positive. However, GDP per capita is not homogenous across the country although the pattern of distribution has been similar during the past 20 years with the capital region having the highest level.

In the Romanian health system, most health expenditures are financed by public sources. The estimated budget for health care in 2012 was US$1.65 billion (4% of GDP), which almost all stakeholders regard as insufficient to cover the needs of the insured people and threatening equitable access to high quality care for all categories. Private expenditure refers to either private insurance or direct (out-of-pocket) payments. Direct payments are mainly to private institutions (private practices, clinics and hospitals) although data about private health expenditures are scarce because private practices are not required to report economic data to the Ministry of Health. However, private expenditures are estimated to be one quarter and one third of total health expenditures (Presidential Commission 2008; World Bank 2012).

7.2 HEALTH RESOURCES

In 2000, according to Eurostat data, Romania had the lowest level of practicing physicians in the European Union. The level increased slightly in 2005 to 218 physicians per 100,000 inhabitants. Although the number of practising physicians has increased, Romania remains an important provider of health professionals for Western European countries. In 2007 one-tenth of Romania's practising medical doctors requested a diploma verification certificate from the Romanian College of Physicians (Gălan *et al.* 2011), although less than one third (28.7%) of those requesting the certificate actually emigrated (Dragomirișteanu *et al.* 2008). Without official estimates of Romanian health professionals who are working abroad, the need for a strategy on human resources in health is evident.

Table 7.5 enumerates Romania's professionals working in health care organizations, academic health centres and medical research organizations. The figures include professionals

Table 7.5 Health Professionals

	2000	2005	2010
Physicians (excluding dentists)	45 786	47 388	52 204
Family physicians	11 466	11 487	14 510
Physicians/100,000 inhabitants*	193	217	—
Dentists	8 307	10 249	12 990
Pharmacists	7 189	9 283	13 624
Medium health care personnel	119 446	123 455	126 656
Midwives	—	5 328	3 796
Auxiliary health care personnel	57 459	59 199	62 838

Sources: Romanian National Institute of Statistics; *Eurostat 2011.

working in institutions that have their own health care networks such as the Ministries of National Defense, Justice and Transportation. Medium health care personnel include nurses, pharmacy assistants, nursing sisters and midwives. Auxiliary health personnel include stretcher-bearers, ambulance drivers and workers responsible for disinfection. Auxiliary personnel ensure the cleanliness of health care organizations, preparation of materials requested for treatments and transportation of patients. While all categories of health professionals other than midwives show increased numbers, there are no aggregated databases about health professionals who have left the health care system. Despite the professionals leaving the country to work abroad, the positive trends could be partly explained by the increased numbers of places available in training programs.

Romania's relatively high number of hospital beds per 100,000 inhabitants indicates its focus on hospital care rather than on primary and secondary care; the budget allocated to hospital care is 40% higher than the European average. Reforms addressed the issue by gradually decreasing the number of beds, an effort visible in the reduced ratio of beds per population. The measure has also been accompanied by introducing family

Table 7.6 Hospital Beds

Year	1990	1995	2000	2005	2010
Total number of beds	207 001	173 311	166 817	142 377	132 004
Total beds/100,000 inhabitants	892	763	743	657	615

Source: Romanian National Institute of Statistics, Tempo-online database.

physician-coordinated centres in order to decrease the burden on the hospitals and emergency services. This trend is positive, decreasing towards the average in the European Union, and is indicative for a stronger focus on primary care, as well as on outpatient care. However, unless strengthening the primary and secondary care sectors continues, the reduced number of hospital beds may limit access to care for a population that has historically used hospital services as a first encounter for health care needs.

7.3 Normative Issues

As a nation with more than 40 years under an oppressive regime, Romania has carried its history into the present. Although the communist regime was formally characterized by efforts to achieve equal rights and equal standards of living for all, there were significant gaps between different socio-economic and professional categories. While solidarity was promoted in the public arena, the regime initiated and perpetuated suspicion among citizens by persuading people to provide information to local communist leaders about other people who were considered dangerous to the party and, by extension, to the whole nation – which led to betrayals among colleagues, friends and even family. Consequently, despite the official state ideology, individualism was the dominant characteristic of the era. The orientation towards individualism and refusal to adopt solidarity in front of a regime that ignored people's basic rights and privileges led to the long duration of communism in Romania (Deletant 1999).

The communist period in Romania was characterized by an aversion towards educated people because education was regarded as an instrument to undermine the regime. Yet education provided by communist leaders was valued to disseminate communist ideas and to attain a high adherence among the population to communist principles. Under vigilant control, visits abroad were strictly limited since a visit to a foreign country was seen as an opportunity to be influenced in the direction of betraying the state. Those who managed to go abroad were often interrogated in depth to provide information about the reasons of their visits or activities undertaken during their stay. These conditions influenced people and their behavior, their way of relating to themselves and to others. This pattern continues today through people who spent most of their lives under communism. As a result, both individually and collectively, democratic principles are hard to appreciate and even harder to adopt. Moreover, rapid change proved to be difficult to adapt to by a significant part of the population. Uncertainty at several levels – economic, social, political – translated into increased levels of stress, which affected health both mentally and physically.

While the majority of policies in place after 1990 in the health sector tried to ensure access by the population to a wide range of medical services, ensured access would require an important amount of resources – human, material and informational. Although universal access to health care services is a stated policy, the last two decades have been characterized by a chronic lack of funds to maintain the health sector at a level that would satisfy patients' expectations. Furthermore, political instability led to a rapid change of the Health Ministers so that 19 individuals have occupied this position between 1990 and 2011. As a consequence, much of universal coverage tends to be formal rather than effectively translated into the reality of health care (Vlădescu *et al.* 2008).

According to current Romanian law, the state offers social protection to less advantaged categories such as unemployed people, retired people, single parent families, disorganized families or homeless individuals. Depending on the political party that is governing, these categories may be more or less targeted by policies meant to reduce disparities as well as to increase the electoral capital of the party. Among the disadvantaged categories, Roma receive considerable attention because they experience problems with documentation, discrimination and marginalization. To address these needs, an Open Society Institute report in 2005 suggests measures such as examining laws that are not traditionally considered in Roma health programs, funding innovative health promotion partnerships, and facilitating information sharing across municipalities.

7.4 Health Sector Governance

In 1998, Romania changed its system of health sector financing from the Semashko model to a social insurance model. As Table 7.7 indicates, money now enters the system through taxes, payroll-based social insurance, and direct payments (fee-for-service, out-of-pocket payments, informal payments).

Table 7.7 Public Sources of Health Financing in Romania, 1990-2000

Source of Financing	1990	1995	2000
Taxes	100	94.7	15.1
General	100	58.5	12.2
Local	—	18.0	0.3
Specific health fund	—	18.3	2.5
Statutory insurance	—	—	77.0
External loans	—	5.3	7.9

Source: Vlădescu *et al.* 2008.

The central role in the current system is occupied by the National Health Insurance House (NHIH), which is represented at county level by 42 County Health Insurance Houses – for the 41 counties in the country plus Bucharest. Although long an autonomous institution, NHIH was placed under the Ministry of Health in August 2011. Contributions are collected by the National Agency for Fiscal Administration (NAFA) within the Ministry of Finance. The level is established at 5.5% payroll tax paid by the employee and 5.2% paid by the employer.

From the NHIH, funds are redirected at county level by taking into account the number of insured people in a county. Several categories – children under the age of 18 years, students between 18 and 26 years, the unemployed, social security beneficiaries and war veterans as well as victims of the 1989 revolution – are exempted from paying. Based on contributions, the population is entitled to receive a basic package of services that is defined individually for each level of care (primary, secondary, tertiary). While this package covers most health services provided by the system, officials have recently been preoccupied with defining a set of procedures and tests to be included in the package because, although everyone who pays a contribution is entitled to the same level of care, substantial differences occur at an individual level. That is to say, some individuals benefit more than others from these services (National Strategy for Hospital Rationalization 2011). This change is intended to prepare for the introduction of private insurance in the Romanian health system. Every insured person would have access to services in a basic benefit package while supplementary insurance would need to be purchased for advanced services.

Money originating from contributions is complemented by money from taxes. Although a special tax on cigarettes and alcohol was introduced in 2006 in order to build eight regional emergency hospitals, the objective has never been realized. From its introduction until early 2011, the tax collected about 1.3 billion euro. In comparison, the 2010 budget of the Health Ministry was about one billion euros. Another tax – the fast food tax – was to be introduced in the country, but strong resistance arose against the initiative (Holt 2010). Eventually the tax was not adopted although similar taxes have been introduced in Hungary and, more recently, in Denmark (Holt 2011).

Out-of-pocket payments, defined as payments for health services borne directly by patients or their households, represent an important source of money for the health sector (Belli and Shahriari 2002). Yet informal payments remain controversial in Romania. Research by the Central and Eastern European Health Network revealed that informal payments account for 41% of out-of-pocket payments in Romania (Belli 2004). These payments have their roots in the communist era when, due to a chronic lack of resources, patients were forced to pay in order to obtain better and/or faster access to care.

Given the current scarcity of resources, patients pay informal fees and also provide medical supplies on their own. A World Bank study revealed that informal payments in Romania were €300 million a year, accounting for 41% of total cash payments (Legicon 2005). In June 2009, the president of NHIH estimated the amount at about €500 million a year. Although the figures should alarm stakeholders responsible for the situation, the phenomenon seems to impress no one. Informal payments have been present in the system for a long time, yet no policies were devised to address them. In an attempt to offer solutions to current problems in the health care system, the recent National Strategy for Hospital Rationalization recognizes informal payments as a problematic issue, but the topic receives significantly less importance than its real magnitude. The document lists a series of possible causes and solutions that have proved to be beneficial in other settings, but fails to provide an in-depth analysis. Given the available data, informal payments in Romania are a barrier when people try to access health care services (Belli 2004). Informal payments have been identified as a major factor in the way of reforming the health care system (Holt 2012; Chereches and Ungureanu 2012).

Contracting and payment models are negotiated annually between the NHIH and health care providers at three levels of care: primary, secondary and tertiary. The terms of entitlement are included in a document called *The Framework Contract*, which is adopted after all the stakeholders involved have reached a consensus. The contract contains regulations that apply separately for primary, secondary and tertiary care. For each level of care, rights and responsibilities are established as well as solutions to address the situation when these rights and responsibilities are violated. Moreover, a package of health care services is associated with each category of providers.

Primary care funding has shifted from a model based exclusively on per capita payment (for each person ensured on the list of a family doctor) to a mixed method of payment, per capita combined with pay for service. In 2011, the distribution of the two methods of payment was equal: half per capita and half pay for service. The package of services to be provided in the primary care sector is structured according to the following categories: insured individuals, optional insurance package, and basic. For insured people, the package includes emergencies, surveillance and diagnoses of diseases with epidemic potential, pregnancy care, vaccination, family planning activities (counselling while choosing the most suitable contraceptive method) and support activities (medical documents). The obligations of primary care services providers, as stipulated by the contract, are curative and preventive. However, the document does not offer details about what the preventive activities are, what strategies are suitable to deliver these activities or how to evaluate the outcomes in terms of patients' health status, patients' satisfaction or resources invested.

Secondary (ambulatory) care receives payment as fee for service. The minimal package of services includes emergency care and detection of diseases with an epidemic potential. For those who have a facultative insurance, the package of services includes the above services as well as curative services. The basic package includes specialty consultation based on referrals by a family physician. The consultation package differs according to each doctor's training.

Hospital services are reimbursed based on diagnostic-related groups (DRGs). Until 2011, the original DRG version was used. After numerous complaints from within the system, the DRG system was updated to a Romanian version to be used in hospitals – RO DRG (Order No. 1199/26.07.2011). Rules for the validation of cases introduced in the DRG system were also changed in order to account for validation entry errors.

Primary care physicians are self-employed and sign yearly contracts with the County Health Insurance House. Private practice is usually provided in single-practice offices. Ambulatory services as well as most hospitals are public. The number of private hospitals is low, one reason being that the law does not offer proper conditions for them to develop. Recently considerable private investments have been made in new hospitals. Some of the services offered by private hospitals can be contracted by the County Health Insurance Houses, which make them more available for the population. However, access to more expensive services, not covered by the social insurance, is limited, although the quality provided is frequently higher than in public facilities. Dental care, on the other hand, is totally private except for emergencies that are treated in public settings.

At the level of primary care, the activity of family doctors is decentralized and regulated by the Framework Contract that they sign each year with the NHIH. However, they own the private practices that they administer. Most practices are organized around one family doctor with a minority of practices being organized by two or more family doctors who share personnel and affiliated costs. In the early 1990s primary care had been reshaped; since then, minor changes occurred in the organization of services. Generally regarded as gatekeepers, many family physicians do not accomplish this role. The situation has drawn the attention of the government and different strategies have been utilized to reinforce this characteristic. Co-payments, formally introduced in the system in the first trimester of 2011, have been regarded as a measure to reduce visits to GPs, apart from their stated purpose of limiting informal payments. However, some voices claim that co-payments limit access to care by the poor.

Secondary care is organized in ambulatory offices, usually grouped to form a polyclinic. Employed by the government, physicians do not own the offices where they practice. Ambulatory offices are based in hospitals, too.

Tertiary care is delivered by over 400 hospitals that, until July 2010, were administered directly by the Ministry of Health. After the de-centralization law was passed, the hospitals became the property of county councils. However, 35 hospitals – many of them pursuing academic activity – remain under the direct coordination of the Ministry of Health.

Although moving from a highly centralized to a more decentralized model, the Government controls most of the health care system. While institutions in the system as well as individuals are periodically consulted about the direction of reforms, little input is obtained from various stakeholders. One reason is that most professionals in the system know too little about its functioning and, as a result, are unable to argue reasonably for one option or another. Another reason is that situations have been rare when the position of various stakeholders was really considered and put into practice. This pattern has negative consequences because the Government is ignoring valuable information from professionals within the system.

7.5 History of Health Reforms

Although health is always on the agenda of politicians before elections, it has never been a priority for the political class. The proof is evident by the many ministers of health in Romania during the past 20 years, by the refusal to continue reforms that were started by other people and by the refusal to address problems in the system that are flagrant and about which strong voices raise concerns.

Since 1990, Romania's health care system has gone through extensive attempts to reform with consistent support from external organizations such as the World Bank. Several aspects characterize the efforts to reform a system that needed to recover after the communist period. These aspects include the strong influence of politics, a lack of commitment from all stakeholders in the reforms that were begun, and no continuity for the ideas included in the reform process. All these aspects affected the way the reforms were designed, implemented and evaluated. Moreover, as a whole, the Romanian health sector has been regarded with distrust and suspicion. This attitude was cultivated especially towards doctors and other categories of health professionals because, during the communist era but also thereafter, informal payments were common practice in ambulatory and hospital settings. The fact that a significant number of the health professionals received or even asked for payments from the patients (whether money or of gifts or both) created and then cultivated the idea that health professionals are the most corrupt category of professionals.

The main change after 1990 was the adoption of social insurance to fund the health sector. Immediately after 1990, the first measures looked for short-term results such as the trust of health professionals in the authority of the Ministry of Health, ensuring their free mobility across the country, addressing the HIV and hepatitis B epidemics, and reducing the rates of maternal and child mortality (Vlădescu *et al.* 2008). In 1994, general practice began to be reorganized, starting with changing the way general practitioners were paid. Instead of a fixed payment, their salaries were calculated using age-adjusted capitation, fee-for-services and bonuses. The program offered 86% coverage with general practice care in the population in only two years. In 1997 the Chamber of Deputies adopted a Social Health Insurance Bill in an attempt to increase the resources available in the health sector. The newly created National Health Insurance Fund (HIF) was a self-governing body until 2002 when was placed under the Ministry of Public Health (Vlădescu *et al.* 2008). In 2006 the law of Reform in Health was issued that governs the organization and functioning of Romania's health system. Selected milestones in health system reforms in Romania are listed in Table 7.8.

Given the global financial crisis, more changes in the system occurred in 2010 in an attempt to reduce costs and increase accountability. The first measure concerned the decentralization of hospitals in order to shift responsibility for hospitals from the Ministry of Health to local and county communities. The second measure focused on the selection of hospital managers. The new law sets standards for anyone who seeks to be a candidate for this position and establishes the procedure through which a hospital manager is selected (based on testing both knowledge and practical skills). The third measure of co-payments – proposed to address the overcrowded waiting rooms of family physicians and to reduce informal payments – has not yet been introduced in the system.

At the end of 2011, after broad consultations with the International Monetary Fund (IMF), the Ministry of Health proposed a new law to regulate the health sector. At its core, the proposal introduced the idea of private insurance. The intent was to develop a basic benefit package that would include all the health care services to which an individual was entitled, based on his/her monthly contribution to its chosen insurance house. For services not included on this list, the individuals were responsible to pay them individually. Another novelty was that hospitals could decide by themselves to be organized as public institutions, foundations or societies. This choice would have allowed a greater autonomy of the hospitals, translated into more customized services for the population served, as well as more consistent methods of raising money, spending money and motivating health care personnel. As a whole, the proposed package would have opened perspectives for competition among diverse health care providers in their attempt to sign contracts with the private insurance houses.

However, after its publication on the website of the Ministry of Health, the proposal generated controversies related to the fear that, once services are contracted and based on competition, the results would not necessarily reflect the differences in competence and quality but rather would be the results of corruption. Different stakeholders argued that

Table 7.8 Selected Milestones in Health System Reforms in Romania

1992-1994	Simulation testing of primary care reform (to financing) in four districts
1993	A Healthy Romania, produced by team of experts funded by World Bank
1994	Social Health Insurance Bill approved by the Senate
1994	Government Decision (No. 370/1994) to pilot primary care reform in eight districts (ended in 1997)
1995	Legislation to establish the College of Physicians
1997	Social Health Insurance Bill approved by the Chamber of Deputies (implementation started in 1999)
1998	Public Health Law (No. 100/1998)
1999	Ministerial Order (No. 201/1999) placed restrictions on number and distribution of pharmacies (amended in 2005)
2002	Emergency Ordinance (No. 70/2002) decentralized ownership of public health care facilities from central to local government
2002	Emergency Ordinance (No. 150/2002) modified initial National Health Insurance Law
2002	Law on Mental Health Promotion and Protection of Persons with Psychiatric Disabilities
2002	National Anti-Poverty and Social Inclusion Plan, Government Decision (No. 829/2002)
2005	Government Ordinance removed National Health Insurance Fund from coordination by the Ministry of Public Health
2006	Health Reform Law (No. 95/2006)
2007	Ministry of Public Health strategic plan for 2008-2010
2010	Hospital decentralization legislation
2010	Co-payment law
2010	Legislation regarding hospital managers selection process
2011	National strategy for hospital rationalization
2012	Drafting of the health care reform law

Source: Adapted from Vlădescu *et al.* 2008.

this change would destroy the emergency system that currently performs at high standards. The civilized dialogue was transformed into street protests and violent expression of opinions. Eventually the Government decided to withdraw the package and initiated discussions with all interested stakeholders in order to design another proposal.

Although every Health Minister intended for his reform to be implemented and offer great results, most of the reforms achieved only short or medium-term results. However, one positive result is the universality of care – meaning that all categories in Romania, including the most marginalized, formally have the right to care. In reality, access to care is inequitable (ethnic, geographic, economic and quality-related inequalities) and heterogeneous as highlighted by the 2008 Report of the Public Health Presidential Commission for Public Health and the National Strategy for Hospital Rationalization. Bara *et al.* (2002) report on inequities based on insurance status and rural/urban divide as well as on significant differences in per capita expenditures for health care across different regions.

The fact that health has low priority on the agenda of politicians is reflected by the small percentage of GDP annually allocated to health. Chronic underfunding is probably the first thing that an average Romanian would say about the health care system that lacks a proper mechanism for accountability, too. Huge amounts of money leave the system without anyone knowing anything. Prescribing expensive drugs for people who then do not receive them is one mechanism used by some doctors to extract money from the system; others have agreements with the pharmaceutical companies for which they receive expensive gifts or trips to exotic locations.

Although quality is a mark of the services delivered, the system lacks a culture of quality – understood as quality assurance, evaluation and improvement. At national level, no mechanisms are in place to acquire the desired quality. Even the legislation is poor; the 2006 health reform law (No. 95) provides insufficient guidelines to address the quality of services despite three articles specifically stating that "the criteria for the quality of services delivered to patients are elaborated by the Ministry of Health and NHIH and are related to diagnostic and medical, surgical and dental treatment" and that "the criteria are compulsory for all health care providers which have a contract with the NHIH".

In March 2011, the Ministry of Health issued a document entitled *The National Strategy for Hospital Rationalization*. Using some of the results provided by previous reports (such as *The National Strategy for the Rationalization of Hospital Services*, a World Bank project, and the 2004 GVG Project for Planning and Regulation of Health Care Services), the document aims at identifying key issues that need to be reformed in the Romanian health care system as well as providing solutions and a calendar with activities meant to address the problematic issues.

The general principles guiding the proposed solutions are equity, people-centeredness, quality and responsibility. Although the name of the document suggests that it is only concerned with hospitals, the document in fact provides an analysis of the entire health care system.

However, equity is difficult to achieve in the present context. Equitable access to care would mean that people from different regions of the country, either rural or urban, within different socio-economic categories, with different cultural and education backgrounds, all have the same chances to access high quality care. All these differences are strong barriers to equitable care. A people-centred health care system is organized in a way that recognizes and values the people's input in their care. But apart from focus on people, people-centeredness places responsibility on them – responsibility for their behavior and resulting consequences as well as responsibility that derives from their consumer status. While the principle of quality refers to the adoption of established standards in order to improve performance, the Romanian health system lacks a history of quality-driven services. Until now, quality was not formally assessed or imposed. Responsibility should apply to all levels of care and to all individuals involved – health care professionals, policy-makers and patients. It is responsibility that enables a system to progress and achieve outcomes beyond the state of the art.

The 2011 document presents solutions on two main directions – the first one concentrating on hospitals and the second one on complementary priorities. For each direction, a set of proposals has been issued, together with their calendar of implementation. From the perspective of the expected law that will promote a new reform process, the 2011 document appears as another wasted opportunity to address important topics in the Romanian health system – lack of accountability, informal payments, lack of human resources policy.

In the 2007 strategic plan for 2008-2010, the Ministry of Health identified the weaknesses, strengths, opportunities and threats of the system. Perceived weaknesses are the lack of responsibility, poor teamwork, numerous coordinated institutions; strengths are the presence of young personnel, each with a different background. The availability of European funding and the willingness of local authorities to share responsibilities with the Ministry of Health are opportunities, while the migration of health care professionals, the ageing of the population, and the lack of training in health issues at the level of local administration are threats.

While a SWOT analysis is necessary to set the characteristics of a baseline situation, this assessment needs to be done thoroughly with a high degree of objectivity and responsibility. Too frequently the problems in the system are minimized or not awarded enough resources to be tackled. If it were for the Romanian health care system to reform, only a deep and objective analysis of what is inside would provide a prerequisite for its success. The next steps involve bringing together the stakeholders and identifying reliable and realistic strategic solutions to address the problems identified. Finally, support from all those involved – health care professionals, policy makers, politicians, and patients – needs to be obtained in order to achieve satisfactory long-term results.

After a failed attempt in November 2011, the Ministry of Health seemed to have learned the lesson that a valuable and sustainable reform process will proceed only if all stakeholders in the system agree. During January 2012, the Ministry website announced extensive consultations with a broad range of stakeholders. Having fulfilled this mandatory condition for general acceptance and commitment, the Ministry is expected to prove that it has learned from mistakes and to draft a law that sets new and revolutionary directions for the Romanian health care system. Time will prove whether this opportunity will be fully exploited. In May 2012, the Government changed, which means that Romania has had three health ministers in three years. Given this context, it is not difficult to answer why so little has improved in the Romanian health care system during recent decades.

7.6 Impact of Informal Payments on Universal Access

Among issues that impact the overall health system performance and have not been properly tackled are informal payments. During the past 20 years, informal payments have been either ignored or treated superficially despite strong signals from international bodies such as the World Bank that identify informal payments as a weakness of the Romanian health system (Legicon 2005). But informal payments are a *taboo* topic for researchers of health services in Romania. In the few articles on the topic, respondents strongly disagree with informal payments but still offer informal payments to health professionals. Fărcăşanu (2010) reports on a quantitative study on the attitudes towards informal health care payments in Romania: 82.8% of respondents do not agree with offering either money or gifts to health personnel. As for why informal payments persist, the reasons most frequently mentioned were the culture of bribery (73.4% of respondents) and the lack of penalties (70.9%). Overall, 20.5% of the respondents believe that corruption is the weakest point of the Romanian health system.

The effect of informal payments is felt at two distinct levels. First, at a system level, informal payments offered by patients to health professionals are not distributed equally; the majority of payments go into doctors' pockets (Belli and Shahriari 2002; Radin 2009). Among doctors most of the money goes to those treating inpatients and surgical cases. Nonetheless, informal payments have been argued to have positive effects. Hungarian experience shows that informal payments may act as a strong incentive for doctors not to leave the public system or the system at all. They may also serve as an attractor for those choosing to practice medicine. But no matter how positive the effects may be on the health professionals, the effects on patients are not positive at all. Although it is argued that informal payments may arise as a sign of gratitude, the international experience shows that gratitude is overrated as an explanation for informal payments (Gaal *et al.* 2006).

Indeed, there are several issues when deciding whether a payment is due to gratitude or an indicator of coercion. First it is difficult to verify empirically the patients' motivation to offer informal payments. When patients report gratitude as a motivation for behavior, gratitude is not always behind the behavior. A growing body of literature (although not in a Romanian setting) shows contradictions among patients when they mention gratitude as a reason for paying informal fees (Mossialos *et al.* 2002; Radin 2009). Another reason is that coercion should not be limited to external coercion, such as the situations when health professionals ask directly for informal payments. Coercion may be also present when health professionals delay necessary care until the patients eventually pays, or when the health professionals' behavior and attitude suggest that informal payment is needed for a patient to receive adequate care. Even if none of the above is present, the patients who are aware of previous situations when they were not treated adequately until they offered informal payments or when the same had happened to relatives or acquaintances still may feel coercion.

The above patterns of behavior negatively affect access to care and the quality of care due to demotivated doctors with low salaries and poor working conditions. Patients, knowing that they will be requested to pay or feel obliged to pay, delay visits to the doctors' office. These factors influence the moment when the doctor eventually consults the patient.

7.7 Conclusions

At a formal level Romania is struggling to reform its health care system. While the process is not as smooth as expected nor does it follow commonly shared principles, the restless process is drafted and redrafted by those who occupied leading positions in the system. Although the history of health reforms is lengthy, some efforts have reached completion. The lack of strategic thinking and planning, major and frequent radical political changes and lack of consistency are among the factors contributing to the phenomenon. Strategic thinking has been frequently disregarded by most of the reforms since only the present and the near future have been taken into account.

The appetite for rapid results was one causal factor. To get a reform right involves a huge amount of resources, both material and human, and requires attachment to it and a strategic planning to allow for it to become reality. The many health ministers who have occupied this function during the last 20 years are another factor that slowed reform. Although a number of projects have been contracted to help the Romanian health sector to find its way through the reform process, little has been put into practice.

8 Patterns of Health Care Reform in Economies under Transition: The Case of Russia

Tatiana Chubarova and Natalia Grigorieva

The chapter analyses Russia's health care system in order to understand why, after almost 20 years of reforms, it still fails to deliver good outcomes. The problems manifest in three areas: poor health status of the population and poor state of the health services; negative demographic trends and the high economic cost of poor health; and people's dissatisfaction with health system performance, including inequalities in health status and access to health care. These problems are largely due to the way health policy is worked out and the assumptions that underline the ideology of health reforms. Although the latter are not always stated explicitly, they nevertheless inform health policy decisions. Consequently modern Russian health policy is problem-making rather than problem-solving. Analysis reveals a divergence between the stated aims and the mechanisms that are used to reach them.

The chapter explores myths that underline health policy decisions and paradoxes that occur when they are used to justify political decisions. The authors suggest that high inequality might destroy the integrated health system and that Russia is likely to end up with two separate streams – one for rich people who can pay and another for poor people for free. The case of Russian health policy demonstrates that health reforms (especially during times of great transformation) should be designed very carefully by placing health issues in a wider societal context and by using the potential of already established models that have social roots in society.

8.1 Russian Health Care: The Necessity for Change

After nearly 20 years of health care reforms, Russian health care is still not in 'good health'.[1] The gloomy picture of Russian health care is well documented by both Russian

1 For details see *Economic Science in Modern Russia* 2007.

and foreign research (Rimashevskaya *et al.* 2011; Bochkareva 2009; Grigorieva 2008). The problems in Russian health care manifests in three major dimensions:

- poor population health status and poor state of health services;
- negative demographic trends and high economic cost of poor health; and
- people's low 'health-esteem' and wide spread dissatisfaction with health system performance, including equity considerations.

As reflected in both statistical and sociological indicators, the health of Russians has declined. Mortality and morbidity levels – the most widely used statistical indicators – are high in Russia. In 2008 the mortality rate reached 14.6 people per 1,000 in 2008, while maternal mortality was 20.7 per 100,000 live births. Compared to European indicators, the latter rate is quite high, although it has been declining from 54 in 1985 and 39 in 2000. Child mortality is also high by international standards – 8.5 per 1,000 live births in 2008. It is important to note that the leading causes of child mortality are those that arise in prenatal period and to a large extent depend on maternal health. The share of newly born with some disease or developing illness during the postnatal period increased from 15% of live births in 1990 to 37% in 2008.

The level of morbidity in Russia is soaring with cases of heart disease, cancer, trauma and poisoning steadily rising since 1990. The same applies to drug addiction and HIV. In the structure of morbidity, cardiovascular diseases occupy the first place (28%), followed by diseases of the respiratory system (24%) and sensory organs (13%). 9.2% of the total population was registered as disabled in 2008.

Russia has a well-developed system of primary, secondary and tertiary care health services. In many cases, however, these units are poorly equipped which affects the quality of services they provide. 45% of hospitals and 24% of polyclinics need serious renovation; 30% of hospitals and 36% of polyclinics lack hot water (RSA 2009). Russia lags behind developed countries in the application of modern health technology and the number of procedures performed. For example, aortic coronary shunting does not cover all needs. There are gaps in the quality of medical care and the availability of medical staff between rural and urban areas and between regions of Russia.

Sociological research confirms the statistical data. Surveys show low self-evaluation of health. According to the National Survey of Household Welfare and Participation in Social Programs, half of respondents think that their health status, is satisfactory, while 18% say it is bad or very bad. "Public Opinion" Foundation data reveal that 46% of respondents think they have satisfactory health status while 23% consider it to be poor and very poor (FOM 2010). Studies also confirm the low level of people's satisfaction with health care services. In August 2010, only 15% of the Levada Centre survey respondents said that they were satisfied with health care system in the country while about 60% of respondents expressed the opposite view. 70% of respondents believed that they would not be able to obtain quality medical care if they needed it (Levada 2011).

When evaluating health care reform, Russians are skeptical because no principal improvement has occurred in the Russian health system. The survey conducted by the Levada Centre revealed that:

- Most respondents (76%) had little information about health reforms;
- 44% thought the reforms would not affect their lives; and
- 31% said their lives would be worsened by reforms.

The negative attitude to health reform initiatives dominated the people's responses: reducing hospital stays (90%); reducing the volume of free medical care and paying money to low-income patients (85%); and closing local children's polyclinics and turning pediatricians into general practitioners (77%).

Today health care systems face problems of a global character that to a large extent will shape their organization in the future. The development of modern medical technology raises new expectations and leads to increased demand for medical treatment. Patterns of morbidity are changing with chronic diseases coming to the front that requires relevant changes in organization and financing of health care systems with strong emphasis on prevention and continuity. The evolution of viruses leads to the emergence of new infectious diseases and re-emergence of old ones in situations aggravated by increased global mobility.

Experts note the growth in health inequality despite the attention that this issue attracts at all political levels. Threats to health come from the interaction with nature and its environment, consequences of people's industrial activities and natural disasters (WHO 2007). Demographic and economic aspects reflect the relations between health and the economy and the influence of health on development. Health expenditures should be an investment that brings economic results rather than mere expenditure. The relation between health and economy is not one way but mutually reinforcing. Investment in both economy and health brings more gains than investment of the same resources either in the economy or in health (World Bank 1993).

Combined with high mortality levels, the decline in Russia's population has had serious political, economic and social consequences (World Bank 2005). In 2008, life expectancy

Table 8.1 Demographic Indicators

	1990	1995	2000	2005	2008	2009	2010
Population (thousands)	147 665	148 460	146 890	143 474	142 009	141 904	141 914
Urban	108 736	108 322	107 419	104 719	103 773	103 690	103 705
Rural	38 929	40 138	39 471	38 755	38 236	38 214	38 209
Under working age	36 101	34 252	29 580	24 095	22 497	22 541	22 854
Working age	83 943	84 332	87 172	90 218	89 752	89 266	88 360
Above working age	27 621	29 876	30 138	29 161	29 760	30 097	30 700
Life expectancy (years)	69.2	64.5	65.4	65.3	67.9	68.7	N.A.
Men	63.7	58.1	59.1	58.9	61.8	62.8	N.A.
Women	74.3	71.6	72.3	72.4	74.2	74.7	N.A.
Births per 1,000 population	13.4	9.3	8.7	10.2	12.1	12.4	12.5
Deaths per 1,000 population	11.2	15.0	15.3	16.1	14.6	14.2	14.2
Infant mortality (up to 1 year) per 1,000 live births	17.4	18.1	15.3	11.0	8.5	8.1	7.5
Rate of population change	2.2	(−) 5.7	(−) 6.6	(−) 5.9	(−) 2.5	(−) 1.8	(−) 1.7

Source: Statistical Yearbook, respective years.

at birth was 66.6 years with a big gender gap: 73.2 for women and 60.3 for men – compared to 69.2 years in 1990 (64.3 and 63.7 respectively). This situation is unique for an industrial country and has attracted the attention of the international research community because it questions the extent to which gains in the health of a modern population are irreversible (Cockerham 1999). The high levels of working-age mortality are increasing not only for men (which is widely acknowledged) but for women as well. During 1990-2006 mortality among working-age men increased from 759 to 1,172 per 100,000 and among women from 198 to 304 (RSA 2009). Cardiovascular diseases (56%), accidents and trauma (14%), and cancer (12%) are the leading causes of death.

Health status is important in terms of ability to work. Decreasing adult mortality from chronic diseases and trauma can bring the following macroeconomic benefits:

- The static economic benefit (*i.e.* value of a life-year gained by one Gross Domestic Product (GDP) per capita) of gradually bringing the Russian Federation's mortality rates for adult non-communicable diseases and injury down to the most recent rates for the EU member states (those in the EU prior to May 2004) by 2025 is estimated to be between 3.6% and 4.8% of the 2002 Russian GDP.
- The broadly defined "welfare" benefits (*i.e.* using a "value of life" measure) from achieving the rates of EU Member States (those in the EU prior to May 2004) by 2025 are estimated to be as high as 29% of the 2002 Russian GDP.
- The dynamic benefits (the effect on economic growth rates) are massive and growing over time. Even if the future returns are discounted to the starting-year value (2002), they represent a multiple of the static GDP effects (Suhrcke *et al.* 2007:ix).

Social and moral dimensions of any health care system are connected with how it incorporates equity issues, on the one hand, and the influence of health status and access to health care on people's perceptions and attitudes, on the other. According to generally accepted social approach to health, it is "a state of complete physical, mental and social well being but not just absence of disease" (WHO 1946). This WHO definition considers health as a social phenomenon rather than only physical abilities. It stresses the importance of both individual biological and behavioral factors as well as social and economic conditions in securing people's health. The social model of health indicates that health issues contain strong social and ethical aspects. The organization of a health care system – the way resources are mobilized and distributed – is influenced by social values such as solidarity and equity. Health care is not merely economic or medical but, first of all, a social system that reflects the relation between the state and society and is a matter of national identification. Research data indicate that health inequalities in Russia are large and associate with income levels (Table 8.2).

In sum, Russia's health system faces specific problems stemming from the social and economic situation in the country as well as general problems of a global character. For Russian people the reforms do not eliminate – and in some cases create – difficulties in access (both financial and territorial) to quality and timely medical care.

8.2 Causes of the Health Care Crisis: Ideology and Practice

The way health reforms in Russia are developed and implemented as well as assumptions on which reform programs are based should be named as one of the major reasons for the poor functioning of health care system in the country leading among other factors to the

Table 8.2 Morbidity Levels by Income Group (Percentage of Respondents)

	Income Level			
Diseases	**High**	**Middle**	**Low**	**Total**
Osteochondrosis	27.2	36.6	35.6	32.2
Hypertonic/heart diseases	21.5	32.2	41.2	27.0
Arthritis	7.1	12.9	21.2	10.5
Cholecystitis	7.6	13.4	12.8	10.0
Bronchitis	6.9	9.2	20.8	8.9
Stomach ulcer	5.0	8.5	8.4	6.7
Urolithiasis	4.6	7.2	7.5	5.8
Diabetes	1.4	5.3	7.5	5.8
Asthma	1.2	2.7	7.5	2.5
Other diseases	14.7	20.0	23.9	17.6
Have no disease (ill health)	32.9	17.3	15.9	25.5
Difficult to say	7.2	6.3	4.9	7.3

Source: Russian Statistical Agency survey 2008.

poor health of the Russian population. The measures undertaken do not seem to contribute to solving existing problems. These problems persist and, as a result, are aggravated.

8.2.1 Normative Issues

Russian society is often considered to be in transition. For health care, transition means that on the one hand the health system is unstable and fragmented while on the other hand there is room for new non-standard decisions. However, a general 'mainstream' trend has already emerged. In the transition from a state-directed to a market-oriented economy as well as to a democratic political system, the priority of the individual over the collective was declared. This implies that health becomes, first of all, an individual responsibility that sits well with a market economy. Therefore, there is a shift – at least in policymaking – towards individualism on the solidarity-individualism continuum. This runs contrary to the Soviet past as Soviet society has been positioned as a collectivist one where collective achievements were valued more than personal ones.

State health policy is influenced by dominant values and welfare principles. In Russia the liberal approach dominates, which is based on ideas of freedom and natural rights. The welfare state is considered to be a burden for the economy because high taxes collected by the state to finance social programs lower the potential for personal initiative and thus improvement in personal well-being and elimination of poverty. It is argued that expansion of the welfare state leads to negative social consequences, including dependency and lack of personal effort. Therefore, extending personal responsibility, introducing a residual welfare model through targeted programs and cutting public social expenditures are justified. Social-Democratic social policy that seeks a balance of social interests, leveling of social inequality and negative social consequences of a market economy is ignored or criticized as not conforming to modern realities.

In economic terms these cause chronic underfunding of health care through public means, the introduction of fee-for-service and co-payments. State social and health services are discredited as little is done to improve the quality of care they provide. It seems that Russian social policy consciously divides the rich and the poor, thus undermining the basis of social solidarity. As social inequality is widening, perceptions of various groups in the society about equity differ and sometimes conflict.

Programs of all Russian political parties encompass the same rhetoric about 'decent and affordable health care' but only two political parties – the Communist and the Right – have a well-defined ideological stand. Other parties – including the ruling United Russia – try to position themselves above ideology so they neither clearly articulate nor openly state their vision of the future.

Promotion of a healthy life style is a good case of distorting political accents. Russian health policy makers generally acknowledge the idea of health determinants and health prevention, but they promote behavioral factors at the expense of social and economic ones. The stress is placed on improved individual behavior and healthy lifestyle ignoring that a healthy lifestyle is expensive and depends on people's social and economic situation (income, education, housing etc.). This is a good example of 'policy closure' when problems are formulated in a way that restricts alternative means of handling them. It excludes the possibility of other ways of thinking and talking about the issues (Sinfield 2005).

In addition, there is a problem of poor quality of health care laws (HCLs) and other documents that are produced by the legislature and the government. State health policy often confuses aims and means that, in many instances, seem to reflect low qualification of politicians and state officials rather than political ideology. For example, in the 'Concept of Long Term Social and Economic Development of Russian Federation for the period up to 2020' the development of a health care system rather than improvement of the health status of the population is stated as an aim of health policy. It is common to introduce amendments into the law already in force. The more amendments are introduced, the more difficult it is not only for a layman but also for an independent expert to understand the direction sought by the legislation.

The general drawback of Russian health reforms is that measures implemented are not subject to proper evaluation. Russian case is a good illustration of re-disorganization theories. Reform measures are often carried during a short period of time so it becomes difficult to assess them. There is little scientific research that assesses the effectiveness and efficiency of selected policies, and often government develops policies on the basis of limited cases that are promoted as success stories (Cutler 2007). Russian health reforms seem to become an endless process that never reaches the stated goals. Feedback from both the medical community and patients is weak. Policy is often formulated behind closed doors and recent initiatives to put draft laws on websites for people to discuss cannot be considered as a real consultation mechanism.

8.2.2 Governance of Health Sector

Health reforms in Russia have two dimensions in terms of financing and organizing health care delivery: the introduction of compulsory health insurance (CHI) and regional decentralization of the health care financing and delivery. The health care system in Russia is financed from both private and public sources. Public sources include budget allocations (the Federal budget plus regional budgets) and compulsory health insurance that was introduced in Russia in 1993. CHI funds are formed by employers' contributions for their employees (3.1% of payroll in 2010) and contributions by regional governments for those who are not employed. The organization of CHI funds parallels the federal budget system – one federal CHI fund and separate CHI funds in the regions. Employers' contributions are split into two parts; the major one goes to the relevant regional CHI fund, the rest — to the Federal CHI fund (2.0% and 1.1% of payroll respectively in 2010). In 2010 62.7% of public money came from budgets – both federal and regional – while CHI amounted to 37.3% of public means.

It should be mentioned that Russian regions – 83 all together – have budget autonomy. The share of regional budgets in total public financing reached about 36% in 2010.

Private means include voluntary health insurance and out-of-pocket payments both official and informal. In 1990s, state health expenditures declined substantially (by almost one-third) while private – mostly out-of-pocket – expenditures increased. As documented by official statistics and sociological surveys, services to be paid by the patient are growing. Voluntary health insurance increased in post Soviet period reaching 68 billion rubles in 2008. The official data indicate that fee for service increased from 48 billion rubles in 2000 to 283 billion rubles in 2008. Informal 'envelop' payments are difficult estimate but according to some experts they increased from about 25 billion rubles in 2000 to 107 billion rubles in 2008 (<www.rodmedstrah.ru/news>). Official statistics are scarce or nonexistent for a number of indicators such as the scope of the private sector or amount of fee-for-service payments. WHO provides the most comprehensive data on health care financing in Russia (Table 8.3).

Geographical (spatial) factors play an important role in Russia's economy and politics for two reasons. Russia is a vast country of 17,076,260 km^2 with an average density of 8.4 persons per square kilometre – five times lower than the world average. However, there are huge variations in population density among Russian regions – from 360 persons per km^2 in Moscow and the Moscow region to 62 in the Kaliningrad region and 0.3 in Yakutia (a region in north-east Russia that amounts to about one-sixth of the Russian territory) – so the problem is how to deliver health services to remote and less populated areas. Because Russia is a federation, regional budgets are autonomous, separated from the federal one. Thus, health responsibilities – both financial and organizational – are divided between different layers of administrative power.

The main tendency in public policy is to shift more responsibilities to regions in general and in health care in particular. The idea is that federal authorities set basic standards while regions can, depending on resources available, supplement them for their residents. However, due to social and economic differences between Russia's regions, the volume and quality of health care they provide to their populations differs. While these differences create a serious problem for securing equal access of all Russian citizens to good health services, the trend of strengthening regional health responsibility continues. Recent initiatives of the government to modernize Russian health care are to be implemented through regional programs of modernization.

In 2009 the Ministry of Health and Social Development conducted its first comprehensive assessment of implementation and effectiveness of regional programs. This assessment analyzed accessibility and quality of care based on evaluation of the dynamics of basic indicators of health status and a poll about satisfaction with quality of medical health services. According to experts, all Russian regions were divided into four groups. The leading group included nine regions (11% of all regions) while 20 regions (about one-quarter of all regions) lagged behind.

The health system developed in Russia is often referred to as 'dual-finance'. The state budget finances medical treatments specified in the Program of the State Guaranties of Free Health Services (mostly expensive hi-tech) while CHI-financed treatments are specified in the CHI Program. Currently, CHI covers medical staff salaries, payroll taxes, consumable

Table 8.3 Health Care Financing in Russia

	1995	2000	2003	2005	2008	2009
Total expenditure on health as % of GDP	5.3	5.4	5.6	5.2	4.8	5.4
General government expenditure on health as % of total expenditure on health	73.9	59.9	59.0	62	64,3	64.4
Private expenditure on health as % of total expenditure on health	26.1	40.1	41.0	38	35.7	35.6
General government expenditure on health as% of total government expenditure	9.0	12.7	9.3	11.7	9.2	8.5
External resources for health as % of total expenditure on health	0.1	0.2	0.2	0	0	0
Social security expenditure on health as% of general government expenditure on health	34.5	40.3	43.7	42.0	38.7	38.7
Out-of-pocket expenditure as % of private expenditure on health	64.7	74.7	71.1	82.4	81.3	80.9
Private prepaid plans as % of private expenditure on health	6.0	8.1	6.6	8.2	10.6	11.0
Per capita total expenditure on health at average exchange rate (US$)	96	96	167	252	568	475
Per capita government expenditure on health at average exchange rate (US$)	57	57	98	202	365	306
Per capita total expenditure on health (PPP in US$)	369	369	518	517	985	1,038
Per capita government expenditure on health (PPP in US$)	221	221	305	415	633	669

Source: WHO Statistical Information Service 2011.

supplies, drugs and food. All other expenses – heating, electricity, transport, communications, work safety, staff retraining – are covered directly by the budget. Health services that are owned by the federal authorities are financed by the federal budget; health services that are owned by the regions authorities are financed by regional budgets.

In Russia the state health services are allowed to charge fee-for-service. To be precise, in certain circumstances, state health services can charge fees for their services rendered above the compulsory state and CHI programs. This issue is controversial because, in

Table 8.4 Health Resources

	1990	1996	2000	2005	2008	2009	2010
Hospitals	12 800	11 800	10 700	9 500	6 500	6 500	6 300
Hospital beds	2 037 600	1 812 700	1 671 600	1 575 400	1 398 500	1 373 400	1 339 500
Beds per 10,000 population	137.5	123.9	115.0	111.3	98.6	96.8	93.7
Doctors	667 300	669 200	680 200	690 300	703 800	711 300	715 800
Doctors per 10,000 population	45.0	45.7	46.8	48.8	49.6	50.1	50.1
Other medical staff	1 844 000	1 648 600	1 563 600	1 529 800	1 511 200	1 517 600	1 508 700
Other staff per 10,000	124.5	112.7	107.6	108.0	106.5	106.9	105.6

Source: Социальное положение и уровень жизни населения России, соответствующие годы. (*Social Status and Level of Living of Population in Russia*, Moscow, Russian Statistical Agency. Respective years).

practice, patients are often manipulated by health professionals who try to increase their income. Public facilities are used to treat patients for money; as a result the quality of free services deteriorates.

The private sector in Russian health care is developing but statistics on the issue are scarce. According to some estimates (Kolesnikov 2010) there are about 30,000 private clinics in Russia – mainly situated in big cities. A study of private medicine in Moscow carried out by the Moscow branch of the First All Russian Association of Private Doctors discovered that the majority of private clinics were dental (59%), gynecology/midwifery (13%) and polyclinic multifunctional (10%) (Kuzovlev and Goncharova 2008). Official statistics indicate that only about 5% of those employed in health care work in the private sector.

Public-private partnerships (PPPs) in health care are a hot issue on the current health political agenda although real progress is not as fast as might be expected. PPP is often understood quite loosely as any interaction or mutually beneficial cooperation between private and state organizations. Sometimes it includes any measure of state support of business. In 2005 the Law on Concessions was adopted but there is no evidence that it has been implemented in health care. Some Russian regions – e.g., in St. Petersburg or Tatarstan – adopted regional legislation on PPP. The prenatal centre in the city of Kazan (Tatarstan) is a widely cited case of PPP in health care. The local administration will contribute land and an old building while private companies will renovate the building, train personnel and introduce new medical technology. It is expected that the project will achieve pay-off in five years.

8.2.3 History of Reforming the Health System in Russia

Historical traditions in Russian health care were not properly incorporated in modern health reforms. Although the notion of public health used to be strong (*zemstvo* medicine or factory doctors in late 19th century), insurance mechanisms have never been well developed. In the 20th century Russia pioneered in establishing an integrated health care system (the *Semashko* model) that eliminated financial barriers in access to health services and secured continuity of care. It should be noted that reforms of health care started in late 1980s under the *Semashko* state system. The experiments aimed first of all to introduce new methods of financing polyclinics, hospitals and medical staff. Unfortunately, they coincided with the beginning of market reforms and were stopped without full evaluation. However, the limited data available indicate that there was a potential to improve the state system itself without changing its basic financing and organizational principles. Twenty years later this experiment is being implemented in some regions – Perm, Kaluga and Samara – where, at their initiative, polyclinics become fund-holders. It still remains unclear whether this model could and should be used all over the country.

The main reasons for introducing CHI in Russia were political and ideological rather than social and economic. The aim was to create markets everywhere because health insurance was associated with capitalism while budget medicine was considered to be socialist. Since Russian health policy is in transition, three stages can be distinguished according to government attitudes to health issues and the structural impact of measures undertaken.

Stage 1 began in the 1990s when transition sought to create a market economy and political democracy. Societal reforms affected all spheres of Russian life, including health care. The decision was taken to shift from the budget model to a social insurance model on the belief that the introduction of market mechanisms would solve all the problems – not only economic but social as well. The Law on Compulsory Health Insurance was adopted in 1993 with new institutions established – CHI funds and health insurance organizations – while other (old) institutions remained almost intact. The economic decline led to a decrease in health care financing by public sources that, in turn, generated fee-for-service in state organizations as well as informal payments. Accompanied by the decline in population numbers, general health status began to deteriorate.

Stage 2 appeared during the mid-1990s to the beginning of the 21st century when the 'dual' budget-CHI system developed. While health reforms continued, these were fragmented with no principal changes introduced. Due to the 1998 economic crisis, emphasis was placed on securing stability rather than improving the situation. The main indicators of health system – including morbidity and mortality rates – continued to worsen while personal spending on health care was growing quickly. At the same time awareness was rising that, without an active state policy, health care problems were unlikely to be addressed. In 1997 'The Concept of Development of Health Care and Medical Science in Russian Federation' was adopted that stated four main aims of health reforms: to improve population health status, prevention and healthy style of life; to develop primary health care based on family practice; to decrease the role of secondary care; and to improve quality of care. In 1998 the first Program of State Guaranties of Free Medical Care was adopted.

Stage 3 started when the 2005 session of the Presidium of the State Council of the Russian Federation was devoted to health care issues. It commissioned the special report 'On Increasing Access and Quality of Health Care'. Health issues were put high on the political agenda – a shift caused, it seems, by negative demographic trends such as the steady decline in population. The shift pushed the government to activate health reforms to improve access and quality of health care. A number of initiatives were introduced in health care such as the special National Project on Healthcare in 2005 that increased state financing of selected priority measures and a program in 2007 to overcome the demographic crisis. After 2008 population indicators such as birth rates and life expectancy slightly increased (see Table 8.1).

The main trend in health policy during these 20 years of transformation continued the switch from budget to social insurance medicine. The strategy of reform led to the development of a hybrid model that combines both budget and insurance mechanisms with budgets (both federal and regional) still playing the major role at least in term of financing. Current reforms aim to strengthen insurance elements while promoting individual responsibility and private initiative. This aim requires the adjustment of legislation in force so in 2010 a new Law on CHI was adopted that envisaged the gradual decrease of direct budget appropriations and transfer to one-channel financing via CHI. The Law on Fundamentals of Health Protection in the Russian Federation has been adopted in 2011. From 2010 the word 'modernization' in official documents is understood mainly in technical/technological terms instead of 'reform'.

8.3 Russian Health Policy: Myths and Paradoxes

To understand health reforms, it is important to analyze theoretical assumptions that underline policy decisions. The analysis reveals two myths and two paradoxes of Russian health reforms that, although not always stated explicitly, influence health policy decisions.

Myth 1: Private (for fee) provision is always better than public (free of charge), and private organizations are more effective than the state organizations.

This myth presents free medicine as a charity by a paternalistic state. It should be noted, however, that services rendered in the public sector – although free at the point of delivery – are prepaid by people through the tax system. Economic theory acknowledges that social taxes that are formally paid by employers at the end are passed to employees (Stiglitz 1986). There is also no clear empirical evidence that state organizations are always less effective than private ones or provide services of a lower quality (Hall and Lobina 2005; Afonso *et al.* 2005). Methodological problems make it difficult to compare productivity in public and private sector – *e.g.*, measuring performance or defining to what extent the success of treatment should be attributed to health services. Quality of auxiliary services is usually better in private sector. Patients definitely prefer positive medical treatment results rather than a comfortable environment. Besides, private health services can choose whom to treat whereas public services are usually required to help any citizen of the country.

Myth 2: Well-off people always prefer to pay for services, including medical care.

The idea that the well off always pay – even more they should pay – is promoted implying that if one does not pay, he or she cannot expect to get quality care. Despite the differences in organization and financing of health care, two basic principles are generally accepted (at least in Europe). First, medical treatment is considered as a social good as its provision to an individual brings benefits to the whole society rather than a purely private good sold to get profits. Second, social solidarity assumes redistribution from the rich to the poor, from the healthy to the sick, from the young to the elderly. An important role in formulating health strategies belongs to the middle class. In the end the main line of social policy becomes not only securing minimal social standards to support the poor but social quality for all (Grigorieva 2007).

Promoting overspending by the rich does not contribute to social solidarity. Today the private sector is marginal in Russian health care, but health policy that aims to promote it is likely to lead to separating health care for the rich from that for the poor, with all the negative health and social consequences to follow. These assumptions in turn help to understand two paradoxes of Russian health policy that are otherwise not easy to explain.

Paradox 1: Lack of funds for health care versus choosing a costly model of health care.

The aim of health reforms in the 1990s was to switch from the Soviet state system of health care that provided medical care free of charge in state-owned health services in order to secure equal access by all groups of population to health care based on an insurance model. The major reason stated in official documents was the lack of state funds and the necessity to raise more money for health care. Paradoxically, while the Russian people are constantly told that there are insufficient means for health care, and while budget medicine is acknowledged to be the best in containing costs, Russian reformers chose the more costly insurance model while less costly public model is rejected. Budget medicine secures relatively high health outcomes in population in general at relatively lower cost. For example, comparisons of financial and health status indicators in developed countries shows that the USA spends almost twice as much on health care as European countries; the USA is characterized by a higher share of private expenditures but its health status indicators are comparable to those countries where the share of public (state) funds is larger (Table 8.5). Maternal mortality in the USA is higher than in the UK while the health life expectancy is lower. In the USA almost one-third of the population older than 15 years of age suffer from obesity, which has become a serious health problem.

Paradox 2. Decrease in state expenses versus uncontrolled growth of personal spending.

Modern health systems in developed countries divide health care expenditures into public and private. Many developed countries aim to optimize not only public but private health spending as well. In Russia the state is concerned only with savings in public health expenditures; it does not seem to care about how much people must pay from their pockets or, if they can, about taking widespread poverty into account. The second paradox of Russian health policy is that the state tries to minimize public expenses on health care (including CHI) while additional personal expenses are left to the people's discretion (Chubarova 2008).

In current reform proposals the idea of co-payments is popular. It is assumed that people should pay a certain amount, usually a fixed sum per doctor's visit in the state health services. Several countries – Italy, France, Germany – have attempted to introduce co-payments but these usually cover marginal services such as subscription charges and dentists, and they are combined with a system of discounts and exemptions. It should be noted that other financing mechanisms in the countries that introduced co-payments did not change.

In theory and practice two main arguments in favor of co-payments can be found – to raise additional funds and to reduce demand for health services. The latter is based on an assumption that free consumption of services stimulates demand. In order to perform these functions, co-payments should be relatively high to cover expenses to administer them as well but the need arises to introduce exemptions for low income people to secure access to health services. Taking into account the modern tendencies in Russian health care mentioned above, state health care would cover mostly poor people. Introduction of

Table 8.5 Selected Health Care Indicators in Selected Countries

	USA		Canada		UK		Germany		France		Russia	
	2000	**2006**	**2000**	**2006**	**2000**	**2006**	**2000**	**2006**	**2000**	**2006**	**2000**	**2006**
Total health expenditures (% GDP)	13.2	15.3	8.8	10.0	7.1	8.2	10.3	10.6	10.1	11.0	5.4	5.3
Share of public expenditures as % total health	43.7	45.8	70.4	70.4	80.9	87.3	79.7	76.9	79.4	79.7	59.9	63.2
Share private expenditures as % total health	56.3	54.2	29.6	29.6	19.1	12.7	20.3	23.1	20.6	20.3	40.1	36.8
Years of life expectancy	77	78*	79	81*	78	80*	78	80*	79	81*	65	66*
Mortality (15-60 years)/1,000	114	108*	81	72*	88	89*	94	80*	100	89*	309	312*
Tuberculosis morbidity per 100,000	4	3	5	4	9	12	9	5	13	11	168	125

Source: WHO Statistical Information Service 2009 (* = 2007 data).

co-payments is likely to affect prevention as there is a possibility that people will seek doctors' help only at later stages of disease. Improvement in quality of care is sometimes cited as a reason to introduce co payments. This may be true if copayments are spent within the health service and if the staff has incentives to turn them into improvements in quality rather than just to increase income. Besides, improvement in quality might be too costly and often requires serious changes in the whole health production process.

8.4 Russian Health and Social Policy: Threats to the Health Care System

Two factors potentially cause problems in designing a health care system. One is connected with the volume and method of health financing. The question of how much to spend on health care remains open. There are different approaches about how to determine the share of health expenditures, taking willingness to pay into account among other things. For example, the minimal amount of health spending as a share of GDP can be legally bound (Savedoff 2007).

In creating new mechanisms to finance health care, Russia is likely to enter the 'health expenditures growth trap'. If the health finance model chosen in the course of reforms under the resource constraint is in principle costly, it will inevitably lead to future increase in spending. But mechanisms used to collect and distribute health money are no less important than its amount. The situation in Russia differs from that in the developed countries. The Russian health care system is 'sustainably underfinanced', so there is a need to increase the amount of resources allocated to it, while in developed countries the main health policy aim is cost containment. However, Russia needs to take into account the experience of other countries that face the spiraling growth of health expenditures. From the beginning, Russia should choose a health financing model that will allow it to turn health appropriations into an effective system of health care provision rather than constantly increase health money without evident positive outcomes. The budget system has a relative advantage over other models of finance. It would be more rational to allocate more money to the budget model than to change it to the social insurance one that will inevitably cause an increase in spending.

While performance results of the two systems are comparable, the social health insurance model is more expensive than the budget one. An OECD study demonstrates that between 1960 and 2006 the adoption of social health insurance led to per capita expenditure growth by 3%-4% and lowered employment in health care system by 8%-10%. Usually the adoption of social health insurance has no significant impact on amenable mortality but for one case – breast cancer among women – social health insurance systems perform significantly worse with 5%-6% more potential years of life lost than the system financed through taxes (Wagstaff 2009).

Inequality is the main threat in the health care system but it is not properly addressed in the proposals for health reform. Inequality in Russian society – its Gini coefficient is 0.43 – is wellknown. Several recent studies investigated the influence of inequity on health status and access to health care, including gender inequality (Shkolvikov *et al.* 2000; Rimashevskaya 2007). Patients differ according to income and social status; the poor and the rich have different demands as well as financial resources to pay for health care. Rich people who can pay for health care stimulate the growth of private sector, which currently serves to increase choice. However, if it expands beyond certain limits, the well-off and usually more demanding and politically active people will leave the state sector and thus reduce pressure on the government to improve public health care services and to increase appropriations for health. As such a development is likely to destroy the integrity of health care system and marginalize the poor Russia might end up with two separate sub-systems: one for the rich people who can pay and another for the poor people that is free.

8.5 Interests in Russian Health Care: In Search of Consensus

The Russian government declares that reforms of health care are carried out in order to secure population access to medical care, but the measures implemented or planned do not solve the declared tasks. Instead they lead to worsening the situation that contradicts the understanding of reform as an improvement. This situation suggests that other driving forces for change may be stronger than those officially declared. The question of 'in whose interests are the health reforms implemented' is relevant because health system accumulates substantial resources – economic, material, financial and human – that are the subject of competition among various interests groups. These can be divided into two broad groups: internal and external stakeholders.

Internal stakeholders include institutions that organize and provide medical services. Russia today has five main players in the health system: the Ministry of Health and Social Development of the Russian Federation; regional health ministries or departments of regional governments; federal and regional CHI funds; health insurance companies; and health services. Relations among them are not easy and division of responsibilities is not always clear. Recent tendencies indicate an increasing role for regional bodies in health policy. Health is becoming the responsibility of regional authorities while the federal agencies retain general control functions. This trend has produced regional variations in health care, including its organization and financing, the formation of different models of CHI in Russian regions and problems of interregional mobility by patients. Financial control in the system is a problem, too, the major issues being corruption and spending money on purposes other than provision of medical care, thereby violating the rules for state purchase of services.

The current position of Russian doctors in the health care system is controversial. On one hand, official salaries of medical staff are low and doctors use any possibility to increase their income, including 'envelop' payments. On the other hand, doctors in Russia have traditionally been on the front line in the fight for the health of population; many prominent public leaders in Russia had medical backgrounds. Because doctors monopolize leading administrative positions in health care system, they are in the people's eyes directly associated with the commercialization of Russian health care (Chubarova 2004). Health reforms are often discussed within the medical community without involving experts from other disciplines; therefore corporate interests often influence final decisions. In 2010, the National Medical Chamber (NMC) was established as a self-governing organization of doctors. The idea of medical community is to introduce licensing of doctors by the NMC as opposed to state licensing of a health service.

External stakeholders include patients, but their position in Russia's health policy process is weak. First, due to high inequality, interests of patients diverge substantially. People with different social and income status have different access and different demands on health care system. Second, illness is a private matter; in order to influence political decisions, patients should be well organized but that is not the case in Russia. Third, the process of development and implementation of health reforms leave little space for the majority of citizens to express their opinions.

Employers are another group of interests in the Russian health care system. Their power is limited to paying contributions to CHI, which they aim to lower. Russian employers are well organized and have been successful in lobbying a decrease in CHI contributions. Employers are more interested in voluntary health insurance because they have tax advantages and can recoup part of the amount used to insure their employees. Many Russian and foreign firms offer health insurance to their staff as a part of their packages of social benefits.

Health policy should definitely be discussed as an integral part of social policy. On one hand, in a market economy and political democracy, many interests arise with each interest having the right to express itself and it is very difficult to reconcile all of them. On the other hand, this creates a possibility to manipulate interests. However, democracy has its price: while the strongest interest wins, it does not necessarily express the concerns of society at large. When corporate interests prevail over the process of reaching agreement between various interests, it is unlikely that a technocratic decision – a 'professional' decision in the language of Russian officials – is adopted.

8.6 CONCLUSIONS

Russia is in the process of changing the model of health care itself — from the integrated state *Semashko* model to basic (limited) social insurance with a strong emphasis on individual responsibility. Evidence suggests that health reforms do not bring many positive results in terms of access and quality of health services, which cause doubts whether they are going in the right direction. The situation in Russian health care is complicated because health reforms are part of greater societal transformations – the main problem being to reconcile the old and the new.

Currently, Russian health policy is being developed and implemented in a way that contributes little to improve the health situation. Analysis reveals the divergence between stated aims and mechanisms that are used to reach them. Taking Russian realities into account, the shift from collective to individual responsibility contributes to wider inequalities in both health status and access to health care. Modern Russian health policy can be characterized as problem-making rather than problem-solving. It needs major revisions that incorporate the historic experience of pre-transition Russia as well as to draw lessons from 20 years of 'new' health reforms under transition. The significance of collectivist values, the role of the state and potential of the government sector to improve its performance should be reassessed in order to ensure that the limited resources allocated to health care today are used efficiently and effectively.

The case of Russian health policy demonstrates that, when designing health reforms (especially those carried out in times of great transformations), health issues should be positioned within a wider societal and historical context. Social and economic conditions of people's lives are among the most important determinants of their health. Growth of social inequality and social exclusion in Russia makes it essential to devise a strategy of social integration in the market economy because the prospects of economic growth and human development are linked to social equity. A system of health for all might yet become a cornerstone for social consensus and social integration in Russian society.

9 Health Reforms in Slovakia

Juraj Nemec

For 20 years, as a successor state of the former Czechoslovakia, Slovakia has sought to improve health outcomes. The main goal – universal and fair access – remained the target for all governments in power but reform strategies and associated policies have often differed. Better health outcomes have emerged but at great cost because efficiency proved to be elusive.

The chapter has three sections. After describing a profile of Slovakia, it examines the processes of health care reform. Limited continuity of health policy and an imbalance in the system's finances represent core problems in the history of reform. The final section presents outcomes and investigates selected examples of limited success, especially how political instability neutered reform and politicized health issues, sometimes causing policy reversals.

Although Slovakia has made progress towards western European standards, much remains to be done. While the costs of health care will continue to rise, it is unclear whether the current political, policy-making and implementation systems can deliver either efficiency or responsiveness to patients.

9.1 Country Profile

Slovakia was established on 1 January 1993 after an amicable division of Czechoslovakia. Since the medieval era, Slovakia had been a part of the Austro-Hungarian Empire. After the latter's defeat in the First World War, Slovakia became part of the first Czechoslovak state that was established on 28 October 1918. In 1939, the first formally independent Slovak state was established, which was closely linked to Germany.

In 1945, after the Second World War, Czechoslovakia was reestablished as a unitary state. The Communist Party of Czechoslovakia won the elections of 1947 and in February 1948 took over all powers in the state. After the Velvet Revolution in 1989, the process of gradual transition towards a pluralistic public administration system began in Czechoslovakia. After successful transitions in social, political and economic life, Slovakia became a member of the European Union on 1 May 2004 and joined the Euro zone on 1 January 2009.

Slovakia is a small country of 49,036 km^2. As Table 9.1 reveals, an emergent problem since 1990 has been the slow growth in the number of inhabitants. In 2000, the natural increase

Table 9.1 Population

	1995	2000	2005	2010
Population total	5 378 932	5 402 547	5 389 180	5 435 273
Population density	109.7	110.2	109.9	110.8
Urban population (%)	57	56	56	55

Source: <www.statistics.sk>.

Table 9.2 Health Status Indicators

		1985	1990	1995	2000	2005	2010
Life expectancy	Men	66.9	66.6	68.4	69.2	70.1	71.6
	Women	74.7	75.4	76.3	77.2	77.9	78.8
Death/1,000 inhabitants		10.2	10.2	9.8	9.8	9.9	9.7
Neo-natal mortality		11.1	8.4	7.9	5.4	4.1	3.2
Infant mortality		16.3	12.0	11.0	8.6	7.2	5.6

Source: <www.statistics.sk>.

was only 2,427 persons compared to 4,821 in 1999, 72% less than in 1995 and 90% less than in 1990. In only a few regions of the country does the number of live births exceed the number of deaths. In relative terms, the population of Slovakia is stable.

During 1989-2010, indicators of health status in Slovakia improved as in more developed CEE countries such as Hungary and the Czech Republic. No data exist to assess the factors behind this positive trend or the extent to which this is caused by increased quality of health care and other factors like changes in living style or an improved environment. Table 9.2 indicates that the life expectancy has significantly improved but remains below EU levels. The difference in life expectancy between men and women is large, but it diminished after 1990. Mortality is slowly declining but remains higher than the EU average.

Indicators of health status show that negative factors connected with transformation (stress, decreasing living standard of many inhabitants, increased consumption of drugs) were over-weighed by positive factors. The medical quality of health services might be one of the latter due to significant improvement of equipment among providers and available medications.

Despite minor problems in 1995-1996 and 2009-2010 due to financial and economic crises, economic development trends in Slovakia were relatively positive for the entire period.

Table 9.3 Economic Indicators (SK = Slovak Crowns; € = Euro)

	1993	1995	2000	2005	2010
GDP current prices (billions)	SK 411	SK 577	SK 934	SK 1 450	€ 65.9
			€ 31.2	€ 49.3	
GDP per capita (thousands)	SK 76.4	SK 107.3	SK 172.9	SK 269.1	€ 12.1
			€ 5.8	€ 9.2	
Unemployment rate	12.2	13.1	18.6	16.0	14.4
Average monthly income	SK 5 379	SK 7 195	SK 11 430	SK 17 274	€ 769.0
			€ 379.4	€ 573.4	
Inflation (%)	23.2	9.9	12.0	2.7	1.0

Source: <www.statistics.sk>.

Table 9.4 Resources for Health Care (billions, 1€ = 30,1 SKK)

Expenditures	**1995**	**2000**	**2005**	**2008**	**2010**
Health Insurance	SK 20.1	SK 35.1	SK 72.2	SK 99.3	SK 102.3
			€2.4	€3.3	€3.4
General Taxation	SK 11.2	SK 15.7	SK 12.0	SK 3.0	SK 6.0
			€0.4	€0.1	€0.2
Direct Payments	SK 1.8	SK 5.9	SK 21.1	SK 30.1	SK 33.1
			€0.7	€1.0	€1.1
Total	**SK 33.1**	**SK 56.7**	**SK 105.3**	**SK 132.4**	**SK 141.5**
			€3.5	**€4.4**	**€4.7**
% of GDP	**5.7**	**6.1**	**7.2**	**6.5**	**7.3**

Sources: Zajac and Pazitny 2002 – data for 1995 and 2000; Szalay *et al.* 2011 for other data.

Health care in Slovakia is predominantly financed by public funds – a combination of health insurance and budgetary resources (transfers to the health insurance system for social groups financed by the ministry of health and local self-governments). Although marginal at the beginning of transformation, private expenditures began to grow significantly after 2000.

Despite limited resources, many indicators of health resources are higher than standards in developed countries. In Table 9.5 data for 1995 and 2000 are full employment equivalent; data for 2005, 2008 and 2010 are physical persons. The methodology for calculating the number of beds also differs in the two sources.

The approaches of all actors influencing health care reforms and trends mirror societal values of European Union members. The heritage of the socialist period remains visible as citizens prefer to rely on "state" help rather than develop individual responsibility for their welfare. Data from different sources highlight absolute and relative situations; Table 9.6 gives examples.

Bunčák *et al.* (2008) confirmed the lack of a sense of individual responsibility as well as a preference for paternalism. According to their data, two-thirds of respondents believe

Table 9.5 Health Resources

	1995	2000	2005	2008	2010
Total work-places in health establishments	77 137	71 605	98 829	109 874	106 233
In private establishments			53 932	67 915	63 818
Total work-places in health establishments per 100,000 inhabitants	0.77	0.72	0.99	1.10	1.08
Doctors (total)	10 567	9 761	19 237	20 866	20 431
Doctors in private establishments			12 823	14 200	11 819
Nurses (total)	30 334	28 037	32 319	33 778	34 477
Nurses in private establishments			16 726	19 585	19 479
Other medical staff (total)	13 036	12 644	21 918	24 508	23 053
Other medical staff in private establishments			13 139	22 326	21 276
Administrative and service staff	21 329	19 982	23 191	28 552	26 072
Administrative and service staff in private establishments			11 244	11 804	11 244
Other staff	1 871	1 181	2 164	2 170	2 200
Hospital beds (total)			48 622	46 742	46 878
Hospital beds per 1,000 inhabitants	7.5	6.5	9.0	8.7	8.8

Source: Zajac and Pazitny 2002 (data 1995 and 2000), Zdravotnicka rocenka 2010.

Table 9.6 Citizen Opinions (Percentages in Selected CEE States)

Country	**Agree with democracy**		**Agree with market economy**		**Comparison to pre-1989**		**Three most critical problems**		
	1991	**2009**	**1991**	**2009**	**Better**	**Equal**	**Corruption**	**Criminality**	**Drugs**
East Germany	91	85	86	82				47	50
Czech Republic	80	80	87	79	45	51	71	55	51
Slovakia	70	71	69	66	29	66	52	55	46
Poland	66	70	80	71	47	47	58	49	49
Hungary	74	56	80	46	8	88	76	69	
Lithuania	75	55	76	50	23	63	78	76	66
Bulgaria	76	52	73	53	13	80	76	76	74

Source: <www.pewglobal.org>.

their problems need to be solved by the state. Fiscal illusion (higher than in developed countries), low level of tax compliance (Orviska and Hudson 2003) and paternalism generate a fiscal trap in which citizens demand large scale public services (free of charge) while total government revenues cannot meet the high demand. Slovakia is among the EU members with the lowest proportion of public revenues to Gross Domestic Product (GDP) – slightly above 30%.

Since Slovakia signed the European Charter of Human Rights, there has been little discussion by citizens, the non-profit sector, think-tanks or political parties about deviations from its principles. Slovakia's health care system is based on the principle of free access at the point of delivery for most services, with costs financed predominantly through compulsory social health insurance. Discussions about health care are mainly connected with the ratio between the state and the market but not about lowered access. Whatever the type of government (left-wing, right-wing, centre or coalitions) the promises of newly elected governments remain stable: universal coverage, high quality for everyone and financial consolidation of the health care delivery system. (The analytical section below demonstrates that such proclamations are only rhetorical; while there is no chance to fulfill them in reality, citizens like and want them).

As indicated above, the core issue of different "own" reform proposals – whether right-wing governments of Prime Ministers Dzurinda (1998-2006) and Radicova (since 2010) or the left-wing government of Prime Minister Fico (2006-2010) – is the level of marketization of health care. Reforms after the Velvet Revolution were predominantly influenced by foreign advice.

From the point of view of finance, the proportion of private payments began to increase significantly during the Dzurinda government at the beginning of this century. Such a trend was inevitable to cope with large financial deficiencies, but citizens have not welcomed it. The Fico government, elected in 2006, promised to reverse the trend but found it to be impossible because of fiscal constraints. The decision about social health insurance as the base for health care financing had been made at the beginning of transformation and was subject to some "academic" discussions, but there was no formal attempt to change the general taxation-based system that functioned under socialism. No political party wants to be connected with that history.

The scale of privatization is a more frequent topic for discussion. The structure of the health care system developed into a public-private-civil sector mix and ways to approach it depend on normative values. Right-wing governments promise that private ownership of medical establishments and health insurance companies will facilitate efficiency and quality improvements – although this claim has not been confirmed by any health care reforms in developed countries. Nemec *et al.* (2010) suggest that the form of hospital ownership is not the main determinant of its performance. Such stress on privatization is linked more with private than public interests.

The left-wing government of Prime Minister Fico did not change much in the system's organization. It managed to stop the privatization of academic hospitals that had already begun. It also passed a law forbidding profit creation by private health insurance companies. However, several weeks after the Radicova government was elected in 2010, Slovakia's Constitutional Court ruled that such a law is unconstitutional.

From the point of view of its administration, the Slovak health care system can be described as decentralized. Given their mixed ownership, the delivery and the financing systems are administered and regulated at all levels of government, with a focus on guaranteeing universal access and good quality. The Ministry of Health (<www.health.gov.sk>) is responsible for health policy development and implementation. It defines the network of health establishments, coordinates central health care programs, and establishes academic hospitals and other specialized units. It is also responsible for training medical staff and for categorization of drugs.

Established in 2004 as a legal entity with responsibility for surveillance over the provision of health care and public health insurance, the second central body is the Healthcare Surveillance Authority (<www.udzs.sk>). The main tasks of the Authority are health care supervision, public health insurance supervision and arbitration on the following levels of relationships:

- health insurance company ↔ provider
- policyholder ↔ provider
- policyholder ↔ health insurance company

Regional governments are responsible for local hospitals and for maintenance of a minimum network of health care providers in the region – including licensing all local and regional providers such as general practitioners, group practices, specialized ambulances and dental care establishments. Local self-governments (municipalities) have limited responsibilities concerning the local network of providers.

9.2 History of Health System Reforms

The objective of the pre-1989 health care system in Czechoslovakia had been to provide a comprehensive system of health care for all members of society. Decisions about medical care provision were made by the Federal Government and by the national Czech and Slovak Ministries of Health, generally on political or administrative grounds. The only accountability in the old system was to the Communist Party.

Under the old system both services and medicines were free to the patients but, until 1987, there was no individual choice of practitioner. The supply of services was constrained by plans, while purchasers and providers were not differentiated. Economic resource allocation had no role in determining services whose level and distribution, although influenced by social, medical and administrative considerations, were determined by political decisions. No cost-benefit calculations were undertaken. There were no economic incentives either for individuals or for the system to improve performance, yet there was a chronic and sometimes acute excess demand for services.

However, when the transition began, the Czechoslovak system was far from the crisis conditions that characterized the Polish and Soviet systems (Davis 2001). When necessary, everyone was able to get appropriate health care at a relatively high international medical standard. Most considerations of equity were achieved although special medical institutions provided higher quality care for high-ranking officials. The old system is often described as obsolete and inefficient but, with approximately 5% of GDP spent on health care expenditures, most of the demand was covered without waiting lists. Despite insufficient quantity and quality of equipment, relatively high quality of care characterized the system.

9.3 First Phase of Reforms

The processes of reforming the Slovak health care system started immediately after the Velvet Revolution in 1989. They introduced important changes into the system – especially privatization and a shift in financing health care from general taxation to social health insurance – changes that are far from completed. Failures in policy-making and implementation during the reform created additional problems, many of them connected with finance.

Since 1968 health care had been the responsibility of the national Slovak level and not of the federal Czechoslovak state. Aspirations in Slovakia's health policy after 1989 were defined by Programmatic Statements of Government and the main reform documents – the first of which was published in 1990. The most important goals of the reform were:

- creation of a system of "health care for everybody" as described by the document 'National Public Health Program',
- universal access to defined scope of health services and benefits,
- the creation, realization and control of health policy as free decisions of citizens,
- cancellation of the state monopoly in health care, plurality of provision of health care, privatization, and increased participation of self-government in the health care system,
- public health as a dominant part of the health care system,
- dominant position of primary care in the health care system,
- the right of citizens to choose providers,
- compulsory health Insurance,
- citizen participation in relation to protection and improvement of health,
- multi-resource financing of health care.
- improved economic and financial management in health care establishments,
- stop the impairment of health status of citizens.

To achieve the proclaimed goals, new legislation was adopted. The most important legal documents that provided the basic frame for the initial phase of the health care system in Slovakia were the Constitution of the Slovak Republic, the package of laws related to the creation of insurance scheme, the Law on Treatment Order, and the Law on Health Care.

The *Constitution of the Slovak Republic* is the highest guarantee of human rights in Slovakia. Adopted on 1 September 1992, the Slovak Constitution provides a standard system of human rights in a democratic society. Its section on economic, social and cultural rights provides that everyone has the right to protection of health and, based on an insurance system, citizens have the right to free medical care according provisions of the complementary law. No article of the Constitution has been amended during reforms of the health care system in Slovakia.

The *Law on Treatment Order* identifies the principles related to qualifying conditions for benefits, their scope (cash and in-kind) and the organization of health care. It regulates the extent of health care to be provided under compulsory health insurance, the conditions under which it is to be provided, the reimbursement schedule, categorization of drugs (for different levels of co-payment) and rules on health insurance coverage of medical aid. It also defines the indications for reimbursement of spa treatment. To summarize the most important parts of this law:

- Health insurance provides health services, medications and medical aid as indicated on the basis of health needs. These indications are based on achievements of medical and biomedical sciences, and guarantee effective treatment, following therapeutical and pharmaco-therapeutical rules.
- Insurance companies reimburse to contractual health care establishments the costs of health care provided according the list of treatments, medications and medical aids. The prices of services, medications and medical aids are defined by regulations issued by the Ministry of Finance.
- Specialized health care is provided to patients only on the basis of referral by general practitioners or referral by other specialists.
- On the basis of health insurance, patients get only the defined daily dose of medications.

In 2004, as part of the liberal reforms announced by the Dzurinda government, this Law was significantly amended.

The *Law on Health Care* deals with provision of health services, their organization and management, definitions of rights and obligations of legal and physical persons. It delegated the main regulatory, planning and managerial tasks to the Ministry of Health. Relevant parts of the law include:

- "Everyone has the right to health care, including medications and medical aids. Health care is provided by state health establishments, municipal health establishments, medical establishments run by legal or physical entities, and is provided on the base of existing accessible know-how of medical and other biomedical sciences".
- "Health care is provided for citizen: (a) free, based on compulsory health insurance; (b) based on additional insurance contracts; (c) free, from the state budget resources; (d) based on financial resources of charities, legal or physical entities; and (e) based on co-payment or full participation by the receiver of health care".
- "A citizen, getting health care, has the right to care according the kind and level of health problem. She/he has the right to choose a doctor or health establishment. In the case of emergency she/he has the right to get medical care at the nearest medical establishment available to handle appropriate health care".

This original Law was significantly amended in 2004 as part of the liberal reforms by the Dzurinda government.

Like most CEE countries, Slovakia switched to the so-called 'Bismarck' system of social health insurance to replace old general taxation system of financing health care. However, together with the Czech Republic, it decided to introduce a competitive/pluralistic social health insurance system as well. (Most CEE countries started with only one public health insurance company.) The main *laws on health insurance* were passed in 1994, which created the base for establishing health insurance companies (two of them public). Most of these have since disappeared from the 'market'; in 2002 five existed but by 2010 only two private and one public remained.

Changes in the health insurance system were supported by the typical arguments of plurality, independence and competition. However, the Constitution and a consecutive set of laws guarantee to any citizen universal and free, at the point of delivery, access to health care; and this package must be delivered by all insurance companies for the price that is regulated by the Ministry of Finance. Therefore some level of plurality and competition was visible only during the initial phase of the insurance system, when the services to the insured were to some extent different.

The introduction of a pluralistic health insurance system is frequently considered an imperfect state decision during the health care transformation process in Slovakia. Arguments for a plurality of insurance providers, for their independence from government and for competition between them have been strongly questioned by several authors (see Björkman 2004). Because the evidence for these doubts comes from advanced market systems, it seems likely that their potential to improve health care in transitional countries may be even more limited. Simple data indicate that this reform idea did not achieve its objective. Many resources were withdrawn from the system when several private insurance companies collapsed, and better quality was not achieved.

9.4 "Next steps" – From Proclamations to Liberal Reforms

Programmatic Declarations of subsequent Slovak governments repeated the key aims of the 1990 Declaration, but increasingly reflected a preoccupation with financial problems. In 1994, the Moravcik government's Declaration sought to reduce health budget deficits, change reimbursement systems, and resolve salary problems of health care employees. The 1995 Declaration repeats the resolve of the then Meciar government to pursue a pluralistic system of health insurance, improve the salaries of health care professionals, and find resources to finance high priority programs. By the time of the 1998 Programmatic Declaration of the Dzurinda government, the deepening financial crisis dominated all priorities. The government again guaranteed general access to as well as high quality of outpatient and hospital care, but it also wanted to implement new pricing measures to prevent wasteful prescriptions and promised to put health activities on a rational economic basis. Interestingly, for the first time there was a longer-term aim to raise the level of spending as a proportion of GDP to European Union levels, although no precise targets were given. However, the policies and goals of the 1998-2002 government were declaratory, non-measurable and therefore non-controllable.

As a result of "reform by proclamation but not effective action," the Slovak system was by 2002 heavily indebted – especially its hospital and insurance sectors. Chronic weaknesses included low economic efficiency; a lack of evidence-based decisions; low relative pay with associated problems of labor retention; excessive drug bills, poorly managed capital programs and a general underdevelopment of preventive medicine. The autumn 2002 elections extended the mandate of Dzurinda's coalition government, which published its proclamation in early November 2002. The wording of this document differed slightly from its predecessors as it indicated plans for new financial rules, downsizing the role of the state and compulsory social health insurance in financing the system, and increasing patients' financial participation.

The semi-radical shift to marketization of the health care system in Slovakia was concluded in June 2004 when health minister Zajac prepared a set of new laws that Parliament approved and that became valid on 1 January 2005. The law on emergency service stipulated that every citizen has the right to rapid emergency service within a maximum of 15 minutes. In order to respect the principle of public-private-civil sector mix, any legal person with a license may provide emergency service. The law on health care and health-related services and the law on the scope and scale of health care financed by compulsory social health insurance and on financing of health related services are linked. The first is the basic law; the second sets the rules of implementation. This new legislation incorporated the principle of rationing into the health care system; by establishing the following structure of health services, it distinguished between what is and is not available free at the point of use:

a. Emergency health care – delivered to all threatened, independently of individual ability to pay
b. Health care services divided into two groups:
   - B1: Basic package of health services fully covered by compulsory social health insurance
   - B2: Other health services, subject to co-payment by the patient
c. Heath-related services (accommodation and catering in hospitals) delivered for a fee.

The law on health insurance provided new rules. For the first time, two layers of health insurance were formally created:

- Compulsory social health insurance, providing insurance services according to specific health care legislation (above mentioned laws).
- Individual (private) health insurance, providing insurance services according to general business law (a Business Code) that was never implemented.

The social health insurance system remained broadly defined to maintain guaranteed access of citizen to a basic package of health services and remained based on fixed-rate contributions from employers, employees and from the state for the economic inactive citizen. The law on health insurance companies transformed them into shareholders companies, with 100% share of the state in two of them (General Health Insurance Company and a Joint Health Insurance Company). The rights and responsibilities of insurance companies significantly increased to allow them to function as real regulators of the health care system. Insurance companies became formally co-responsible for securing the minimum network of health facilities in their region and for contracting health providers.

The law on health providers, health professionals and their professional bodies enlarged the list of types of health providers (*e.g.*, by including home care, one day care), set the principles of minimum network and provided for transformation of all health providers to non-profit or shareholders companies.

However, Slovak citizens did not appreciate such radical reform changes. According to public opinion surveys, health care reform was the least successful reform of governments during 1998-2004. Reflecting such opposition and based on left-wing normative ideas, Fico's socio-democratic government in power after 2006 tried to change several elements of this reform. After less than two years of functioning by the new system, several systematic changes were introduced that favored paternalistic over market approaches.

Three main areas of contention were privatization, co-payments and health insurance. Privatization or denationalization began in the mid-1990s, mainly in outpatient care and pharmacies, and is almost completed. In 1995, the state system accounted for 58% of expenditures in primary care, in 1996 only 8%, and by 2001 5%. For pharmacies the trend was similar: the proportion in the state sector decreased from 97% in 1995 to 5% in 1996 and 3% in 2001. Privatization of specialized ambulatory care was slower but by 2001 the state sector accounted only for 26% of facilities, a proportion that is currently about 15%.

The objective of privatizing in-patient care has been repeatedly proclaimed, but by 2001 there were still only three non-state hospitals in the whole country. The process of hospital privatization began during the second term of the Dzurinda government. In 2002 the management of hospitals was decentralized, and some hospitals were given self-governing status. By 2003, all regional hospitals had been transferred to regional self-governments or converted into non-profit bodies. The Ministry remained responsible for university hospitals. Although the latter were expected to be transformed into shareholder companies, such a transformation did not occur during the Dzurinda government period and the Fico government terminated the idea. Table 9.7 displays the current structure of hospitals in Slovakia.

Table 9.7 Hospital Ownership by Region (2009)

Ownership	Western Slovakia			Central Slovakia		Eastern Slovakia		Bratislava	Total
	TT	TN	NR	BB	ZA	PO	KE		
State – Ministry of Health establishments	4	3	6	13	6	8	11	10	61
State – other state bodies' establishments	0	1	0	0	1	2	0	2	6
Public – regional or local self-governments	4	4	2	2	5	3	1	1	22
Other (profit and non-profit companies)	4	8	6	14	5	21	11	14	83
Total	**12**	**16**	**14**	**29**	**17**	**34**	**23**	**27**	**172**

Abbreviations of regions: TT – Trnava, TN – Trencin, NR – Nitra, BB – Banska Bystrica, ZA – Zilina, PO – Presov, KE – Kosice.
Source: Ministry of Health.

In the area of health insurance, strict governmental control was re-introduced that produced an improper mix of market-based regulation (pluralistic insurance) but strict state control over all aspects of the system. Several changes were realized. The state significantly lowered the limit for "overhead" expenditures (management/administration costs) of health insurance companies with different limits for public and private companies. As noted above, the law prohibiting profit in private health insurance was passed but then found to be unconstitutional. The Radicova government had to settled legal cases connected with this law; one private company ceased operations and others claimed costs due to violation of their entrepreneurial rights. A law on compulsory transfers of all public employees to public insurance companies was prepared but not passed. Two public companies merged, as did two private companies. The result is an oligopolistic structure with two major players (public Vseobecna zdravotna poistovna – <www.vszp.sk> for about 60% of inhabitants; a large private company Dovera – <www.dovera.sk> for about 30% of inhabitants) and one small private company named Union.

While almost all co-payments introduced by the second Dzurinda government were abolished, Table 9.5 indicates this reversal did not impact the trend towards increased private financial participation, which shifted to the area of drug expenditures. The level of the state budget's contribution to the health insurance system to cover the non-working population (pensioners, students, the unemployed) rose from 4% to 5% to provide extra resources, but only in the first quarter of 2007. To lower the costs for drugs, VAT in this category was reduced from 19% to 10%.

In 2010, the liberal coalition returned to power but, because of the economic and financial crisis, health care was no longer a core issue. However, although no comprehensive reform strategy was published, the government resumed privatization of major hospitals in 2011 – but it was stopped by Parliament in late autumn. Some successful attempts were realized in the domain of drug management. After 2009, the referencing system for pharmaceuticals has been related to prices in all EU countries because the reference price is the average of the six lowest prices. Adopted in 2011, the new law on drugs and drug management also requires the prescription of substance but not of the specific medication.

Calendar 2011 was an active period in the Slovak health care system. In September about a quarter of medical doctors (dentists were not counted) submitted their resignations according to rules of the Labor Code. Organized by the medical trade unions, the arguments of this 'protest' were:

- stop the transformation of public hospitals into shareholder companies,
- increase salaries of medical doctors,
- respect the Labor Code rules on maximum workload for doctors as well as others.

Compared to the Czech Republic where a similar protest had been settled through effective dialog, the Slovak Government did not react before late November. Because no solution was found during a very brief period of negotiations, the government on 28 November announced an "emergency situation" and forced doctors to return to their ambulances. Many of the latter did not respect this decree (by claiming to be ill) and for several days the system almost collapsed. Even emergency care did not operate full-scale while routine treatments were not provided in many hospitals. After days of chaos a memorandum was signed and most doctors accepted new contracts. Necessary legislative changes were submitted to Parliament, which were passed with votes from the opposition. The Prime Minister signed the Memorandum but simultaneously motivated MPs in the coalition not to vote for the changes. This Slovak case requires in-depth policy analysis in order to investigate the country-specific environment that led to such developments.

9.5 Selected Outcomes of Reforms

To contextualize the current situation of Slovakia's health care system after almost 20 years of chaotic reforms, Table 9.8 presents comparative indicators in the 2001 World Health Report.

As noted previously, health status in Slovakia has improved although decomposition of causal factors is not possible. Improved health technologies and better focus on prevention are likely to have contributed to the trend. By law, access to most services is free at the point of delivery. There is no evidence that any group or citizen has been denied access to any service to which it has a right. General practitioners, dentists and opticians cannot

Table 9.8 Ranking of Health Care Systems: Selected Countries

	Health		**Attainment of Goals (Responsiveness, Fairness)**	**Expen-ditures**	**Performance**	
	DALE	**Distribution**			**On Level of Health**	**Overall**
France	3	12	6	4	4	1
Italy	6	14	11	11	3	2
United Kingdom	14	2	9	26	24	18
Germany	22	20	14	3	41	25
USA	24	32	15	1	72	37
Slovenia	**34**	**23**	**29**	**29**	**62**	**38**
Czech Republic	**35**	**19**	**30**	**40**	**81**	**48**
Poland	45	5	34	58	89	50
Slovakia	***42***	***39***	***39***	***45***	***88***	***62***
Hungary	62	40	43	59	105	66
Lithuania	63	48	52	71	93	73
Estonia	69	43	48	60	115	77
Macedonia	**64**	**85**	**89**	**106**	**69**	**89**
Romania	**80**	**78**	**72**	**107**	**111**	**99**
Bulgaria	**60**	**53**	**74**	**96**	**92**	**102**
Armenia	**41**	**63**	**81**	**102**	**56**	**104**
Russia	**91**	**69**	**100**	**75**	**127**	**130**

Source: World Health Organization 2001.

refuse to treat patients. However, as there are no formal rules of precedence for access, waiting lists exist for specialists so unequal treatment may occur. And in the hospital sector additional non-legal payments are common for extra services such as a separate room.

Corruption and other factors undermine equality of access. According to Transparency International (<www.transparency.sk>), more than 25% of Slovak households have had to pay bribes to ensure good care. Bribes have been estimated to amount to about one-tenth of health costs (unpublished study financed by the World Bank). Formally the health care system in Slovakia provides equal and universal access but, in reality, hidden inequality exists and may be increasing – due, to large extent, to the deepening financial crisis. The problem of inequality of access to health services in Slovakia has been recognized (see fairness rank in Table 9.8).

It is difficult to assess developments in the quality of care after 1989 because no indicators are available. But there have been improvements in quality on the supply side, specifically in the structure and quality of equipment available in health establishments as well as medications for treatment. After 1989, several barriers limiting the import of 'Western' technologies were dismantled, and regulation of what can be prescribed and purchased has been weakened. Such trends deliver contradictory outcomes; on the one hand, there are improvements in technical aspects of quality services while, on the other hand, relative 'oversupply' of technologies and expensive drugs, which are among the causes of the health system's financial problems.

Compared to positive technical developments, the trends in other aspects of health care quality are more controversial although difficult to prove. Despite many promises, no government has been able to introduce systematic medical and organizational audits of health providers that would provide more information about how care is delivered by doctors and the conditions under which it is delivered to patients. The mistreatment of the Slovak President in 2000 (Zajac and Pazitny 2000) revealed basic weaknesses in the daily delivery of care, but the case was not used as an impetus for changes.

The organizational quality of patient care has improved, albeit slowly. Compared to the old system, there is choice of provider, but patients remain far from being the central subject of the system. In 2000, a document on 'Patient Rights' was prepared and published but queuing without the chance for an exact appointment is typical among a large proportion of providers, including private ones. The quality of care (in any of its dimensions) is not systematically evaluated in Slovakia. Formally the Health Care Surveillance Authority and insurance companies are responsible for evaluations and benchmarks. When Nemec *et al.* (2010) sought to evaluate the performance of Slovak hospitals, the following occurred.

The original idea was to prepare a comprehensive evaluation of the purposes of complaints and the addressees of complaints submitted to the Health Care Surveillance Authority. No problem had been anticipated because the full list of complaints and the Authority's opinions on them was originally publicly available. However, during the Fico government, this practice had been discontinued so the Authority had to be asked for data. The response from the office responsible for regulating the health system and its quality was a refusal to provide any data. The office claimed that such data were not held in a form that allowed

Table 9.9 Complaints received by the Health Care Surveillance Authority 2006-2008

	Complaints Received	Authority Decision		Number of Complaints Against Academic Hospitals
		Valid	Invalid	
2008	1431	148	613	901
2007	1226	146	530	720
2006	1263	209	535	664

Source: Health Care Surveillance Authority 2009.

comparative so only a limited sample of partial data could be obtained. The information in Table 9.9 indicates that a majority of complaints is related to the quality of care in academic hospitals and that the Authority is unable to provide timely decisions.

According to current legislation, quality rankings of health establishments in Slovakia are compulsory, and health insurance companies are required to construct them as a basis for contract negotiations with providers. Under such regulation it may seem obvious that ranking systems provide effective quality benchmarks, but again reality is different. Health insurance companies respect the law and construct rankings, but their attempts are uncoordinated and their criteria differ.

Table 9.10 provides examples of such rankings that, because of different criteria, produce very different results and therefore are of no use for comparisons of performance in hospitals. The first ranking is for the company Dôvera in 2007. Its criteria are the general level of health service quality; the complexity of services and departments; personnel; equipment and the position of the hospital in its region. (This approach focuses on capacities and availability of services; real clinical quality is not effectively incorporated.) The second 2007 ranking is by the largest provider – the General Health Insurance Company. It was constructed by using indicators on the management of chronic diabetes; the management of chronic pneumonia; non-planned readmissions of patients after day surgery; and surveys of patients' satisfaction. The final ranking was constructed in 2008 by a consortium of insurance companies – Apollo, Dôvera and Union. It was based on surveys of patients' satisfaction with twelve questions focusing on satisfaction with medical staff approaches and behavior, satisfaction with care and its results, and satisfaction with support services (catering, accommodation and cleaning).

Table 9.10 shows that different quality indicators tell different stories. If service complexity is the issue, academic hospitals are superior. However, patients feel better in smaller non-state hospitals. The negative message is that current rankings of quality cannot be used to produce a comprehensive comparative analysis of performance.

Table 9.10 Selected Hospital Quality Rankings

	Ranking by Dôvera	Ranking by VšZP	Ranking by Apollo, Dôvera and Union
1	FNsP Bratislava	Ľubovnianska nemocnica, n. o.	FNsP Milosrdní, s. r. o. Bratislava
2	FN J.A. Reimana Prešov	Nemocnica Zdravie, s. r. o. Púchov	Nemocnica, a. s. Šaca - Košice
3	FN L. Pasteura Košice	Nemocnica, s. r. o. Krompachy	Nemocnica Zdravie, s. r. o. Púchov
4	NsP Žilina	NsP Dolný Kubín	Ľubovnianska nemocnica, n. o.
5	FNsP Nové Zámky	Nemocnica Stropkov	Nemocnica, s. r. o. Bánovce
6	FN Nitra	Nemocnica, s. r. o. Handlová	Nemocnica, n.o. Kežmarok
7	MFN Martin	VšNsP. A. s. Levoča	Nemocničná a. s. Malacky
8	FNsP F. D. Rooswelta BB	Nemocnica, n.o. Kežmarok	Nemocnica, s. r. o. Handlová
9	FN Trnava	Nemocnica, a. s. Šaca - Košice	NsP Hnúšťa
10	FN Trenčín	NsP Ilava	NsP Snina

Source: author's compilation from web pages of selected health insurance companies.

9.6 ECONOMIC PERFORMANCE OF THE HEALTH CARE SYSTEM IN SLOVAKIA

The main problems of the system after 1989 are connected with finance. Under-financing of the system and the decline of economic performance as a result of transition are factors that lie behind the financial insufficiencies of Slovakia's health system. A combination of poor design of reforms and implementation-connected factors has brought the system close to collapse. Table 9.11 describes financial performance of the health system during 1995-2002. (Data differ slightly from data provided earlier due to different sources and methodology.)

Although the necessity to improve the poor economic performance of the system was on the agenda of all Slovak governments, the results have been unsatisfactory. From 1997, the system systematically consumed 10%-15% more resources than the resources available, and this trend did not change despite many implemented measures.

Table 9.11 Economic Performance of the Health Care System (Billions of Slovak Crowns); 2009 Data are Millions of Euros but Only Expenditures Paid by Insurance Companies (1 Euro = 30 Crowns)

	1995	1998	2000	2001	2002	2005	2009
Total health insurance system resources	26.3	41.4	45.3	49.6	57.0	72.3	3305
Resources from the Ministry of Health	4.1	4.7	4.5	4.9	4.2	3.6	174
Resources from Social Insurance Company	0.9	1.3	1.0	1.1	0.5	0.5	15
Direct payments from inhabitants	1.8	4.1	5.9	6.3	8.4	17.6	1142
Total resources	**33.1**	**51.5**	**56.7**	**61.9**	**70.1**	**94.0**	**4 835**
Primary care costs	1.3	4.2	4.7	4.9			
Secondary ambulatory care costs	0.0	1.5	1.9	2.1	7.3	13.3	776
In-patient care costs	25.3	25.6	26.0	28.1	20.5	27.1	1 298
Medicaments and health aids costs	2.0	16.1	20.6	22.8	32.2	34.2	1 075
Other costs	0.9	5.0	6.9	7.7	12.0	17.3	167
Ministry of Health costs	4.1	4.7	4.5	4.9	4.7	4.1	x
Total costs	**33.6**	**57.1**	**64.6**	**70.5**	**76.7**	**96.0**	**x**
Balance	**–0.5**	**–5.6**	**–7.9**	**–8.6**	**–6.6**	**–2.0**	**x**
Debt settlement	0.5	5.6	7.9	8.6	119	0	199
External debt	0.5	5.6	4.4	5.2	5,0	1,6	n.a
Privatization grants	0.0	0.0	3.5	3.4	0	0	0

Sources: Zajac and Pazitny 2002; Pazitny *et al.* 2006; Szalay *et al.* 2011.

One core problem connected with increased debts is that the system penalizes private sector suppliers for problems caused mainly within the public system by health professionals and health establishments. This solution of shifting the debt burden out of the health care sector shows that the level of relations between the state and other sectors remains far from international standards. There is too much space for the state to manage its own problems (imbalance between resources available and scale of 'free' services promised to citizens) at the costs of others – mainly the private sector and patients who are pushed to bribe in order to obtain appropriate services. Table 9.11 shows how the deficit had developed while Table 9.12 provides older data about its coverage because recent data are not available.

Table 9.12 Scale and Structure of External Debt of the Health Care System

(December)	1995	1996	1997	1998	1999	2000	2000	2001	2001	2002
Non-paid drugs delivered by pharmacies	0.9	0.8	2.1	3.8	3.6	4.0	4.7	5.9	6.6	8.0
Credits and other similar resources	0.6	0.7	1.7	1.9	4.4	4.0	4.4	4.4	5.8	5.9
Non-paid social contributions	0.4	0.4	0.7	1.8	3.0	4.5	4.4	3.1	4.2	4.1
Non-paid drugs from other suppliers	1.2	1.2	2.3	3.6	3.7	3.8	3.8	3.9	3.8	4.5
Non-paid food and other material supplies	0.6	0.7	1.0	1.9	2.6	2.7	2.2	3.5	3.7	4.6
Non-paid energies	0.4	0.4	0.6	1.0	1.1	1.5	1.7	2.0	2.5	2.9
Total	**4.0**	**4.2**	**8.4**	**14.0**	**18.4**	**20.5**	**21.1**	**22.7**	**26.6**	**30.0**

Source: Zajac and Pazitny 2002.

Table 9.13 Development of Debts in the Inpatient Care Sector (millions of Slovak Crowns)

Health Establishments	31.12.2005	30.6.2006	31.12.2006	30.6. 2007	31.12.2007	31.12.2010
– under Ministry of Health	2 033	2 887	4 435	5 155	5 842	6 960
– private companies	x	15	14	21	6	
– under self-governments	2 384*	2 342*	2 275*	2 094*	1 960	2 525
– non-profit organizations	x	x	x	x	194	
Cumulative debt	5 634	5 523	6 821	7 292	8 074	9 505

*including non-profit organizations.
Source: <www.health.gov.sk>.

After the reforms in 2004, the system deficit situation improved slightly but Table 9.13 indicates that the positive trends have been very short-term. (Data comparative with Tables 9.11 and 9.12 are not possible due to changes in the methodology of reporting.)

9.7 Resources in Slovakia's Health Care System

Slovakia spends about 7% of its GDP on health care (see Table 9.4), which is below the average of developed countries. WHO (2010) reports that, as a share of GDP, average expenditures for health care in the world in 2007 were 9.7%; for European countries 8.8% and for Slovakia 7.7%. In nominal terms (purchasing parity) the situation is slightly better: Slovakia US$1,555 per inhabitant, world average US$863, and Europe US$1,875. However, the figure for developed EU countries ranges between US$3,500 and US$5,700.

The core problem is the base. The performance of Slovak national economy is far below the EU average (and in purchasing parity terms as well). In such a situation the promise to deliver 'European' quality of health care to everyone independent of the ability to pay could only be achieved via extremely high efficiency of the system.

In relative terms, compulsory social health insurance premiums are similar to many developed countries. Initially the level of the insurance premium was set at 13.7% of an income-related base and increased to 14% from 2002 onwards. Limited collections in monetary terms are the result of two limits:

- The state budget is expected to pay into the health insurance scheme for a large group of persons without regular income – a group representing about 3.5 million from a total of 5.5 million inhabitants. The state funds this group of citizen at a very low level; Parliament sets the amount to be paid on a yearly basis when voting on the state budget. Formally it was expected that the rules for 'state' and 'private/self' insurers would be similar (14% of the base). However, the state never contributed the full amount (the level of transfer ranged from 3% to 5% of the minimum wage) so the system is not provided with expected amount of resources from the state budget.

Table 9.14 Contributions from the State Budget to the Health Insurance System

	1995	**2000**	**2005**	**2010**
Contribution per 'state' insured person (Slovak Crowns)	181	283	690	€35.4
Total contribution (billons Slovak Crowns)	7.1	11.2	21.1	€1.1

Source: <www.finance.gov.sk>.

- The insurance premium is derived from an income-related base. For employees the maximum base is 300% of average salary two years previously (€2,233.50 in 2011), which is very low. Many self-employed taxpayers pay contributions from a minimum base that is 44% of an average salary two years previously (€329.60 in 2011).

9.8 Costs of the Health Care System

Limited revenues require the system to focus on cost-containment measures, efficiency and economy in order to balance demand with supply of available resources. However, little has been done in this respect since 1989. The most important inefficiencies are over-employment, low economic performance of hospitals and ineffective policies for the regulation of drugs.

Table 9.5 highlighted issues of employment. Although 'over-employment' was accepted as a significant problem from the beginning of the post-1989 reforms, the total number of health personnel changed very little during the entire period. Overstaffing of physicians and accompanying health staff in relation to EU-15 has been a key issue (Verhoeven *et al.* 2007). The relatively low salaries of medical staff compensate for such overstaffing since doctors receive only about 150% of average wage, but this is only a short-term solution. In the Czech Republic, a successful strike by doctors in 2011 produced a massive wage increase.

Ineffective drug management is another core deficiency. The costs for drugs doubled between 1996 and 2002, and the trend continues. As Table 9.15 indicates, the share of pharmaceuticals in total health expenditures is high and current trends are similar. Although

Table 9.15 Expenditure on Pharmaceuticals 1999-2002 (Averages)

Country	Public Expenditure (% of Public Health Expenditure)	Public and Private (% of Public & Private Expenditure)	Public Expenditure (PPP$ per Capita)	Public and Private Expenditure (PPP$ per Capita)
Slovak Republic	31.8	34.8	180.8	220.8
Czech Republic	19.0	22.2	178.5	232.0
Hungary	24.9	28.1	165.3	293.0
Poland	15.0	28.4	67.5	208.0
NMS-10 average	22.7	26.1	148.0	238.4
EU-15 average	13.4	15.4	200.4	334.6
OECD average	14.1	17.4	184.9	330.9

Source: Verhoeven *et al.* 2007.

partly explained by the changing structure of drugs used (import of more effective but also more expensive medications at international market prices), the trend is also caused by ineffective regulation of drug prescriptions. Tools of evidence-based medicine are still not used for setting the rules for medications, to whom and under what circumstances to prescribe, leaving the space open for lobbying of pharmaceutical firms that bribe doctors to prescribe more expensive drugs as well as larger amounts of drugs than necessary. Insurance companies have no mechanism to handle such over-prescriptions.

The ineffective regulation of prescriptions is currently the core negative factor in this area. Regulation of prices and reimbursement rules improved significantly during last decade and now approximate international practice. During the second Dzurinda government, electronic auctions became the tool to set prices. While subsequent governments did not adopt this method, its replacement with internationally refereed prices is acceptable and may be even more transparent (benchmark are lowest prices in EU). After 2012 a doctor's prescription may only indicate the effective substance; the choice of the concrete drug will be at the pharmacy.

The most costly and financially complicated part of Slovakia's health care system is inpatient care. The hospital system regularly generates debt as older data reveal in Table 9.16 while Table 9.13 provides more recent information. Fixed costs remain the most important problem. At 60-70% occupancy, current bed capacity is not utilized well while costs to operate poorly constructed and excessively large buildings are not acceptable. In 2011 the Slovak government 'navigated' insurance companies towards significant reductions of reimbursed beds, thus pushing hospitals to close selected wards.

Table 9.16 Performance of Hospitals (Millions of Slovak Crowns)

	1996	**1997**	**1998**	**1999**	**2000**	**2001**
Number of patients	**1 055 757**	**1 090 672**	**1 109 210**	**1 059 533**	**1 063 611**	**NA**
Change %	2.6	3.3	1.7	(–) 4.5	0.4	NA
Costs						21.6
Fixed costs	15.4	17.7	19.3	19.3	19.7	6.5
Variable costs	6.1	6.4	6.3	5.7	6.3	28.1
Total costs	21.5	24.1	25.6	25.0	26.0	8.1
Total costs – % change		12.1	6.2	(–) 2.3	4.0	24.9
Revenues	**19.8**	**22.9**	**22.3**	**20.2**	**22.5**	**(–) 3.2**
Balance	**(–) 1.7**	**(–) 1.2**	**(–) 3.3**	**(–) 4.8**	**(–) 3.5**	

Source: Zajac and Pazitny 2002.

Low quality procurement and outsourcing are other important sources of ineffective hospital financial management. Vlach *et al.* (2004) indicate sources that remain valid. In 2011 a new public procurement law introduced compulsory e-auctions as the main method to purchase goods, but results from this change remain unclear. Based on a sample of medium-sized hospitals, the process of public procurement was investigated.

Concerning the organization of public procurement, one hospital lacked qualified staff – *i.e.*, legally certified as responsible for public procurement – and no hospital prepared a public procurement plan nor an audit of public procurement outcomes. Public procurement processes in hospitals are not supported by effective software and data are of very low quality. Most hospitals have their own web pages but these rarely display procurement information. Joint procurement and frame contracts are not regularly used. Based on these indirect indicators, the quality of the organizational system for public procurement in Slovak hospitals is low.

In order to evaluate the quality of financial management in hospitals via public procurement processes, outcomes were evaluated by benchmarking the final prices of goods and services procured compared to standard market prices. This approach to evaluate public procurement was used in Slovakia for the first time. Data obtained by benchmarking indicate significant differences between unit prices under which hospitals procure medications, medical equipment, daily goods and services. Since all data were obtained directly from the account books of hospitals they are fairly reliable. Results show the quality of public procurement in hospitals measured by outcomes to be very low. Strangfeldova (2008) investigated hospital performance in Slovakia. Despite a limited sample (many hospitals refused to provide data), findings indicate important reserves both on the level of public and private providers.

9.9 Dimensions of Health Policy

Many sources argue that there is no consistent health policy in Slovakia (Slovensko 2001, 2002). The main problems of the health care system are well known, described, and publicly named. These include misbalances between the amount of resources available and the scale of care provided free at the point of delivery. However, no Slovak government before 2002 reacted to them and the Fico government largely reversed the 2004 reforms.

Mazmanian and Sabatier (1989, summarized by Pavlík 2008) list preconditions for successful policy-making. Table 9.17 assesses the level of their achievement in Slovakia as these policy arguments partly explain Slovakia's limited success in reforming its health care system.

While some experts may argue that the statements above have a normative character, the picture is clear.

Table 9.17 Preconditions for Implementation of Health Care Reforms in Slovakia

Assumption	Evaluation
Main actors support effective health care reforms and their implementation	– Hospitals are normally unconstrained by hard budgetary constraints. Their managements are able and frequently like to channel part of institutional finance into private pockets because official salaries are low. – Doctors are normally unconstrained by hard budgetary constraints and professional regulations. Many utilize the potential for supplier-induced demand by ordering extra treatments, equipment and drugs. They have job control over shadow incomes to compensate for low official salaries. – Politicians benefit from providing their voters with "free" universal coverage and from many (albeit unrealized) promises. – Bureaucrats with extra resources increase their power. – Patients are not well informed and can be persuaded to opt for better (more expensive) drugs or treatments, even if not needed. They accept the fact that they are not customers, but "slaves" of the system. – Insurance companies are not independent and do not serve as regulators, but only as resource distribution channels. For them more resources means a higher level of overheads for their own use. *Conclusion: Preconditions for successful reform never existed.* Only one main player might be willing to change the system – the 'clever and responsive' government of elected politicians; the 2004 reform was partly such an example. Data indicate that a left-wing government's main goal is universal access, independent of the system's financial situation. Thus the potential of any populist government to change the system is almost zero because cost containment-based health reform is too painful.
Replacing politics with evidence-based policies	In Slovakia real public policy does not exist and may not appear in short term perspective. Decisions of political parties are based on rent-seeking principles (rent has different forms, like extra votes or financial gain). Without databases and benchmarking systems, evidence-based policy is technically impossible. Independent advice is rarely available and not requested. *Conclusion: Preconditions for successful reform never existed.*
Strong position of government in the Parliament	During all periods of modern Slovakia, coalition governments have been in power, many of them with a marginal majority. *Conclusion: Full preconditions for successful reform never existed. The best situation was in 2006-2010.*

Table 9.17 Preconditions for Implementation of Health Care Reforms in Slovakia

Assumption	Evaluation
Co-operation within the governing coalition	In most cases, the party leading a coalition has not been supported by its partners on issues of health care reforms; during the Fico government, his party was the 'lead' party. *Conclusion: Full preconditions for successful reform never existed. The best situation was in 2006-2010.*
Support of changes by voters	Slovak voters (with paternalistic attitudes and fiscally 'deluded') are not ready to support radical changes in the health care system. *Conclusion: Preconditions for successful reform never existed.*
Sufficient resources to realize the reform	Slovak health care is underfinanced and extra public resources are difficult to find. The main way to increase resources is connected with the mobilization of private funding. *Conclusion: Preconditions for successful reform never existed.*
Stability	On average there were at least two health ministers per each electoral period. Continuity and stability do not exist within election periods nor between them (even with the same leader). *Conclusions: Preconditions for successful reform never existed.*
Well formulated reform targets and paths to achieve them	All governments formulate new reform strategies, but such documents were mainly proclamations unsupported by realization documents. The exception is the second Dzurinda government. *Conclusion: Preconditions for successful reform partly existed in 2002-2006.*
Existence of "professional" policy making capacity, local knowledge and skills	– During the 1990s, when most reforms began, there was lack of general and specific expertise to set effective health reform policy. No country in the world had previous experience with transformation from a centrally managed and planned society to a market-based democratic one. The main driving force behind reforms was to depart as quickly as possible and to detach as much as possible from past. – Persons responsible for health reforms were mainly medical doctors with limited economic background and, in some cases, protected the interests of the medical profession. – Many governments have been unstable and short-lived coalitions of different political groups while ministers of health changed frequently. – The relation between politicians and bureaucrats was not standard. A professional and sustainable system of bureaucracy was not established. Administrative structures changed when the government or the minister changed (OECD 2009). *Conclusion: The precondition of effective "internal and professional" policy formulation was not fulfilled.*

9.10 Conclusions

This chapter explored the development of Slovak health policy and its health sector across two decades. The initial post-Velvet Revolution reforms showed no sign of popular influences but a desire by the new elite to mark a clean break with the past, plus some foreign advice, led to the choice of the pluralistic health insurance model. Together with the Czech Republic this approach was unique in Central and Eastern Europe. The most visible change has been the substantial increase of expenditures on health care both absolutely and as a proportion of GDP, although these remain below EU expenditure levels.

Many positive improvements have been achieved during reforms of the Slovak health care system after 1989. The health status of inhabitants shows significant progress due to more resources, improved technologies, and better life styles. The maintenance of largely universal access is another advantage. Yet problems remain such as chronic financial imbalances; an inability to fashion an effective prescription policy; limitations in insurance companies' regulatory performance, stemming from an unwillingness by left-populist governments to delegate authority; the primacy of politics over health policy; economic decisions influenced by local interest groups, ideologies or coalition politics; and the inability of left-wing governments to implement necessary reforms.

10 The Health Care System in Slovenia, 1980-2011

Stanka Setnikar-Cankar and Veronika Petkovšek

The chapter describes facts and changes in the field of health care in Slovenia from 1980 to 2011. The aim of the analysis is to study and analyze significant data, trends, changes and open issues within Slovenian health care. The conclusions were achieved by synthesizing data from statistical and health databases. After describing demographic and national economic data, the chapter examines public and private expenditures on health care and their proportion of Gross Domestic Product (GDP). The largest share of spending on health care is public through compulsory health insurance but the share of private spending is rising due to voluntary health insurance funds (HIF) and direct payments. Most expenditures on health care are allocated for curative services, medicines and medical goods. The factors of production are then presented through trends in the numbers of medical staff, hospital beds, and the value of equipment. During the period studied, the number of nurses increased significantly while the number of doctors increased slowly. The number of hospital beds declined year by year.

The next section describes the nature of Slovenian public health care. The Slovenian health care system is based on a network of public and private health care providers at primary, secondary and tertiary levels. Private providers can work within the public network with a concession or outside as 'purely private'. Compulsory health insurance assures the basic rights to health services for Slovenian citizens and other insured parties. The financing system for health care is based on a public-private model. Health care is financed by public and private sources of compulsory and voluntary HIFs and by direct payments.

The results of previous health reforms and the plans and aims of future reforms are presented. Despite the changes introduced by two reforms during the period studied, the Slovenian health system faces a number of problems. A new reform of health system was planned in 2010 but was not implemented. An upgrade of Slovenia's health care system is expected in the near future. If Slovenia wants its health care to remain sustainable in future, it needs to modernize the health system and amend its laws about health care.

10.1 Introduction

Over the past decade the Slovenian health system has faced increasing needs and expectations from the general public. Slovenia inherited a relatively sound health system from the former Yugoslavia, and it has maintained the high level of social solidarity. Nonetheless Slovenia has experienced several negative trends that have made health care conditions more difficult and reduced both solidarity and fairness.

Providing adequate funding is an increasing problem within the Slovenian health system. The biggest challenge comes from demographic, socio-economic, medical, pharmaceutical and technological trends that cause growth in health care costs. The ageing of the population is a major trend as it has changed both the need and the demand for health services. Another challenge to maintaining health service provision at an adequate level within the public sector is the pressure to modernize medical procedures. Technology can mean greater financial investment as well as greater effectiveness. The result of these pressures is increased growth in health costs (*Poslovno poročilo ZZZS za leto 2009* 2010:14-15, 18). The key question within the Slovenian health system is how to maintain a suitable level of access and quality in conditions while financial resources remain fixed or are even reduced. The health system must provide citizens with equal access to health services and a level of care appropriate to their health regardless of age, income, sex, employment or place of residence. At the same time, the system must ensure that all members of society contribute to health care funds on the basis of fairness and solidarity (Tajnikar 2009:6).

The geographical size of the Republic of Slovenia is 20,273 km^2 and its population in 2010 was 2,048,951. Since 1980, the population has grown by 139,385. The population grew from 1980 to 1990, fluctuated until 1999 and since then has grown consistently. As Table 10.1 indicates, life expectancy in Slovenia is increasing for both males and females. The life expectancy of a boy born in Slovenia in 2010 is 76 compared to 83 years for a girl. Over the past three decades, life expectancy has increased by eight years for females and nine years for males. Similar progress has been evident in the rate of infant mortality. Between 1984 and 2010 the number of infant deaths has declined year by year. In 1985 infant deaths per 1,000 live births were 13.1, ten years later 5.5 and in 2010 2.5 per 1,000 live births.

The population of Slovenia continues to grow, primarily due to immigration, but Slovenia faces negative natural growth and an ageing population. These trends represent a direct threat to the long-term financial stability of the health system. The reduced working population has a smaller income potential while the ageing of the population exacerbates pressures leading to the growth of health care and other costs. Demographic projections indicate that Slovenian population will continue to age. This development is due to

Table 10.1 Demographic Data, 1980-2010

Year	Year-End Population	Life Expectancy at Birth		Infant Mortality Rate (Per 1000 Live Births)
		Male	Female	
1980	1 909 566	67	75	–
1985	1 975 273	68	76	13.1
1990	1 999 945	69	77	8.4
1995	1 990 266	71	78	5.5
2000	1 990 094	72	80	4.9
2005	2 003 358	75	82	4.1
2009	2 042 335	75	82	2.5
2010	2 048 951	76	83	2.5

Sources: Statistični letopis 2009; Statistični letopis 2010; European Health for All Database 2011; *Poslovno poročilo ZZZS za leto 2011*, 2012: 14.

Table 10.2 Economic Indicators, 1995-2011

Year	GDP€ Million (Current Prices)	GDP € Per Capita	% GDP Growth	Inflation Rate (Percentage)
1995	10 294.3	8 101	4.1	12.6
2000	18 480.7	10 858	4.4	8.9
2005	28 749.6	14 369	4.5	2.5
2010	35 415.8	17 300	1.4	2.1
2011	35 638.6	17 400	−0.2	2.1

Source: Eurostat 2012.

increased life expectancy at birth, lower fertility, lower infant mortality as well as population emigration (*Obvezno zdravstveno zavarovanje v Sloveniji: danes za jutri* 2007:23).

Slovenia has also been affected by the global economic and financial crisis. The lowest rate of economic growth in Slovenia during the period studied was minus 7.8% in 2009 when GDP per capita declined by €1,275 in comparison with the previous year and reached €17,092. Between 1995 and 2011, the highest rate of economic growth was 6.8% in 2007.

In 2010, the rate of economic growth increased to 1.4%, but in 2011 it was minus 0.2%. In 2011, GDP per capita grew to €17,400. In 2009 the inflation rate fell to 0.9% compared with the previous year but increased to 2.1% in 2010 and stayed at the same rate in 2011.

10.2 Health Expenditures in Slovenia, 1995-2011

Public spending at all levels grew between 1996 and 2001 and fluctuated between 2002 and 2008. After 2008, public spending at all levels grew again and in 2011 it was 50.9% of GDP, with public expenditures on health care at 6.4% of GDP. The latter figure includes general, specialist and hospital health services, the supply of medicines and medical products, aids and equipment, applied research and development, and other health activities (*Prva statistična objava* 2009). Table 10.3 indicates that the share of total expenditures on health care in 2011 was 9% of GDP with the public share at 71.4% (6.4% of GDP) and the private share 28.6% (2.6% of GDP).

Most funding of health care in Slovenia is provided by public sources. Most of these public funds come from compulsory health insurance, which represented 66.7% of total health spending in 2011. The remainder of public expenditures is provided by municipal and national budgets that together represented 4.8% of total spending in 2011. Meanwhile, a significant proportion of health spending comes from private funds that, according to 2011 estimates, were worth 28.6% of total health spending. The insurance companies that offer voluntary health insurance contribute most of the private funds. The other private

Table 10.3 Expenditures (Percentage of GDP or Total Health Expenditures), 1995-2011

Year	All Public Spending (% GDP)	Total Health Spending (% GDP)	Public Spending on Health Care (% GDP)	Public Spending on Health Care (% Total)	Private Health Care Spending (% GDP)	Private Health Care Spending (% Total)
1995	52.6	7.5	5.8	77.7	1.7	22.3
2000	46.7	8.3	6.1	74.0	2.2	26.0
2005	45.3	8.7	6.3	71.9	2.4	28.1
2010	50.3	9.1	6.6	71.9	2.5	28.1
2011	50.9	9.0	6.4	71.4	2.6	28.6

Sources: Statistični letopis 2010; European Health for All Database 2011; *Poslovno poročilo ZZZS za leto 2010,* 2011: 146; *Poslovno poročilo ZZZS za leto 2011, 2012:144.*

expenditure comprises spending on various goods and health services that people in Slovenia pay directly "from their own pockets" (Table 10.4).

Since the introduction of voluntary health insurance in 1992, the proportion of public spending on health care in Slovenia has declined while private spending has increased with intermediate fluctuation. The burden of additional financing for health care has shifted to private spending by the population in the form of voluntary health insurance and direct payments, *i.e.* payments from "patients' own pockets". Access to health services is increasingly achieved via direct payments. In 2011 direct household spending accounted for 13.7% of total health expenditures or 47.9% of all private health expenditures (Table 10.5).

As Table 10.6 reveals, half of total health expenditures (50.8% in 2003; 52.5% in 2010) were used to finance curative health services, followed by medicines and medical goods (23.3% in 2003; 22.4% in 2010) and long-term care (7.2% in 2003; 8.3% in 2010). Between 2003 and 2010, the proportion of health expenditures on different types of services changed little in the total share of health expenditures but has changed in sources of financing. The share of health expenditures for rehabilitation services, auxiliary services, medicines and

Table 10.4 Total Health Expenditures in 2010 and 2011(*estimate)

	2010		2011*	
	Structure in%	**% of GDP**	**Structure in%**	**% of GDP**
Total health care funding	**100.0**	**9.1**	**100.0**	**9.0**
Public funding	**71.9**	**6.6**	**71.4**	**6.4**
National budget funds	3.8	0.4	3.9	0.3
Municipal budget funds	0.9	0.1	0.9	0.1
Compulsory health insurance	67.2	6.1	66.7	6.0
Private funding	**28.1**	**2.5**	**28.6**	**2.6**
Voluntary health insurance	13.4	1.2	13.7	1.2
Direct payments	13.4	1.2	13.7	1.2
Companies (excluding insurers) and non-profit institutions	1.2	0.1	1.2	0.2

Sources: Poslovno poročilo ZZZS za leto 2010, 2011:146; *Poslovno poročilo ZZZS za leto 2011,* 2012:144.

Table 10.5 Direct Payments (Percentages), 1995-2011 (*Estimate)

Year	Private Health Care Expenditures (% Total Health Care Spending)	Direct Payments (% Total Health Expenditures)	Direct Payments (% Private Health Expenditures)
1995	22.3	11.2	50.3
2000	26.0	11.5	44.2
2005	28.1	12.5	44.5
2010	28.1	13.4	47.7
2011*	28.6	13.7	47.9

Sources: European Health for All Database 2011; *Poslovno poročilo ZZZS za leto 2010,* 2011:146; *Poslovno poročilo ZZZS za leto 2011,* 2012:144.

Table 10.6 Health Expenditures (Types of Service and Sources of Financing)

	Percentages in 2003			Percentages in 2010		
Type of Service	**Total**	**Public Sector (% of Total)**	**Private Sector (% of Total)**	**Total**	**Public Sector (% of Total**	**Private Sector (% of Total)**
Curative care	50.8	79.1	20.9	52.5	80.0	20.0
Rehabilitation	2.1	57.3	42.7	2.2	48.9	51.1
Long-term care	7.2	94.3	5.7	8.3	96.8	3.2
Auxiliary services	2.5	71.8	28.2	3.3	68.2	31.8
Medicines and goods	23.3	55.9	44.1	22.4	49.9	50.1
Preventive health	3.4	77.1	22.9	3.7	75.6	24.4
Health care and health insurance management	4.5	59.2	40.8	3.4	60.0	40.0
Investment	6.2	59.5	40.5	4.2	84.3	15.7
Total	**100.0**	**72.0**	**28.0**	**100.0**	**72.8**	**27.2**

Sources: Prva statistična objava 2011; *Prva statistična objava* 2012.

medical goods and preventive health services grew in the private sector and fell in the public sector. The opposite occurred for curative health services, long-term care, health insurance and investment where the share of health expenditures grew in the public sector and fell in the private sector.

The principal factors influencing the growth in health expenditures are demographic changes, development of medical technology and medicines and growth in income. Demographic projections indicate that the proportion of the population aged over 65 will increase. Health spending on those above 65 years of age was several times higher than on the younger population. The development of medical technology and medicines requires significant funding for research and development. The costs of modern technology are reflected in the rapid growth of treatment costs (Kranjec 2007:1-2).

10.3 Factors of Production in Health Care

Until 1999, the number of doctors in Slovenia fluctuated; thereafter the number has gradually increased. Table 10.7 indicates that the number of doctors reached a total of 4,979 in 2010 or 243 doctors per 100,000 inhabitants. The biggest shortfall is among general practitioners, which generates problems concerning adequate regional coverage (*Socialni razgledi 2009* 2010:42). The number of nurses has increased substantially since 1992; in 2010 Slovenia had 16,771 nurses or 818 nurses per 100,000 inhabitants.

In 2010, Slovenia also had 457 hospital beds per 100,000 inhabitants. As Table 10.8 indicates, the number of hospital beds per 100,000 inhabitants declined during 1980-2010 – a

Table 10.7 Health Care Staff, 1992-2010

Year	Doctors	Doctors Per 100,000 Inhabitants	Nurses	Nurses Per 100,000 Inhabitants
1992	4 169	209	11 223	562
1995	4 206	212	12 705	639
2000	4 317	217	13 765	692
2005	4 723	236	15 057	752
2009	4 915	241	16 370	802
2010	4 979	243	16 771	818

Sources: Institute of Public Health 2009; *Socialni razgledi 2009,* 2010:42; European Health for All Database 2011; OECD.StatExtracts, 2012.

Table 10.8 Hospital Beds and Occupancy Rates, 1980-2010

Year	Hospital Beds	Occupancy Rate (%)	Beds/100 000 Inhabitants
1980	13 183	88	695
1985	12 496	85	633
1990	12 081	82	605
1995	11 411	77	574
2000	10 745	71	540
2005	9 666	70	483
2009	9 389	71	459
2010	9 367	71	457

Sources: Institute of Public Health 2009; European Health for All Database 2011; OECD.StatExtracts, 2012.

Table 10.9 Value of Equipment and Tangible Assets, 2001-2011

Year	Equipment Value (€ Thousand)	Proportion of HIIS Funds in Total Assets (%)
2001	8 554	9.4
2005	4 257	2.9
2010	7 077	3.1
2011	5 599	1.9

Source: Poslovna poročila ZZZS za leta 2001, 2005, 2010 and 2011.

decline mainly in acute hospital beds due to shortening the average period of stay in hospitals and using day-visits (*Socialni razgledi 2009* 2010:43-44).

The share of funds for equipment in the total assets of the Health Insurance Institute of Slovenia (HIIS) declined from 9.4% in 2001 to 2.7% in 2009. In 2010, the share of funds for equipment increased to 3.1% and again fell to 1.9% in 2011. Investment is needed to upgrade health sector equipment.

10.4 State of Public Health Care in Slovenia

The basic principles of health care in Slovenia are fairness, solidarity, access, quality and effectiveness. The principles of fairness and solidarity emphasize that the system's users must receive equal treatment, regardless of ability to pay. The solidarity principle is expressed in six different forms relating to illness, income, age, sex, employment status and place of residence (Tajnikar 2009:6). Slovenia has a network of public and private health providers at primary (health centres), secondary (hospitals) and tertiary levels (clinics, clinical institutes and clinical departments). The health system is based on social health insurance that respects the principles of solidarity, non-profit-making and social justice.

Health insurance has a long tradition in Slovenia. In the early 19th century, workers established 'fraternity funds' based on solidarity and mutuality. The first sickness fund in Slovenia was founded in 1889 and similar providers of health insurance followed. Initially health insurance was only compulsory for workers but gradually expanded to other population groups. Despite changes in the organization of health protection, Slovenia has retained the main features of health insurance such as funding by contributions from employers and employees, autonomy and self-governance (*Obvezno zdravstveno zavarovanje v Sloveniji: danes za jutri* 2007:11).

All inhabitants of Slovenia are included in compulsory health insurance. Compulsory health insurance provides insured parties with two basic sets of rights: to health care and to cash benefits or reimbursements. The HIIS provides insured parties with access to health services on the basis of partnerships. Adequate access and appropriate quality of health services are keys to the protection of insured parties. Equal provision of doctors and other capacities to the population is an essential component (*Poslovno poročilo ZZZS za leto 2009* (2010:16, 28, 38).

10.5 HEALTH SECTOR MANAGEMENT

At the end of the 1980s the management of Slovenia's health system passed into the exclusive hands of the state. Health funding became part of the republic's budget, a change that caused financial instability within the health system and led to proposals for new laws. Since the introduction of voluntary health insurance in 1992, Slovenia has had a mixed public-private model for financing health care. Health care is financed by public and private sources of compulsory and voluntary health insurance and by direct payments (*Obvezno zdravstveno zavarovanje v Sloveniji: danes za jutri* 2007:11, 45).

The problems associated with funding health care through compulsory health insurance have increased the pressure for supplementary payments to become usual practice and a source of regular financing for health care. The supplementary payments then force the population to subscribe to voluntary health insurance that has eliminated one mechanism for the promotion of health care effectiveness (Tajnikar and Došenovič Bonča 2010:2-3).

Expenditures on health care staff constitute the largest proportion of health costs. Depending on the level at which health services are delivered, various payment methods are applied. The primary level combines systems of capitation and fee-for-service – each providing about half of the funds. The secondary level (hospital care) uses a diagnosis-related group (DRG) payment method. Hospitals plan the volume of funds according to the number of cases in line with standard average length of stay while a fee-for-service system is used for specialist departments. Standards are defined for specific clinical specializations that define the annual financing plan (Ceglar 2004:26-27; Setnikar-Cankar and Seljak 2006:178, 179).

Plurality within Slovenia's health system is evident in patterns of ownership as well as the relations between private and public property of health providers and those who provide funding. Slovenia has two parallel health systems – public and private. Until 1992 health care was provided exclusively by public health institutions but thereafter private provision of health services within the public sector has been enabled by the award of concessions. Private providers are divided into private providers operating entirely within the market and providers operating within the publicly financed health system. The proportion of private health service providers in Slovenia has increased in recent years, particularly in the public health network. The highest proportion of private practice is among general practitioners (*Socialni razgledi* 2009:43-44).

The number of private concession-holders increased throughout the period from 1993 to 2010, with the exception of 2011 when the number fell slightly. In addition to private practitioners who operate within the public health network with an HIIS contract, 'purely private' practitioners provide services that are not included in the public network. Patients

Figure 10.1 HIIS Contracts with Health Centres, 1993-2011

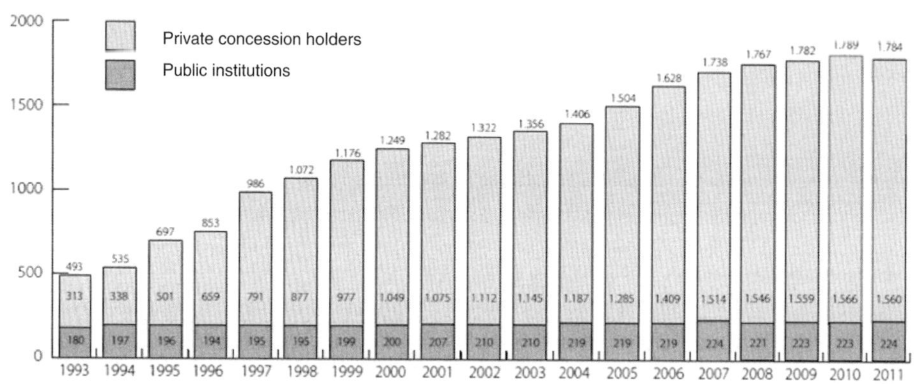

Source: *Poslovno poročilo ZZZS za leto 2011*, 2012:143.

Figure 10.2 Doctors in Health Institutions and Doctors with Concessions in 2011

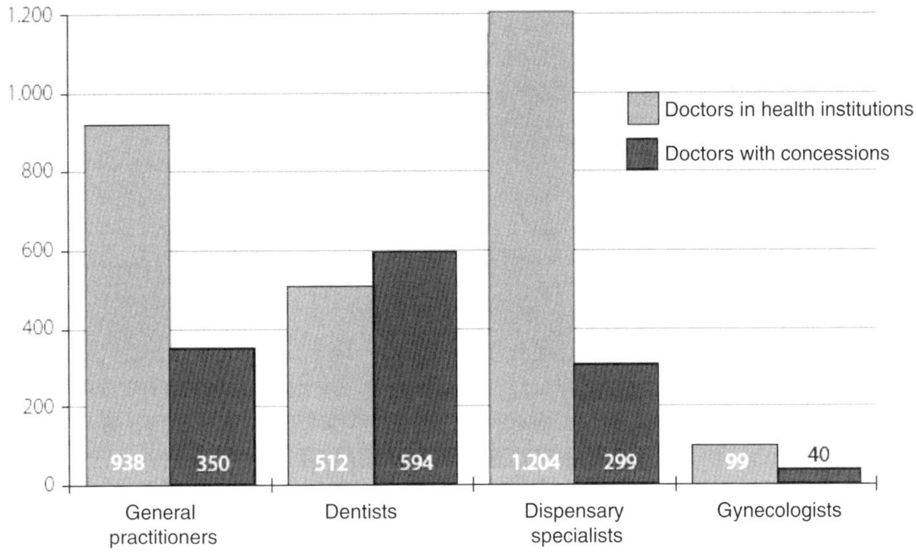

Source: Poslovno poročilo ZZZS za leto 2011, 2012:36.

themselves must pay for all these services except for urgent medical assistance (Gregorič Rogelj 2009:9; *Poslovno poročilo ZZZS za leto 2011*, 2012:143).

Cooperation between public and private health sectors has been primarily organized through concessions. A concession is a transfer of the authorization to provide a service from the state to an authorized body or civil law entity. Co-financing by private capital has been unusual. The main motive of the public sector for engaging in public-private partnerships is to provide funds for investment and better quality services for users within the limits of public funds (Gregorič Rogelj 2008:51-52, 54; Setnikar-Cankar and Seljak 2006:188).

Cases of public-private partnership, including those where private partners invested funds to construct health facilities, are rare. One such case was the construction of a dialysis centre in Sežana Hospital in 2004-2005 with an investment of €2.5 million. Sežana Hospital acquired an investor who was prepared to implement construction work and purchase equipment for the dialysis centre. The next example was the construction of three primary health facilities in the Gorenjska region worth €6.6 million that involved four partners: municipalities, the state (ministries), public health institutions and private investors. Another case was the construction of a new entrance and supporting facilities at the Institute of Republic of Slovenia for Rehabilitation. The investment amounted to €4.7 million and a public-private partnership concession was agreed. The fourth case is a public-private partnership in the field of energy savings assurance and fuel supply in Brežice General Hospital. The object of the project was reconstruction of boiler plants that would lower heating costs (Gregorič Rogelj 2008:97-118). Two other cases qualify as public-private partnerships. One was construction of a garage for the University Medical Centre in Maribor; the other provided parking spaces near Jesenice General Hospital in cooperation with a private partner (Gregorič Rogelj 2011).

10.6 Health Reform in Slovenia

Health care legislation underwent a major revision in 1992. The new act formed the basis for the current system of compulsory and voluntary health insurance, promoted the process of privatization of the health care system and defined in detail the role of the key partners. The changes introduced by the 1992 reform included funding as it reintroduced compulsory and voluntary health insurance that brought new private funds into the health system. The law created a mixed public-private model for funding health care as well as structural changes in the implementation of health services. These changes led to a partial privatization of health providers within the network of public services and introduced the free choice of doctor at the primary level of health care. New roles and partners were defined including professional medical associations, and a new model was promulgated for partnerships and contracts (*Obvezno zdravstveno zavarovanje v Sloveniji: danes do jutri* 2007:11). The second major Slovenian health reform occurred in 2003 that introduced a payment model in which the money was to follow the patient. It was intended to improve the function, management and governance of the health system (Keber 2003).

A reform had been planned in 2010 and 2011 to address the problems in Slovenian health care – inappropriate distribution of capacity, lack of adequate information required for decision-making, problems at different management levels in the health system, and challenges related to the mission of health care – but it was not realized. Only the draft amendment of a new Health Care Act is available that sketched an enhancement of primary health care, a reorganization of secondary health care, the establishment of a quality system and changes in economic conditions.

The current situation in Slovenian health care makes it necessary to introduce legislative changes to adapt to the need for and the development of a flexible health system – one that can effectively meet the needs of citizens. The strategic objective of such legislation is to rationalize and reorganize the health system, and to reorganize health insurance (Gregorič Rogelj 2012). In 2011 the government adopted two laws: the Act Amending the Patients' Rights Act and the Healthcare Databases Act (*Nadgradnja zdravstvenega sistema* 2012).

Another problem that needs to be solved is inadequate definition of the basis for insurance, categories of insured persons and contribution rates – all of which have led to discrimination between different categories. Likewise changes are needed is the basket of rights to health care, which is currently universal. The new basic basket of rights will be funded in full from public resources (compulsory health insurance); private funding will cover the other rights not included in the basket of basic rights.

The aim for development of health care in the future is to increase the share of public funding for health care from 73 to 80% with a corresponding reduction in private funding – the latter now to consist mainly of supplementary health insurance premiums and direct payments. The Ministry of Health has indicated three options on how to increase public funding gradually for the provision of health services. The first option is to increase the contribution rate by two percentage points and maintain the current basket of rights in compulsory health insurance. This would cover all services in full, which means that there would be no more charges and thus no supplementary insurance. The second option also offers the abolition of supplementary health insurance, taking a lesser increase in the contribution rate (1.4 percentage points) but with a reduction in the basket of rights. Candidates for elimination from the basket of rights are primarily services that are currently largely paid from supplementary insurance. The third option does not provide for the abolition of supplementary insurance, but its contraction. In this case, the contribution rate would increase slightly (by 0.57 percentage points) and the basket of rights would be slightly reduced (*Dopolnilno zdravstveno zavarovanje in zdravstvena reforma* 2011: 22).

Changes of a more long-term nature are also proposed, with public institutions for health care at primary and secondary levels beginning to integrate horizontally and vertically into knowledge centres. The goal of integration is to optimize costs and improve the quality and accessibility of health services. It also proposes to establish a clear and transparent definition of the provision of public and private services by public institutions through the provision of separate accounting and record-keeping for individual health services (*Nadgradnja zdrav-stvenega sistema do leta 2020: korak naprej* 2011:8, 14, 17-18; Gregorič Rogelj 2012).

In 2012, when financial measures were accepted to achieve fiscal stability in Slovenia, a number of proposals for the health sector was put forward, such as reduction in the percentage of services covered by compulsory health insurance, centralization of the purchase of medical and technical instruments (public procurement), the classification of drugs to take account of drug interactions, and the working arrangements of health workers under fee-based contracts. However, to a large extent, these proposed measures have not been accepted.

10.7 Conclusion

The Slovenian health system faces the problem of how to provide sufficient financial resources for health care at a time when both the needs and the expectations of the population are increasing. Slovenia's population is ageing – a trend that will exacerbate pressures on the health budget. Total expenditures on health care account for 9% of GDP, of which approximately 70% is paid by public sources and 30% by private sources. Most public money (around 90%) comes from compulsory HIFs. A smaller amount (around 4%) comes from national and municipal budgets. Households pay private expenditures through voluntary HIFs and direct payments. The latter direct payments already account for almost 48% of private health spending. Over three-quarters of current expenditures on health are used to finance curative health services, medicines and medical goods.

The number of doctors in Slovenia gradually increased over the period studied while the number of nurses increased more significantly. The number of hospital bed declined almost every year and by 2010 Slovenia had only 457 hospital beds per 100,000 inhabitants. The proportion of funds for equipment also declined from 9.4% in 2001 to 1.9% in 2011.

The health system in Slovenia needs a radical overhaul in terms of the organization, management and financing of general and long-term care. Particular attention must be paid to the quality and efficiency of performance. Improvements to the health system in Slovenia must be based upon several fundamental principles: the provision of geographical access to health care; the provision of high-quality and safe services; and the provision of financial access to services for specific population categories through a redefinition of the basket of rights to health care. The health system must reduce inequalities in health care services but also become competitive and development-oriented.

The key challenges to achieving and following the basic principles for an upgrade of the Slovenian health system are as follows: prevention and health promotion; sustainable health care system within the financial possibilities; and efficient management of public resources with separation of public and private funding (*Nadgradnja zdravstvenega sistema do leta 2020: korak naprej* 2011:4).

11 Observations, Inferences and Conclusions

Juraj Nemec

After 1989, all Central and Eastern European (CEE) countries implemented large-scale health reforms as they tried to convert the 'socialist' model of a health care system into a 'modern' one. Although differences existed between countries, the starting point was relatively similar (Shakarashvili 2005). The 'old' systems sought to provide a comprehensive system of health care for all members of society, free at the point of use. Decisions on health care were made on political or administrative grounds; accountability was solely to the Communist Party. In terms of results, common but partly different patterns were visible during and especially at the end of the 'socialist' period. Many authors argue that, when transition began, the Hungarian and Czechoslovak systems were far from the crisis state of the Polish system (Millard 1994) and the Soviet system (Davis 1993).

If necessary, everyone was able to obtain appropriate health care at a relatively high medical standard. Although special institutions provided higher quality services for high-ranking officials, most considerations of equity were achieved. While the old Semasko system is often described as obsolete and inefficient, health expenditures consumed approximately 5% of Gross Domestic Product (GDP) and most demands for high quality of care were met. Despite insufficient quality and quantity of equipment, the old system was characterized by relatively high quality care.

Nevertheless the old system emphasized quantitative indicators and had physical overcapacity, excess medical staff and too many hospital beds. National systems were centralized with strong vertical management. Allocation of finances for the system was based on five-year central plans. The State determined the level, composition and mechanisms for allocation of public spending based on national norms in order to ensure the provision of health care services in compliance with certain standards. Strict top-down control over expenditures of public resources characterized the system.

Given such conditions on the eve of transition, many felt that much more could be achieved through a more rationally organized, decentralized and responsible system. Opportunities for improvement existed and reforms were also necessary for political reasons. All governments had to show to their citizens a willingness to change.

Depending on the specific conditions present at the start and during the process, the changes after 1989 vary among CEE countries. However, there are some common issues among their health reforms – notably the introduction of market-based instruments to reform 'socialist' systems for delivering health services. The most important 'market changes' were the introduction of health insurance financing systems to replace a general taxation-based model, privatization and the introduction of private payments as well as co-payments. While much was expected from these changes, recent evidence assessing the outcomes of health reforms in Central and Eastern Europe indicates that expectations of reforms based on 'marketization' of health care were not fulfilled. Our book describes trends, analyzes outcomes and indicates selected barriers for success, especially in health policy-making and implementation.

11.1 Overview of Heath Reforms in Central and Eastern Europe

This book presents a sample of 'post-soviet' countries across several dimensions. In size they range from the largest (Russia) to the very small (Macedonia). In economic terms, Slovenia performs best while Armenia is very poor. Six countries are members of the European Union (Bulgaria, Czech Republic, Hungary, Romania, Slovenia, Slovakia) while two belong to the Commonwealth of Independent States (CIS) (Armenia, Russia). Geographically the countries span Central and Eastern Europe from a classic core (Hungary, Slovakia and the Czech Republic) through the Balkans (Bulgaria, Macedonia, Romania, Slovenia) to the Caucasus (Armenia) and Eurasian Russia. In terms of level at the beginning of health reforms, several countries had relatively well-performing systems under 'socialism' (Hungary, Czech Republic, Slovakia and former Yugoslavia) while others had serious economic gaps (Armenia, Bulgaria, Romania, Russia). This sample of nine countries adequately represents the region and highlights common trends.

11.2 Armenia

After its independence in 1991, the Republic of Armenia took the path from a centralized system of governance towards a market economy. During the course of reforms, radical changes aimed at structural and regulatory changes in the centralized and inefficient health care system inherited from the Soviet era. These changes focused on decentralization, devolution and privatization, new mechanisms of finance, and reforms for effective management. Reforms were externally driven, supported by international financial institutions and bilateral agencies like the World Bank, the World Health Organization, USAID and the UK Department for International Development (DFID). Health reforms sought to increase the utilization of sustainable, high-quality primary health care services, optimize and modernize hospital networks to improve the quality and efficiency of services, and strengthen the capacity of the Ministry of Health to implement effective health sector policies.

New laws enabled privatization of hospitals and health care facilities in the pharmaceutical and dental sectors. New approaches to health financing focused on diversifying revenues for the health sector, improving financial management and sustainability, and linking financing to the quality and volume of services provided. Measures to optimize health system effectiveness were undertaken to rationalize the system through restructuring, reorganization of functions, and redistribution of resources.

The measures implemented have changed the state of Armenia's health system with both positive and negative impacts on key indicators. Raising the role of private providers produced more revenue and increased provider income but it failed to ensure equal access of population to qualitative health care. During the economic transition after independence in 1991 Armenia experienced social and political transformations. A severe economic crisis, sociopolitical problems and a dramatic decline in the level of expenditures on health care undermined the public health achievements of the socialist era, dramatically affected the status of health care service provision and, eventually, caused the collapse of public health activities. The public finances available failed to sustain the inherited system characterized by expensive tertiary curative care rather than primary and preventive medicine. Due to inadequate clinical and managerial skills of health care providers, overstaffed facilities in disrepair, obsolete equipment and insufficient supplies there were long periods of non-payment of wages to medical personnel. Private payments by the population became the main source of financing for health services. Impoverishment of the population led to an inability to pay for basic health care that, in turn, led to a decline in the utilization of health services and ultimately damaged the health status of the population by increasing mortality and morbidity rates.

11.3 Bulgaria

Compared to other countries in our sample, major changes in the Bulgarian health system began relatively late (1998) and are not 'too radical'. Only in 2000 was a National Health Insurance Fund (NHIF) established, and the statute on GPs changed when private choice to supply and demand health services became the main principle of the system. Thereafter, a comprehensive discussion about the introduction of a pluralistic health insurance model ended with a common consensus to retain the existing health system in order to avoid resistance and implementation problems.

The system is based on compulsory health insurance implemented by the NHIF and its territorial divisions (Regional Health Insurance Funds). Voluntary health insurance is optional and is conducted by shareholder companies registered according to commercial law. Compulsory health insurance in Bulgaria is carried out in compliance with the following basic principles: solidarity of insured persons in the use of accumulated funds; a basic package of medical services guaranteed by the NHIF's budget; free choice of medical care provider; and equality of all health care providers in concluding contracts with the NHIF.

Currently Bulgaria's health system is financed through two sources: insurance premiums and taxes. Central and local budgets cover the unemployed, the poor, pensioners, students, civil servants and members of the military. Taxes are allotted for health care services by law. Other sources include voluntary health insurance contributions, subscriptions by employers for specified health services, cash payments by citizens, and co-payments by patients. About 15% of the population lacks health insurance rights due to unpaid contributions and only 1.8% of the population has contracted voluntary private health insurance. From an organizational point of view, General Practitioners control access to specialized outpatient and hospital care. Public and private for-profit hospitals coexist.

Because the current level of revenues is insufficient to cover health expenditures, the core problem of Bulgaria's health system is growing inequality – a trend that should not occur in a member state of the European Union. Although the health system seeks to provide free and accessible comprehensive health care, patients have in practice increasingly paid out of pocket for many health services during recent decades. Despite good intentions of achieving universal and equal access to health care, several factors cause substantial inequalities in access to health services.

11.4 Czech Republic

Based on the relatively well developed 'socialist' system, structural changes in the health system occurred after the 1989 Velvet Revolution that were market-oriented but retained the principle of a public insurance system. Transformations between 1990 and 1993 occurred quickly and were oriented mostly to financial topics. Physicians greatly influenced the approach to these initial changes – even within the citizen participation mentioned above in which physicians sought to increase their social prestige and income. Left-oriented as well as right-oriented political parties accept the principle of solidarity during all phases of changing the system.

Since 1990 many attempts to reform the health system have been initiated; none, however, has been fully implemented and most of the changes were non-systemic. The aims of the reforms were almost invariably the same: to ensure sufficient financial resources, to improve effectiveness of financial resources allocation, and to improve the quality of care.

As a reaction to the long-term state monopoly over health services, the Czech Republic is among the few CEE countries that significantly rely on plurality in the health system. This situation is reflected in many elements of the Czech health system such as freedom of choice for patients, a public-private mix of providers, multi-source financing, and especially pluralistic health insurance executed through several Health Insurance Companies (HICs) that compete for enrollees. However, results show that 'automatic' benefits stemming from plurality (like cost control, quality, and efficiency) did not occur on the scale expected.

From the point of view of finance, the Czech Republic has a multi-source system of financing health care. The sources include health insurance (76.9%), state and municipal (8.3%) and out-of-pocket payments (14.8%). While the Czech Republic has the lowest official private financial participation in our sample, co-payments must significantly increase in order to maintain this level.

From the point of organization about 95% of primary health care was privatized by 2002. Most primary health physicians work alone but groups of them may work together in health centres or in the few polyclinics that provide primary health care in addition to specialist care. Currently the Czech network of health care facilities for secondary and tertiary care consists of the offices of specialized outpatient physicians, hospitals, and specialized bed facilities. While approximately three-quarters of outpatient physicians have become private in recent years, most bed facilities remain public. However, the status of the latter is undergoing changes in relation to reforms in public administration. Hospitals are owned both by the state and by private for-profit and not-for-profit organizations. There are also private hospitals and church hospitals. Faculty hospitals have a special status.

In terms of results, health status indicators have improved due to both better quality of care (based on improved technical equipment) and changing life-style. Health expenditures grew steadily and consume an increasing proportion of private resources. The principle of universal access is evident in real practice.

While the Czech health system demonstrates troubles, inefficiencies and a need for systematic rather than *ad hoc* reform, it is far from failing and certainly not near collapse. During the past twenty years, several 'factors of success' indicate hope for future developments. The most influential actors (health insurance companies and providers) show considerable flexibility as well as an ability to learn quickly. Overall the system has proved its ability to manage crises and solve conflicts of interest in a civilized way.

11.5 Hungary

The starting point of Hungary resembled but also differed from other CEE countries. Prior to the change of regime the exclusive role of the state was evident in the health sector. Being responsible for health services, the state owned all health institutions and facilities as well as managed, provided and financed their services. Coverage was universal and services were provided free at the point of use. Nevertheless, the actual quality of services available to citizens depended on the latter's residence, informal connections, willingness and capacity to offer under-the-table payments and gratuities. The laws of the time did not recognize the concept of patient rights and failed to address ethical issues in health care.

By the 1980s, structural problems (inefficiencies and redundant capacities) in the health sector became apparent when the emergence of private arrangements was officially accepted much earlier than in other CEE countries. While policy management remained centralized and while professional interest groups were tightly controlled, part-time private practices for specialists (dentists, dermatologists, urologists and gynecologists) were permitted. A dual structure emerged in which public services continued to dominate the sector but private services began to gain a share. In 1988, when restrictions on private provisions were completely eliminated, previously existing private practitioners were recognized and full-time private entrepreneurship was legalized. In the same year the financing of the health system switched from taxation to compulsory social insurance contributions. The Social/Health Insurance Fund was detached from the central budget and became the main source for financing health institutions. Also in the late 1980s, university clinics followed international developments and began to address ethical questions as well as the rights of patients.

After the change of political regime in 1989, the roles of regulator, owner, purchaser and service provider in the health sector were fully separated from one another, and the institutional landscape of the sector transformed. From the point of view of finance, a mixed scheme between an NHS and insurance systems was created; governments maintain a certain level of control over the size and operations of the HIF. Moreover, after 1998 Self-government for Health Insurance – a supervisory body of employer and employee representatives – was abolished, and control over the HIF was fully transferred to the government. Proposals to replace the state-run HIF with competing private funds failed to obtain cabinet support.

The HIF finances public health services, ambulances, blood supply, health education, research and the health insurance scheme of social groups exempted from contributions. It also contributes to the health expenditures of citizens with low income; transfers earmarked and targeted subsidies to local governments; negotiates with pharmaceutical retailers on the subsidies of (certain) medicines; and supports the members of voluntary health funds with tax rebates. The services of both public and private operators are equally funded from the HIF. Most hospitals and clinics are publicly owned; the few exceptions are comprised of privately owned institutions and church-sponsored hospitals.

In addition to being covered by the state-run health insurance system, citizens may join voluntary insurance funds. These funds offer both complementary services (which are not covered in the state-run system) and services of better quality (creating the system of universal but not equal access). Although membership in voluntary private funds has expanded, their impact on the financing and the operation of the health system remains limited.

As in the Czech Republic and Slovakia, the imbalance between resources and demand is evident. For some years this problem was addressed through strict limits on performance volume that produced long waiting lists. In 2009, the system was modified but the change only deepened the underfinancing of services and increased the indebtedness of hospitals to such an extent that yet another round of hospital consolidation was required.

Concerning organizational issues, in 1990 local governments obtained broad competences including responsibility for local health services. In order to meet that task, they became owners of most primary care facilities, hospitals and polyclinics – altogether more than 90% of all health facilities. Nevertheless their freedom in capacity planning remained restricted; they could reduce capacities only if the respective (local or county) chief medical officer approved their decision while the expansion of capacities had to be jointly approved by the ministers in charge of health and finance. Responsibility for secondary care was shared between municipal and county governments. While the HIF covered the operational costs of both municipal and county institutions, the owners were put in charge of raising capital/stock, the costs of investments and development. Local governments also received earmarked financial support from the central governmental budget to cover the wage costs of public health employees. This system prevailed until 2011 when the process of re-centralization began.

11.6 Macedonia

Macedonia inherited the former Yugoslavian health system with its widespread and easily accessible health infrastructure, large hospitals and a regional network of institutes of public health responsible for preventive activities as well as the notion of social ownership of health facilities. One characteristic of the Yugoslavian model of health system organization that left its mark on the Macedonian health system was the notion of universal and free access of health services for all citizens regardless of their ability to pay. After independence in 1991, the health system was re-established to protect and promote the values of solidarity, equity and participation. But for many internal reasons these goals have never been achieved.

Since 1991 three main periods are evident in the development of health system reforms: post-socialist (1991-1998), pro-market (1998-2006) and manifesto-driven (2006-continuing). These periods are not sharply divided and some aspects overlap in different periods. These periods are based on reforms developed and implemented during political developments in the country.

The main features of the post-socialist phase in health sector reforms were oriented to prevent the collapse of the health care system (due to lack of finance) and to maintain some characteristics of the old system such as strong prevention, free access, and solidarity in financing. In this phase the HIF was an integral part of the Ministry of Health and all decisions for allocation of resources, financing of health care providers, and planning of investments came from the Cabinet through different Ministers of Health.

The pro-market period in health sector reforms coincides with the first official shift in political power from left-oriented former socialists to center-right conservatives. This period is marked by intensive health sector reforms, mainly initiated and guided by the World Bank's Health Sector Transition Project (HSTP). The influence and the pressure of the World Bank were key in the design of structural and financial reforms in the health care sector. The most important feature of the reforms within this period was the formal separation of the Health Insurance Fund from direct control by the Ministry of Health. The next important developments were preparations for the privatization of primary health clinics. By October 2007, less than three years after the adoption of the first changes in the laws, a total of 3,521 health workers (doctors, dentists, pharmacists and nurses) had been privatized. The pro-market wave of the reforms was also felt in the private health care sector. This period marked the development and opening of large private hospitals for cardio-surgery, gynecology and obstetrics, and one general hospital.

The whole manifesto phase of health system reforms has been influenced by government promises to improve quality in the delivery of services in public hospitals by purchasing medical equipment and renovating their facilities. The reform program divides health reforms in four main components: protect the values of solidarity, equity and participation of the citizens in the decision-making process; advance and preserve the social health insurance system; strengthen public health services; and continue to invest in the health care sector. Whether such improvements really occur remains an open question.

To date, reforms did not deliver much. Over the years, poor maintenance, low efficiency and high operational costs have increased out-of-pocket expenditures for health and reflect the deterioration of public hospital infrastructure. These trends have reduced quality in the provision of health services in public facilities. Parallel to these processes, liberal health care market regulation produced a trend in the commercialization of health care services and investment in new private for-profit hospital services. Long transitions and ineffective reforms in the public health sector impelled many health personnel to move to the private sector. Disappointed in the quality of services provided in the public health sector, many citizens now opt for services in private health care facilities, despite lack of available health insurance. Key problems are poor quality and low efficiency of the services provided in public health facilities, distortion of the social health insurance system and politicization of the health sector.

The health system in the Republic of Macedonia is funded by social contributions deducted from the gross salary of employees. The rate of health contributions is rather low compared to other countries with similar organization of social health system financing. Added to the fact that transfers from the central budget to the HIF are decreasing, the sustainability of health financing is jeopardized.

Apart from public financing of the health system, a significant percentage of total health expenditure comes from private expenditures for health. According to a household expenditure survey, out-of-pocket expenditure constitutes 25% of total health expenditures in the Republic of Macedonia. Due to poor data, however, these figures are probably underestimated so private payments may be as high as 40%-50% of total health care spending.

Limited public resources and the rise in costs of access to health care have direct implications for inequities in the country. Given the lack of complementary private health insurance, a portion of private spending is devoted to the direct financing the health services provided in private hospitals, which are inaccessible for those without private money.

11.7 ROMANIA

During its recent history, Romania has struggled to improve the organization of its health care system. Given the scarce resources allocated to the health sector, the results can be considered partly successful. However, although health is always on the agenda of politicians before elections, it has never been a priority. The proofs are evident by the many Ministers of Health in Romania during the past 20 years, by the refusal to continue reforms that were started by other people and by the refusal to address flagrant problems in the system about which strong voices raise concerns.

Since 1990, Romania's health care system has gone through extensive attempts to reform with consistent support from external organizations such as the World Bank. Several aspects characterize the efforts to reform a system that needed to recover after the communist period. These aspects include the strong influence of politics, a lack of commitment from all stakeholders in the reforms that were begun, and no continuity for the ideas included in the reform process. All these aspects affected the way the reforms were designed, implemented and evaluated.

The main change after 1990 was the adoption of social insurance to fund the health sector. Immediately after 1990, the first measures looked for short-term results such as the trust of health professionals in the authority of the Ministry of Health, ensuring their free mobility across the country, addressing the HIV and hepatitis B epidemics, and reducing the rates of maternal and child mortality. In 1994, general practice began to be reorganized, starting with changing the way general practitioners were paid. Instead of a fixed payment, their salaries were calculated using age-adjusted capitation, fee-for-services and bonuses.

In 1997, the Chamber of Deputies adopted a Social Health Insurance Bill in an attempt to increase the resources available in the health sector. The newly created NHIF was a self-governing body until 2002 when was placed under the Ministry of Public Health. In 2006, the law of Reform in Health was issued that governs main aspects of the current organization and functioning of Romania's health system.

Given the global financial crisis, more changes in the system occurred in 2010 in an attempt to reduce costs and increase accountability. The first measure concerned the decentralization of hospitals in order to shift responsibility for hospitals from the Ministry of Health to local and county communities. The second measure introduced competition-based appointment of hospital managers. The third measure of co-payments and private co-insurance, proposed to address the overcrowded waiting rooms of family physicians and to reduce informal payments, has not yet been introduced in the system. After its publication on the website of the Ministry of Health, the proposal generated controversies and later the civilized dialogue was transformed into street protests and violent expression of opinions.

In March 2011, the Ministry of Health issued a document entitled *The National Strategy for Hospital Rationalization*. The document sought to identify key issues that need to be reformed in the whole (not only on hospital level) Romanian health care system as well as providing solutions and a calendar with activities meant to address the problematic issues. The general principles guiding the proposed solutions are equity, people-centeredness, quality and responsibility. However, the document appeared during a period of political instability – *e.g.*, three health ministers in three years – and the likelihood of implementation of needed measures is doubtful due to both political and contextual limits.

As noted above, Romania changed its system of health sector financing from the Semashko model to a social insurance model much later than other CEE countries. Its social insurance system has been in force since 1998. Financial resources enter the system through payroll-based social insurance (77%), taxes (15%) and direct payments (fee-for-service, out-of-pocket payments, informal payments). Insurance contributions are collected by the National Agency for Fiscal Administration (NAFA) within the Ministry of Finance. The level is established at 5.5% payroll tax paid by the employee and 5.2% paid by the employer.

In reality, the level of private payments is much higher. Given the scarcity of resources, patients pay informal fees and also provide medical supplies on their own. A World Bank study revealed that informal payments in Romania were €300 million a year, accounting for 41% of total cash payments. In June 2009, the president of NHIH estimated the amount at about €500 million a year. Although the figures should alarm stakeholders responsible for the situation, the phenomenon seems to impress no one. The high level of private payments has a negative impact on the most important positive element of health system in Romania – the universality of care. Formally all categories in Romania, including the most marginalized, have the right to care. In reality, however, access to care is inequitable (ethnic, geographic, economic and quality-related inequalities) and heterogeneous.

The policy dimension of health care reforms in Romania is similar to others in the region. Every Health Minister expects his reform to be implemented and to produce great results, but most reforms achieve only short or medium-term results, if any. Although moving from a highly centralized to a more decentralized model, the government controls most of the health care system. While institutions in the system as well as individuals are periodically consulted about the direction of reforms, little input has been obtained from medical staff. Moreover, as a whole, the Romanian health sector has been regarded with distrust and suspicion. The fact that a significant number of the health professionals received or even asked for payments from the patients (whether money or of gifts or both) created and then cultivated the idea that health professionals are the most corrupt category of professionals.

11.8 Russia

Health reforms in Russia have two dimensions in terms of financing and organizing the delivery of health care: the introduction of compulsory health insurance (CHI) and regional decentralization of health care financing and delivery. The main reasons for introducing CHI were political and ideological rather than social and economic. The aim was to create markets everywhere because health insurance was associated with capitalism while budget medicine was regarded as socialist.

Since Russian health policy is in transition, three stages can be distinguished according to government attitudes to health issues and the structural impact of measures undertaken. Stage 1 began in the 1990s when transition sought to create a market economy and political democracy. The decision was taken to shift from the budget model to a social insurance model. Stage 2 appeared during the mid-1990s until the beginning of the 21st century when the 'dual' budget-CHI system developed. While health reforms continued, these were fragmented with no principal changes introduced. Due to the 1998 economic crisis, emphasis was placed on securing stability rather than improving the situation. Stage 3 started when the 2005 session of the Presidium of the State Council of the Russian Federation was devoted to health care issues. It commissioned the special report 'On Increasing Access and Quality of Health Care'. Health issues were put high on the political agenda – a shift caused, it seems, by negative demographic trends such as the steady decline in population. The shift pushed the government to activate health reforms to improve access and quality of health care.

The health care system in Russia is financed by both private and public sources. Public sources include budget allocations (the Federal budget plus regional budgets) and compulsory health insurance that was introduced in Russia in 1993. CHI funds are formed by employers' contributions for their employees and contributions by regional governments for those who are not employed. The organization of CHI funds parallels the federal budget system – one federal CHI fund and separate CHI funds in the regions. In 2010, 62.7% of public money came from budgets – both Federal and regional – while CHI amounted to 37.3% of public means.

Private means include voluntary health insurance and out-of-pocket payments both official and informal. In 1990s state health expenditures declined substantially (by almost one-third) while private – mostly out-of-pocket – expenditures increased and (officially) represent about 40% of total health expenditures. Informal "envelop" payments are difficult estimate but according to some experts they increased from about 25 billion rubles in 2000 to 107 billion rubles in 2008.

The private sector in Russian health care is developing but statistics are scarce. According to some estimates there are about 30,000 private clinics in Russia – mainly situated in big cities. A study of private medicine in Moscow discovered that the majority of private clinics were dental (59%), gynecology/midwifery (13%) and polyclinic multifunctional (10%). Official statistics indicate that only about 5% of those employed in health care work in the private sector.

After nearly 20 years of health care reforms Russian health care is still not in 'good health'. The problems in Russian health care manifests in three major dimensions: poor health status of the population and poor state of health services; negative demographic trends and high economic cost of poor health; people's low 'health-esteem' and wide spread dissatisfaction with health system performance, including equity considerations. As reflected in statistical and sociological indicators, the health of Russians has declined. Russia has a well-developed system of primary, secondary and tertiary care health services. In many cases, however, these units are poorly equipped which affects the quality of services. Russia lags behind developed countries in the application of modern health technology and the number of procedures performed. There are gaps in the quality of medical care and the availability of medical staff between rural and urban areas and between regions of Russia. Experts also note the growth in health inequality despite the attention that this issue attracts at all political levels.

11.9 SLOVAKIA

As noted above, unified Czechoslovakia was characterized by a relatively good position when the transition began. The Czechoslovak system was far from the crisis that characterized other systems in the region. Whenever necessary, everyone was able to get appropriate health care at a relatively high international medical standard. Despite insufficient quantity and quality of high level equipment, relatively high quality of care characterized the system.

The common point of all post-1993 reforms is the fact that Slovakia's health care system is based on the principle of free access at the point of delivery for most services, with costs financed predominantly through compulsory social health insurance. Whatever the type of government (left-wing, right-wing, centre or coalitions) the promises of newly elected governments remain similar: universal coverage, high quality for everyone and financial consolidation of the health care delivery system.

The processes of reforming the Slovak health care system started immediately after the 1989 Velvet Revolution. They introduced important changes into the system – privatization and a shift in financing health care from general taxation to social health insurance – changes that are far from completed. Failures in policy-making and implementation during the reform created additional problems, many of them connected with finance.

Like most CEE countries Slovakia switched to the so-called 'Bismarck' system of social health insurance to replace the previous system of general taxation for financing health care. Together with the Czech Republic, it decided to introduce a competitive/pluralistic social health insurance system. The main laws on health insurance were passed in 1994, which created the base for establishing health insurance companies (two of them public). Most of these have since disappeared from the 'market'; in 2002 five existed but by 2010 only two private and one public remained. The Slovak government intends to switch back to one public social (health, pensions, unemployment) insurance company in 2013.

As noted above, the core issue of different reform proposals is the level of marketization of health care. The scale of privatization is a frequent topic for discussion. The structure of the health care system developed into a public-private-civil sector mix and ways to approach it depend on normative values. Rightwing governments promise that private ownership of medical establishments and health insurance companies will facilitate efficiency and quality improvements; left-wing governments try to limit the scale of privatization – accepting it only in primary and secondary care.

From a financial point of view, two problems have become increasingly obvious. The core issue is fiscal imbalance in the system; almost every year the health care system consumes more resources than available and the total debt increases. Because co-insurance has not really been introduced, the second issue is the fact that the proportion of direct private payments began to increase significantly during the Dzurinda government at the beginning of this century. The Fico government, elected in 2006, promised to reverse the trend but found it to be impossible because of fiscal constraints. As of today, the level of co-payments starts to limit universality of access.

From the point of view of its administration, the Slovak health care system can be described as decentralized. Given their mixed ownership, the delivery and the financing systems are administered and regulated at all levels of government, with a focus on guaranteeing universal access and good quality.

For 20 years, as a successor state of the former Czechoslovakia, Slovakia has sought to improve health outcomes. The main goal – universal and fair access – remained the target for all governments in power but reform strategies and associated policies often differed. Many positive improvements have been achieved during reforms of the Slovak health care system. Since 1989, the health status of inhabitants shows significant progress due to more resources, improved technologies, and better life styles. The maintenance of largely universal access is another advantage. Yet many problems remain such as chronic financial imbalances; an inability to fashion an effective prescription policy; limitations in insurance companies' regulatory performance, stemming from an unwillingness by left-populist governments to delegate authority; the primacy of politics over health policy; economic decisions influenced by local interest groups, ideologies or coalition politics; and the inability of left-wing governments to implement necessary reforms.

11.10 SLOVENIA

Slovenia inherited a relatively sound health system from the former Yugoslavia and to a large extent it has been able to develop the system further. In 1992, health legislation underwent a major revision. The new act formed the basis for the current system of compulsory and voluntary health insurance, promoted the process of privatization of the health care system and defined in detail the role of the key partners. These changes led to a partial privatization of health providers within the network of public services and introduced the free choice of doctor at the primary level of health care.

The second major Slovenian health reform occurred in 2003 when a payment model was introduced in which the money was to follow the patient. It was intended to improve the function, management and governance of the health system. A reform had been planned in 2010-2011 to address problems in Slovenian health care – inappropriate distribution of capacity, lack of adequate information required for decision-making, problems at different management levels in the health system, and challenges related to the mission of health care – but it was not realized.

Health care in Slovenia is financed by public and private sources of compulsory and voluntary health insurance and by direct payments. Slovenia has the highest health care expenditure in Central and Eastern Europe. In 2011, total public spending was 50.9% of GDP with total expenditure on health care at 9% of GDP; public health care expenditures were 6.4% of GDP.

Health insurance has a long tradition in Slovenia. In the early 19th century, workers established 'fraternity funds' based on solidarity and mutuality. The first sickness fund in Slovenia was founded in 1889 and followed by similar providers of health insurance. Despite changes in the organization of health protection in "socialism", Slovenia has retained the main features of health insurance such as funding by contributions from employers and employees and to some extent also autonomy and self-governance (the role of the state significantly increased in "socialism"). From 1992, all inhabitants of Slovenia are included in compulsory health insurance. Compulsory health insurance provides insured parties with two basic sets of rights: to health care and to cash benefits or reimbursements. Adequate access and appropriate quality of health services are keys to the protection of insured parties. Equal provision of doctors and other capacities to the population is an essential component.

Slovenia is one of the few CEE countries to introduce a functional model of voluntary health insurance based on equality of access. However, some private health services establishments operate outside the 'compulsory health insurance market', thereby undermining basic principles of health care such as fairness, solidarity and access. Slovenian commitment to the latter emphasize that the system's users must receive equal treatment regardless of their ability to pay.

Slovenia has a network of public and private health providers at primary (HCs), secondary (hospitals) and tertiary levels (clinics, clinical institutes and clinical departments). All ownership forms (working in the system of public insurance) are treated equally and the cooperation between public and private health sectors has been primarily organized through concessions. A concession is a transfer of the authorization to provide a service from the state to an authorized body or civil law entity.

In terms of reform processes and their results, data indicate that Slovenia is the most successful CEE country – thanks also to better financial inflows. Nonetheless, its system has experienced several problematic trends that have made health care conditions more difficult and reduced both solidarity and fairness. Providing adequate funding is an increasing problem. The biggest challenge comes from demographic, socio-economic, medical, pharmaceutical and technological trends that lead to increasing growth in health care costs. The ageing of the population is another major trend as it has changed both the need and the demand for health services. A major challenge to maintaining health service provision at an adequate level within the public sector is the pressure to modernize medical procedures. A key question within the Slovenian health system is how to maintain a suitable level of access and quality in conditions while financial resources remain fixed or are even reduced. The other questionable issue, noted above, is equality of access regardless to the ability to pay because private insurance schemes undermine formal guarantees.

11.11 Comparative Evaluation of Selected Reforms

This section focuses on comparative elements of health care reforms in Central and Eastern Europe – specifically on health policy-making, implementation and the 'marketization' of health care provision. The core question is why, after so many years of attempted reform, are the results not very positive.

11.12 Health Policymaking and Implementation

As outlined in the introductory chapter, this volume identifies problems linked with the 'quality' of health policy-making and implementation in Central and Eastern Europe where there is a chronic gap between proclamation and implementation, between intent and result, between promise and performance in terms of access, quality and cost of health services. Substantive health policy-making and effective implementation of reform strategies are almost impossible in the CEE region for many reasons (Dunn *et al.* 2006). Changes in the region are difficult because a switch from centrally planned and managed society to modern democratic conditions had not occurred in history before 1989. Many researchers stress that the transition from a centralized to a market-based system is a unique process that cannot be based on a simple transfer of existing 'western' knowhow but needs substantial local potential to adopt and adapt existing practices to local conditions (Coombes and Verheijen 1997). Because such potential does not normally exist, reforms cannot be a straightforward process.

During the 1990s, when most reforms began, there was lack of general and specific expertise to establish effective health reform policy. The main driving force behind reforms was to depart as quickly as possible and to detach as much as possible from the past. Persons responsible for health reforms were mainly medical doctors with limited economic background and, in some cases, sought primarily to protect the interests of the medical profession. The relation between politicians and bureaucrats was erratic. A professional and sustainable system of bureaucracy had not been established. Administrative structures changed whenever the government or even its minister of health changed. From this point of view, little has changed after twenty years of attempts to reform heath care systems in Central and Eastern Europe. Most governments declare their intention to reform the health sector but do not adopt specific steps leading to recovery. Partial non-systemic measures are adopted instead of basic reforms – often because real reforms are expected to exaggerate problems in the health sector in short term perspective. Consequences rather than reasons for the bad conditions of the health sector are addressed (UNDP 2003).

Two country chapters deal in detail with the policymaking issue. The Czech case focuses on the role of political parties and indicates that popularity is more important than real needs to reform the health sector, even during periods when the governing coalition has a sufficiently strong position in Parliament. The introduction of regulatory fees in the Czech Republic is an example of interactions between politics and health policy. Between 1998 and 2006, despite rhetoric about government intentions for health reforms, no appreciable progress occurred. All governments had weak and unstable mandates that inhibited systematic reform. During 2006-2007, the cabinet did achieve a majority in all regions as well as in the Senate and Chamber of Deputies. Based on the criterion of majority control, no cabinet had ever had a better position; hence the space for reform seemed sufficiently large. However, implementation of regulatory fees became controversial and generated public frustration. The government failed to explain the change as a part of a broader, sophisticated, beneficial reform supported by major interest groups. Instead, unity inside the coalition weakened. Opposition parties used regulatory fees in their campaign arguments during the 2008 regional elections and obtained overwhelming success. Consequently coalition deputies did not pass other reform bills in the House of Representatives.

The Slovak chapter compares the list of generally accepted preconditions for successful policymaking with empirical reality – and the results are poor. Main actors do not support effective health care reforms and their implementation. Hospitals and their management prefer 'non-transparent waters'; many doctors utilize the potential for supplier-induced demand for their own benefits; politicians benefit from nice promises but 'pay' politically for painful reforms; patients are not well informed but rather are fiscally 'deluded'; and paternalistic attitudes dominate in society. For all these reasons, patients are not ready to support radical changes in the health care system; moreover they regard themselves not as customers but as 'slaves' of the system. Politics is much more important for political parties than evidence-based policies – and, without databases and benchmarking systems, evidence-based policy is technically impossible. Independent advice is rarely available and not requested. Most Slovak (and most CEE) coalition governments have been in power with a marginal majority and the political party leading a coalition has not been supported by its partners on issues of health care reforms.

All other chapters indicate deficiencies in policy-making capacity, too. Reforms implemented in Armenia focused on the establishment of a cost-effective, equitable and sustainable health system. However, severe economic crisis, sociopolitical problems and a dramatic decline in the level of health expenditures not only blocked the progress but also undermined the public health achievements of the socialist era. These factors dramatically affected the status of health care service provision and, eventually, caused the collapse of public health activities. All this led to a decline in the utilization of health care services and ultimately damaged the health status of the population by increasing mortality and morbidity rates.

In Bulgaria, the impact of political parties on health reforms has been weak since 2003. The political left-wing (Socialist party) seeks to maintain high levels of access to and state support for health care. In 2005, the Socialists prepared a national strategy for health of the nation that was adopted in 2008 without political consensus and without any significant steps in terms of health care reforms. Two parties emerged in political life that became significant during 2002-2006 and 2009-2011. One party (National Movement Simeon Second) did not make any reforms; rather it froze them. The second party – 'Citizens for European Development of Bulgaria' currently governing the country – has no alternative. In such a situation, despite the fact that the health reforms are imperative, almost nothing happens.

The Hungarian case indicates another political problem. Its author argues that political cynicism prevails in the new system; accepted rules are repeatedly violated and loopholes actively sought. Low confidence in the system and its institutions demonstrates the lack of moral support. Moreover, the majority of the population has had an ambivalent attitude towards the state. Polls suggest that a large proportion of citizens like the state as such (*i.e.* in principle) but do not like the state as it is.

The Macedonian case highlights the problem of continuity. During a relatively short period of transformation three sets of health system reforms are evident: post-socialist, pro-market and manifesto-driven. These are based on different reforms developed and implemented during political changes in Macedonia. Non-continuity and lack of resources undermined the chance for successful policy. Public hospital infrastructure deteriorated; the quality of health services in public facilities was reduced. Disappointed in the services provided in the public sector, many citizens opt for services in private health care facilities where they pay out of pocket.

The report on Romania stresses the lack of strategic thinking and planning. Frequent political changes and lack of consistency are among the factors contributing to the limited success of health reforms in the country. Strategic thinking has been disregarded by most of the reforms because only the present and the near future have been taken into account. The appetite for rapid results was one causal factor. The many health ministers who have occupied this function during the last 20 years are another factor that slowed reform. Although a number of projects have been contracted to help the Romanian health sector to find its way through the reform process, little has been put into practice.

Authors of the Russian case argue that current problems are largely due to the way in which health policy is worked out and the assumptions that underline the ideology of health reforms. Problems include the poor health of the population, the poor state of health services, negative demographic trends, the high economic cost of poor health, and popular dissatisfaction with health system performance, including inequalities in health status and access to health care. Consequently modern Russian health policy is problem-making rather than problem-solving. Analysis reveals a divergence between the stated aims and the mechanisms that are used to reach them.

Even in Slovenia, where some continuity of reform and capacity is visible, reforms planned in 2010 and 2011 to address the problems in Slovenian health care (such as the inappropriate distribution of capacity, lack of adequate information required for decision-making, problems at different management levels in the health system, and challenges related to the mission of health care) have not been realized. The draft amendment of a new Health Care Act sketched enhancement of primary health care, reorganization of secondary health care, establishment of a quality system and changes in economic conditions. However, due to difficult economic circumstances, Parliament did not adopt it.

11.12.1 'Marketization' of Health Care Systems in Central and Eastern Europe

Among reforms proposed in the region are elements of 'marketizing' the delivery of health care such as privatization, the establishment of structures for public-private mixes, and the introduction of health insurance. All the case studies indicate that CEE countries underwent massive privatization at the level of health care providers. While views about effectiveness and optimal scale of privatization are often normative, distinctions should be made between levels of providing health services and between 'full' privatization versus the creation of schemes for a public-private mix or public-private partnerships. Although a claim that remains unconfirmed by health reforms in developed countries, rightwing governments promise that the private ownership of medical establishments and health insurance companies will facilitate efficiency and improve quality. Nemec *et al.* (2010) suggest that the form of hospital ownership is not the main determinant of performance. The stress on privatization is linked more with private than public interests.

The theoretical basis for pluralization in the delivery of public services was described in late 1980s (Cullis and Jones 1987). The main principle is that is possible to move from the classical system of delivering public services (public production and public financing) by enabling the private (for profit and not for profit) sector to be involved into all processes connected with the provision of public services. Currently economic theory distinguishes between provision, production and financing; in specific cases public services might be provided by the state but both produced and financed by private actors. The traditional mode of delivery in which services are financed by public funds and produced by public institutions is replaced by a multi-tier system with clear boundaries between financing, procuring and producing functions. The basic principles for public-private (civil sector) partnerships are:

- The state remains responsible for the provision of public services and public infrastructure.
- Financing of public services and infrastructure can be partly or fully switched to private sources (consumers, private firms and financial institutions).

- Potential suppliers of any ownership type have the right to compete for the right to produce and deliver the public service or to build and maintain public infrastructure.
- There is no single uniform solution about how to deliver public tasks that is valid everywhere. Concrete decisions for discrete environments must be made in each case.

Case studies in Central and Eastern Europe indicate that the structure of health care systems developed in two directions. In the less developed countries, 'private medicine' (private production and private payments) plays an important role because access to health care services is based on the ability to pay. The more developed countries have switched to mixed systems of public-private cooperation in which public sources are dominant in financing, private production is dominant in outpatient care, and mixed systems exist in the inpatient sector. Private insurance or cash payments to providers outside the public system are rare and do not (significantly) undermine the principles of universal and equal access. However, the fact that co-payments begin to be a 'too important way of financing services' is a harbinger of future dangers. The introduction of user fees to supplement budgetary resources is critical for governments. But the success of the policy, no matter how logical in theory, has been constrained by the dwindling capacity of citizens to pay for health care.

The introductory chapter noted that comparative experiences throughout the world reveal three basic models for public financing of health care services (Altenstetter and Björkman 1997):

- General taxation – in the UK and Nordic countries as well as in former socialist regimes in Central and Eastern Europe
- Social insurance – Bismarck's model in which state-mandated resources are provided through the insurance market
- Targeted programs – public funds are provided to selected groups such as Medicare and Medicaid in the USA.

After 1989, almost all post-communist countries decided to switch from the general taxation model to social insurance. The change to a health insurance system was supported by arguments about plurality, independence and competition as positive features (Lawson and Nemec 2003). For post-communist countries, the political economy rationale for such a switch from a tax-based to an insurance-based financial model is a mixture of economic, administrative and political considerations.

The economic arguments involve a trade-off between the costs of a public monopoly evident in the previous system, whose efficiency might have been improved by an internal market, and the possibility of excessive administrative costs if there are many competing insurance companies but few economies of scale. Alternatively there would be the general economic welfare problems of oligopolies if the market came to be dominated by a small number of large insurance companies. The administrative arguments for the change were that the new insurance companies would be separate from the main government administration – an arrangement that by itself would improve the quality of administration.

The political considerations for proposing a switch are complex. On the one hand, earmarking taxes for health and sub-contracting their administration to independent insurance funds would have the advantage of distancing government from a contentious area of public policy. And the switch to an earmarked insurance system would have the advantage of reducing pressure on general budgets. But other than the insurance companies, interest groups are not concerned about where extra resources for health will be found. Neither local nor indeed many central policymakers in the health sector are concerned about such trade-offs. They continue to push for increased expenditure whatever the consequences for either taxation or expenditure on non-health items.

The political purposes behind decisions to switch during conditions of transition are straightforward: the need to differentiate a new system from its predecessor as well as to show willingness to change and improve. However, theory in health economics and experience in the history of health systems in the world do not unambiguously favor an insurance-based system. Theory and experience show the positives and negatives of any system and conclude that there is no general prescription. Like other approaches to public sector reform, every decision must be based on careful evaluation of local internal and external situations of the health system (Coombes and Verheijen 1997). The insurance system is not the only alternative and, even if introduced in an optimal way, involves possible problems. Potential problems include:

- Patients with a high probability of requiring costly treatments are usually required to pay a very high premium that may be unaffordable; therefore private health insurance would fail to cover high-risk groups of citizens (Feldstein 1993).
- Insurance companies try to 'cherry pick' by focusing on very low risk customers who have no problems paying the premiums (Cullis 1979).
- For efficiency an insurance system needs competition, but in health care the level of competition is naturally limited (Klein 1992).
- Regulating the insurance system can multiply politicians' possibilities for intervention that, in turn, can negate the advantages of market regulation.
- A specific problem connected with the pluralistic model of health insurance is the possibility of excessive administrative costs – especially if, as initially evident in the Czech and Slovak cases, there are many competing insurance companies but few economies of scale.

- Alternatively, if the market is dominated by a one insurance company (true in most CEE countries) or by a small number of large insurance companies (as in Slovakia), then the usual welfare problems with monopolies/oligopolies will occur.

The problems linked with pluralistic health insurance can be exaggerated in transitional countries due to many factors. There is the issue of improper government interventions in health insurance; despite formal delegation of authority, the state is not willing to lose control. If insurance premiums and benefits are strictly regulated, competition is stifled and insurance companies become redistributors rather than the intended regulators. Implementation problems with pluralistic health insurance can be expected, if undertaken too early in the transformation period when financial markets do not yet perform in a standard way.

Our sample reveals that two main approaches are used by countries in Central and Eastern Europe: establishing a monopolistic public HIF or establishing a pluralistic public health insurance system, each of which is responsible for maintaining equal and universal access to services. However, former members of the Soviet Union are much more reluctant to switch and the result is a "mixed" system.

The Ministry of Health of the Republic of Armenia manages the health budget while the State Health Agency is responsible for purchasing a defined BBP for the population. The main formal financing source is the state budget that generates its funds from general tax revenue. No health funds exist; there is no mandatory health insurance and very little voluntary health insurance. Under such arrangements and because of limited public funds, access is now significantly determined by the ability to pay. Russia is a specific case in which the tax-based model is only partly replaced by insurance.

The issue of switching from tax-based financing to one single public insurance fund is not overly complicated. In reality it may only be a cosmetic change because the state still sets all major 'rules of the game'. Economically such change is questionable due to the need to cover transition costs but, as previously indicated, such change was politically almost inevitable. Taking into the account many possible implementation options, there is no surprise that countries with single insurance body differ. They vary according to the status of the insurance body, the role of co-payments and private co-insurance schemes, and the timing of reforms.

Bulgaria introduced a compulsory and a voluntary health care system as an alternative to central budgeting with its 1998 HIF. Funding for the health care system is financed through the semi-independent NHIF, state and municipal budgets, voluntary health insurance funds (almost insignificant), local and foreign legal bodies, individuals and co-payments.

Hungary introduced a semi-independent HIF soon after political changes in 1989. However, the responsibilities of this fund remained limited as Parliament determined the size and structure of the annual health budget as well as the annual contribution rate to the HIF. Given stable backing in parliament, governments were usually able to maintain control over the size and operations of the HIF. This became evident after 1998 when the Self-Government for Health Insurance – a supervisory body of employer and employee representatives – was abolished, and control over the HIF was transferred to the government. Initially a political state secretary in the Prime Minister's Office controlled the area and proposed to replace the state-run HIF with competing private funds, but his proposal failed to obtain cabinet support. Control over the Fund was then transferred to the Ministry of Finance. In 2001 the Ministry of Health obtained the right to supervise the HIF and it has retained the portfolio ever since.

Like its neighbor Bulgaria, Romania introduced social health insurance in 1998. However, in 2011 responsibility for its "monopolistic" health insurance company was transferred to the Ministry of Health. Collection of fees has always been under the Ministry of Finance.

Slovenia (re-) introduced a system of combined compulsory and voluntary health insurance in 1992. Compared to other countries, the system of voluntary health insurance effectively helps citizens to comply with the increased pressure for co-payments. In order to manage rising private costs, co-payments forced the population to subscribe to voluntary health insurance.

Is pluralistic health insurance effective for small and less developed 'post-socialist' countries? Some cases indicate that the answer is 'no'. The Czech and Slovak health reforms illustrate the implementation problems with pluralistic health insurance, especially if undertaken early in the transformation period (*e.g.*, several HIFs were created to channel money and not to service the citizens) and in an environment of state regulation that is arguably too comprehensive. Pluralistic health insurance may be effective, if not always efficient, in a well supervised but not overly regulated competitive market environment. But it not clear that such preconditions exist in any CEE country. After 20 years of experimentation, Slovakia is now officially ready to return to the system of one single public health insurance company and to pay the costs connected with re-nationalization of existing private actors in EU conditions.

11.12.2 Reform Results: Cluster Analysis

By focusing on the core dimensions of finance, access and quality of care, clusters summarize outcomes from health reforms and developments in nine countries of Central and Eastern Europe.

11.12.3 Finance

Compared to the pre-reform period, a core problem for countries in Central and Eastern Europe has been the lack of resources to maintain universal and equal access. Other than the slightly better situations in Slovenia and the Czech Republic, all CEE health systems are underfinanced and additional public resources are difficult to find. Two primary reasons have been identified.

First, after changes in 1989 or shortly thereafter, all countries experienced serious recessions and the recovery therefrom started much later. Calculated through either exchange rates or purchasing power parity, GCP per capita is lower than in developed countries. If a country's per capita GDP is 60% of the EU average and if it spends 5% of GDP for health care, then health expenditures are far below EU standards (measured in hundreds compared to thousands of Euro). Although reliable data are difficult to find, case studies in previous chapters reveal that many CEE countries spend less than a thousand US dollars per year per capita on public health care expenditures – Armenia (US$100 per capita annual health expenditures), Bulgaria (US$300), Russia (US$500), Macedonia (US$700), Romania (US$800). In a market-based economy, such amounts are not enough to ensure access to cost-effective quality care.

Second, while a gap did exist in formerly 'socialist' systems, it was balanced by manipulating input 'prices' such as non-market wages, medications or medical equipment. Currently most costs are derived from worldwide market prices for drugs, equipment and energy that are imported from abroad. As evident in strikes by doctors in Slovakia and the Czech Republic, lower salaries of medical staff cannot balance such costs.

In all selected countries public health resources are unable to cover needs – even cases of need-realized treatments. Ways to cope with increasing fiscal problems in health care systems differ. An obvious choice is to increase private participation as has occurred everywhere, but this trend impacts on universality and equality of access. Another approach is to allow deficits in the system and to recover them through *ad hoc* principles. However, such an approach undermines motivations for efficiency at the level of large-scale providers. It also may create burdens for private sector suppliers (via non-paid or late-paid invoices by hospitals and other health providers) that impact on economic stability. The Slovak case is a typical example. After 1997, the system systematically consumed 10%-15% more resources than the resources available and, despite many implemented measures, this trend did not change. In 2002 (the last year in which last analytical data on this issue are available), about 60% of the debt burden was shifted out of the government health care sector to private actors (suppliers of drugs, energies, food etc.). This situation shows that relations between the state and other sectors in the economy remain far below international standards.

The pivotal issue for all countries is an effective cost-containment system. Health systems not only suffer from limited resources; imbalances are exaggerated by large-scale waste and the misuse of money. Typical phenomena are illustrated by an oversupply of hospital beds, excessive ratios of staff per patients and too much weight on inpatient care. Standardized data in all country chapters indicate that no country has been able to establish an effective cost-containment system.

Table 11.1 displays three dimensions of health care finance: mode of financing, scale of resources and level of co-payment.

The issue of switching from systems funded by general taxation to different types of health insurance systems was previously analyzed. Most Central and Eastern European countries opted for a monopolistic health insurance system with one insurance body that was provided with different level of independence from the central government. While the Czech Republic and Slovakia selected pluralistic health insurance, in September 2012 Slovakia officially published the schedule about how to switch back to one insurance company. Eastern Europe countries use different patterns; Russia and Armenia have established a mixed system.

The core problem of all systems is the amount of public finance available to finance public health services. While waiting lists may exist, developed countries spend thousands of dollars per capita to provide health care to their inhabitants. But Armenia's economic situation allows only a hundred dollars or thereabouts. With such underfunding, the option of universal access to a standard package of services is a "mission impossible". Slovenia is the only country in the sample where lack of resources (imbalance between needs and resources) is not critically visible.

The final but by no means least issue is official copayments and their management. Because of limited public resources, countries try to mobilize private sources. However, the extent of official copayments is already too high in economically low performing countries. The

Table11.1 Health Finance Clusters

Financing system	
Monopolistic public health insurance fund	Bulgaria, Hungary, Macedonia, Romania, Slovenia
Pluralistic public health insurance	Czech Republic, Slovakia
Mixed system (tax financing in combination with health insurance, regionally different approaches, plus relatively high level of private payments)	Armenia, Russia
Total Health Expenditures (approximation in US dollars per inhabitant)	
Very low	Armenia (100)
Low	Bulgaria (300), Macedonia (700), Romania (800), Russia (500)
Medium – significantly below the level of developed countries	Slovakia (1300), Hungary (1,000)
Medium – slightly below the level of developed countries	Czech Republic, Slovenia (both close to 2000)
Share of private expenditures (official data, without shadow economy)	
45%-60%	Armenia
30%-45%	Slovakia, Russia
Below 30%	Bulgaria, Czech Republic, Hungary, Macedonia, Romania, Slovenia

Source: Construction based on country chapters.

only country where copayments are effectively managed via voluntary insurance schemes is Slovenia. Everywhere else a shadow economy flourishes. The most important issue is that the poor are not protected from unacceptable financial burdens connected with deprived health.

11.12.4 Access

Developments after 1989 delivered significant reforms in service delivery in terms of who gets what, when, where, how. The baseline was almost universal and equal access in CEE countries. The current situation differs significantly as equality decreased (in different levels) everywhere. The issue of universality is more complicated but some countries departed significantly from this goal.

The issue of equality of access is a complicated concept and less relevant for countries that lack of resources. For example, should both rich and poor have the same 'quality' of access and services? For developing countries with limited public resources, the policy of providing extra funds for the poor in order to assure universality of access to the 'basic package' might be acceptable because the well-off already have better services and pay much more.

Among all case-study countries, only Slovenia appears to guarantee universal (albeit not fully equal) access via a workable system of co-insurance. The key principle within the Slovenian health system is to maintain a suitable level of access and quality in conditions while public financial resources remain fixed or are even reduced. The Slovenian health system is expected to provide citizens with equal access to health services and a level of care appropriate to their health regardless of age, income, sex, employment or place of residence. At the same time, the system must ensure that all members of society contribute to health care funds on the basis of fairness and solidarity. A significant proportion of health spending comes from private funds that, according to 2011 estimates, provided 29% of total health spending. Unlike other CEE countries, most private funds in Slovenia are contributed in the official economy through insurance companies that offer voluntary health insurance (covering non-urgent services not included in the 'basic basket'). Moreover, the state officially expresses the goal to retain or even to decrease the share of private expenditures in future.

The typical situation is formally universal access with significantly decreased equality. The wealthy pay relatively the same as other citizens but receive better services. The insurance rate is the same for all and the maximum premium is capped in most countries at a very low level; in Slovakia, whatever the income level, all pay the same contribution above certain (medium level) income. This situation typifies new EU members with limited financial resources. Based on EU membership these countries are expected to provide universal health coverage for a 'basic package' for all citizens; in reality such coverage is impossible due to lack of money as well as ineffective cost containment systems. The typical solution for lack of resources is through waiting lists for specialists and inpatient care. In such situations unequal treatment occurs because there are no effective rules for deciding patient priority; those with contacts or capacity to pay bribes receive faster and better service.

The problematic impact of informal payments on access to health care is described in detail in the Romanian chapter. Citizens strongly object to informal payments but still offer informal payments to health professionals. Health professionals may delay necessary care until patients eventually pay, or the behavior and attitude of health professionals intimate that an informal payment is needed for a patient to receive adequate care. Furthermore patients are aware of previous situations in which they were not treated adequately until they had offered informal payments or when the same had happened to relatives or acquaintances.

The last and least case is the situation when both equality and universality are lost during the transition period. Except for the Baltic countries, this situation typifies the New Independent States area. In our sample Armenia is the most critical case, where state expenditures on health care remain very low, which necessitates direct out-of-pocket payments to fund the system. After 1990 a severe economic crisis compounded by sociopolitical problems affected the provision of health services and eventually caused the collapse of public health activities. Private payments by the population became the main source of financing for health services. However, impoverishment of the population led to an inability to pay for basic health care that, in turn, led to a decline in the utilization of health services and consequently to the dramatic decline of both universality and equality of access to basic health services.

Table 11.2 reveals that of access is a critical topic in Central and Eastern Europe. Other than the best-performing countries (Czech Republic, Hungary, Slovakia, Slovenia), the rest departed from this principle. The link between the decreasing universality of access and decreasing health quality indicators is visible in Armenia and Russia where the ability to pay significantly limits the chance to receive good quality (if any) health services. Surprisingly, from the point of view of EU membership (because universality of access is a formally stated EU value), Bulgaria and Romania suffer limited access by some groups and have problems in finding solutions due to lack of resources.

Table 11.2 Access Clusters

Universality and Equality of Access	
Both almost lost; recent attempts to 'come back'	Armenia, Russia
Significant inequalities on both dimensions	Bulgaria, Romania, Macedonia
Universal access remains the principle; equality of access partly limited and not 'regulated'	Czech Republic, Hungary, Slovakia
Universal access remains the principle, equality of access partly limited and 'regulated' via a functional co-insurance system	Slovenia

Source: Construction based on country chapters.

11.12.5 Quality

It is not simple to measure the quality of health care services because many dimensions exist such as clinical quality, organizational quality and results. Given the lack of comparative data about clinical or organizational quality, comparisons look at indicators of life expectancy, mortality and morbidity. From this point of view, the impact of health care on life expectancy is limited; most estimates are between 10% and 20%. However, the link between deteriorating health systems and lack of universality of access and health outcomes is visible.

The critical situation is in Russia. Its indicators are far below those in developed countries and show negative development trends during the start of transition (especially in the period 1990-1995). Men in Russia live approximately twenty years less than men in neighboring Finland; their life expectancy in 2010 is almost the same as in 1990. The high levels of working-age mortality are increasing not only for men but for women too. During 1990-2006, mortality among working-age men increased from 759 to 1,172 per 100,000 and among women from 198 to 304. This situation is unique for an industrial country and has attracted the attention of the international research community. Such mortality and morbidity trends are undoubtedly caused by many factors, but limited access to health services by citizens must be a key factor. Only half of Russian citizens think that their health status is satisfactory while almost one-fifth (18%) say that it is bad or very bad. Studies confirm the low level of satisfaction with health care services. In August 2010 only 15% of survey respondents said that they were satisfied with the health care system in the country while about 60% of respondents expressed the opposite view. Likewise 70% of respondents believed that they would be unable to obtain quality medical care if they needed it.

A second case is Armenia where life expectancy at birth had been the highest among all the Soviet republics – in 1986 an average of 73.3 years (70.5 for males and 75.7 for females) but it had begun to decline before the transition began. In 1991 life expectancy fell to an average of 70.4 years (67.4 for males; 73.3 for females), then started to grow again and returned to its previous level (73.4 years) in 2004.

For all countries in our sample, Table 11.3 indicates that the main indicators of the heath status of inhabitants are below the level in developed countries (*e.g.*, the EU average). Yet some positive trends are also visible. Many factors contribute to improved quality (especially clinical quality – better equipment, new treatment methods and drugs) in the four Central European countries, especially Slovenia.

Table 11.3 Clusters of Health Outcomes

Life Expectancy, Mortality, Morbidity	
Decreasing after 1989; recent improvements	Russia
Increasing after 1989, but far below developed countries	Armenia, Bulgaria (life expectancy decreasing after 2000), Macedonia, Romania
Increasing after 1989 but a gap compared to developed countries	Czech Republic, Hungary, Slovakia
Increasing after 1989; small gap compared to developed countries	Slovenia

Source: Construction based on country chapters.

In terms of clinical quality, health systems in Central and Eastern Europe have undoubtedly improved their ability to cure diagnoses that were considered terminal not so long ago. The standard of equipment in hospitals and other health providers improves constantly, especially in top-level private establishments for those with the ability to pay. There are also new, more effective drugs and treatment procedures.

The improvements of health care quality are normally based on internal and external quality control as well as on internal quality management systems, but the Slovak case indicates that this dimension has some gaps. Despite many promises, no government in Slovakia has been able to introduce systematic medical and organizational audits of health providers that would provide more information about how care is delivered by doctors and the conditions under which it is delivered to patients. Diagnostic and treatment standards are not used in most CEE countries; the same is true about modern health technology assessment systems.

The organizational quality of patient care has improved, albeit slowly. Compared to the old system, in most CEE countries there is choice of provider, but patients remain far from being the central subject of the system. Queuing without the chance for an exact appointment is typical among a large proportion of providers, including private ones; transparent waiting lists for treatments are also not a rule. While most countries adopted 'Patient Rights' documents, the level of respect to main rights of a patient by the medical staff is limited.

During the past year, the media in Central and Eastern Europe began to pay greater attention to the malfunctions of medical establishments that directly led to health damage or even death of patients. Such increased publicity of clinical problems does not mean that the quality dropped drastically; it only means that the public has finally begun to discuss the existing problems. However, a serious shortcoming in the clinical quality of the health system is that medical establishments are unable to take a stand about failures that simply happen during the process of treating patients, even if documented by media.

In developed countries, if doctors and other members of the medical staff neglect their obligations, fail to observe standard procedures or cause damage to patient's health, medical establishments invoke clearly defined procedures that form part of accreditation criteria and are designed to make up for the failure immediately. The Slovak case indicates that despite the mistreatment of the Slovak President in 2000 that revealed basic weaknesses in the daily delivery of care, there has been no impetus for changes towards increased responsibility of medical staff for any kind of mistreatment.

11.13 Conclusions

The analysis of health care reforms in Central and Eastern Europe shows some improvements but many gaps and malfunctions remain. Compared to 1990, the heath status of inhabitants improved for most although not all countries. Equality and universality of access declined everywhere but with different patterns and scale. The financing of health care and the need for effective cost-containment systems to cope with limited resources, remain real problems.

What are the possible explanations for why, after so many years and so many attempts, reforms in CEE health systems lack systematic positive outcomes? Three factors may play determinative roles: economic and health resources; low quality of health policy-making and implementation; and actors who are not ready to support the changes needed, especially citizens who are not well informed and inactive.

The economic situation in the region is a particularly important negative determinant. In the 1980s CEE countries had modest levels of income per capita in comparison to OECD states, a picture that has only recently begun to change in order to narrow the gap with older members of the European Union EU. Until recently, the hope that improved health outcomes were attainable rested on several ideas. Improvements in efficiency were possible after 1989 that would not be masked by diminished resources due to the transformational recession of the 1990s. And a higher priority would lead to more and/or better resources being spent on health by governments as well as citizens.

Unfortunately, all country case studies reveal that such a pattern did not occur. Expressed as a percentage of GDP, public expenditures for health care in Central and Eastern Europe grow very slowly, if at all, while cost-effective containment measures have not been implemented. Without a proper economic base, all promises of 'top quality health care for everybody' remain just phrases. However, even with limited resources, health systems may function better compared to the countries in our sample. Limited financial resources are important barrier but not the core deterrent to reforms in Central and Eastern Europe.

Based on the country chapters as well as existing knowledge, the lack of systematic reform outcomes is linked with the dimensions of public policy. Potential for reform is conditioned by the limited capacity to prepare and implement effective health policies and by the positions and strategies of main actors about the contents of the reforms. As already indicated, Dunn *et al.* (2006) argue that policy-making and policy implementation are the missing links of public administration reforms in Central and Eastern Europe. Country cases confirm the same for health care reforms. Several chapters deal with details of capacity for health policy-making and implementation in the region but none provides a positive evaluation. Even the 'best' country – Slovenia – was recently unable to realize needed reforms because of political limits. In place of evidence-based policy-making, political factors – such as frequent changes of governments (many with their own new concept of health care reforms), instability of health ministers and corruption – block chances for effective reforms.

It would be unfair to blame only governments about their limited policy-making and policy implementation. Health reforms are possible only in situations where main actors support their implementation. The situation in almost every case-study is complicated. In the Slovak case, analysis of 'utility functions' of main actors revealed negative results – a situation characteristic throughout the region. The chapter analyzed strategies of main players – politicians and bureaucrats on one side; health providers (hospitals, medical staff and insurance companies) on the other side – not to mention the role of hidden players like the pharmaceutical industry. The results of such analysis indicate that the dominant strategies of main actors limit the chance for positive changes.

Under current conditions, public hospitals are normally unconstrained by hard budgetary constraints. Because official salaries are low, their managements are able and frequently do channel part of institutional finance into private pockets. Therefore cost-containment and transparency-based changes are not welcomed by public hospitals. Doctors, too, are lack hard budgetary constraints and professional regulations (*e.g.*, examination and treatment standards). Consequently many doctors utilize the potential for supplier-induced demand by ordering extra treatments, equipment and drugs, or use the chance to earn extra incomes via the 'shadow' economy. Increased cost-efficiency, transparency and standardization endanger their current benefits.

The switch to the health insurance was formally based on expectations that, compared to the state, insurance companies may serve as better regulators of the system. However, most countries opted for one monopolistic health insurance company that is more or less controlled by the state. Even in the Czech and Slovak Republics where pluralistic health insurance has been advocated, insurance companies are neither independent nor serve as regulators; rather they act as resource distribution channels. In such conditions the voice of insurance sector is marginal and without capacity to be a real opponent to the central government.

Important problems also appear at the level of patients. Active and well-informed patients – health care 'consumers'– are essential for the preparation and realization of effective reforms. However, in Central and Eastern Europe most patients are neither well informed about their rights and needs nor ready to protect those rights and needs actively. While Hungary has had some successful patient movements, the capacity of patients to defend their individual rights remains limited in the region. Despite the fall of the old system, most patients see themselves not as customers but as 'slaves' of the system. Moreover, the illusion of 'free' care paid by the state motivates patients to opt for more care and for better (more expensive) drugs or treatments, even if not needed. Path dependency remains visible and blocks positive reforms. Based on the facts and analyses in this volume and elsewhere, reforms of health systems in Central and Eastern Europe rarely achieve success due to a combination of limited financial resources, imperfect health policy-making and implementation, inadequate capacity as well as the strategies of main actors.

References

Altenstetter, C. and J.W. Björkman. 1997. *Health Policy Reform, National Variations and Globalization*. London: Macmillan Press

Afonso, A., L. Ludger, L. Schuknecht and V. Tanzi. 2005. Public Sector Efficiency: An International Comparison. *Public Choice* 123:321-347

Akukwe, C. 1999. The Need for a Closer Working Relationship between Public Health and Public Administration Professionals, *PA Times* 22(4):3-4

ÁSZ (Állami Számvevőszék). 2005. Jelentés az irányított betegellátási modellkísérlet ellenőrzéséről (Summary of the Audit on the Managed Health Care Model Experiment), No. 0508. Budapest: Állami Számvevőszék (State Audit Office)

Annual Reports of the Minister of Health. 2008, 2009. *The Health of the Nation*. Sofia: Ministry of Health, Government of Bulgaria

Armenia Demographic and Health Survey. 2010. *Preliminary Report*. Yerevan: National Statistical Service of the Republic of Armenia. <www.armstat.am/en/?nid=82&id=1253>

ArmInfo. 2011. *Financial Analytic Portal*. <www.finport.am/view-archive-201107072044eng15197.html>

Asian Development Bank (ADB). 2009. *ADB and Armenia: Fact Sheet*. <www.adb.org/Documents/Fact_Sheets/ARM.pdf>

ADB. 2010. Economic Trends and Prospects in Developing Asia. *Asian Development Outlook* 3:105-108

ADB. 2011. Economic Trends and Prospects in Developing Asia. *Asian Development Outlook*. 3:89-92

Atanasova, E., E. Moutafova and T. Kostadinova. 2010. Patient payments in Central and Eastern Europe: The Opinion of Health Care Stakeholders. Policy brief No PB-/2010, The Netherlands. <www.ec.europa.eu/research/social-sciences.pdf>

Auster, R.D. 1975. Some Economic Determinants of the Characteristics of Public Workers. In *Economics of Public Choice* (volume 2) edited by R. Leiter and G. Sirkin. New York: City University of New York. Pages 185-198

Baji, P., M. Pavlova, L. Gulacsi and W. Groot. 2011. User Fees for Public Health Care Services in Hungary: Expectations, Experience and Acceptability from the Perspectives of Different Stakeholders. *Health Policy* 102:255-262

Balaban, L. 2010. Health Care System with Frozen Salaries. *Dnevnik* (25 March)

Balabanova, D., M. McKee, R. Rose, J. Pomerleau and C. Haerpfer. 2004. Health Service Utilization in the Former Soviet Union: Evidence from Eight Countries. *Health Service Research* 12:1-9

Bara, A.C., W.J.A. van den Heuvel and J.A.M. Maarse. 2002. Reforms of Healthcare System in Romania. *Croatian Medical Journal* 43(4):446-452

Baraczka, M. and P. Mihályi. 2009. Egészségügy 2008: A Kontrollok Éve (Health Care 2008: The Year of Control). In *Magyarország Politikai Évkönyve 2008-ról (Political Yearbook of Hungary - 2008)* edited by Péter Sándor and László Vass. Budapest: Demokrácia Kutatások Magyar Központja Közhasznú Alapítvány (Hungarian Centre for Democracy Studies). Pages1120-1151

Bauer, T. 1982. A Második Gazdasági Reform és a Tulajdonviszonyok (Reform of the Second Economy and the Property Structure). *Mozgó Világ* 1:17-42

Belli, P. and H. Shahriari. 2002. Qualitative Study on Informal Payments for Health Services in Georgia. *Human Development Network*. World Bank

Belli, P. 2004. Formal and Informal Household Spending on Health: A Multicountry Study in Central and Eastern Europe. *Central and Eastern European Health Network*. Cambridge, Massachusetts: Harvard School of Public Health

Bihari, M. 2005. *Magyar Politika 1944-2004. Politikai és Hatalmi Viszonyok* (*Hungarian Politics 1944-2004. Political and Power Relations*). Budapest: Osiris

Björkman, J.W. 2002. Health Sector Reforms in Comparative Perspective - An Unending Quest … or Chasing a Chimera? *Ciência & Saúde Coletiva* 14:373-381

Björkman, J.W. 2004. Health Sector Reforms: Measures, Muddles and Mires. In *Health Care Delivery Systems: Opportunities for Public Management* edited by A. Rosenbaum, J. Nemec and K. Tolo. Bratislava: NISPAcee. Pages 11-26

Blasszauer, B. (no date) Egészségügyi Törvény - Betegjogok. Egy Kísérleti Program Hazai és Külföldi Visszhangja (Health Care Act - Patient Rights. National and International Reflection on a Pilot Project). <www.szoszolo.hu/06tanulmanyaink/frindex.htm>

Björkman, J.W. and K. Mathur. 2002. *Policy, Technocracy and Development: Human Capital Policies in the Netherlands and India*. Delhi: Manohar Publishers

Bobak, M., M. McCarthy, F. Perlman and M. Marmot. 2004. Modernizing Public Health in Figures. *Health Systems in Transition: Learning from Experience*. Copenhagen: European Observatory on Health Systems and Policies. <www.euro.who.int/observatory>

Bochkareva, V. 2009. Space Factor and Formation of Effective Health Care System. *Health Management* 3:11-18 (Бочкарева В.К. Пространственный фактор в формировании эффективной системы здравоохранения. Управление здравоохранением. 2009. № 3. С. 11-18)

Bognár, G., Róbert I.G. and J. Kornai. 1999. Hálapénz a Magyar Egészségügyben (Gratuity in the Hungarian Health Care). *TÁRKI Társadalompolitikai Tanulmányok* No. 17. <www.tarki.hu/adatbank-h/kutjel/pdf/a199.pdf>

Boskovska, N. 2010. Hospitals are Drawing in Debts. *Nova Makedonija* (12 January)

Bozóki, A. 2003. *Politikai Pluralizmus Magyaroszágon, 1987-2002* (*Political Pluralism in Hungary, 1987–2002*). Budapest: Századvég

Brainerd, E. 2010. Human Development in Eastern Europe and the CIS since 1990. Human Development Reports Research Paper. New York: UNDP. <http://hdr.undp.org/en/reports/global/hdr2010/papers/HDRP_2010_16.pdf>

Brunnbauer, Ulf. 2002. The Implementation of the Ohrid Agreement: Ethnic Macedonian Resentments. Journal of Ethnopolitics and Minority Issues in Europe *3:1-24* <www.ecmi.de/jemie/download/Focus1-2002Brunnbauer.pdf.

Bunčak, J., R. Džambazovič, M. Hrabovský and J. Sopóci. 2008. Názory občanov na budúcnosť Slovenska (Opinion of Slovak Citizens). *Bratislava: Academy of Sciences*

Caiden, N. and A. Wildavsky. 1980. *Planning and Budgeting in Poor Countries.* New Brunswick, New Jersey: Transaction Books

Cardno. 2010. *USAID – Innovations in Support of Reproductive Health (Project NOVA): Achievements and Lessons Learned.* <www.cardnoem.com>

Castle-Kanerova, M. 1992. Social Policy in Czechoslovakia. In *The New Eastern Europe: Social Policy Past, Present and Future* edited by D. Deacon. London: Sage. Pages 91-117

Ceglar, J. 2004. *Modeli plačevanja izvajalcem bolnišnične dejavnosti v Sloveniji in izbranih državah* (Paying Models for Providers of Hospital Activity in Slovenia and Selected Countries). Master Thesis. Ljubljana: Faculty of Economics

Center for Research and Policy Making. 2005. Macedonian Health Insurance System: Current Analyses <www.crpm.org.mk/Papers/Occasional/Occasional4_mak.pdf>

Central Intelligence Agency (CIA). *The World Fact Book.* <https://www.cia.gov/library/publications/the-world-factbook/geos/am.html>

Cherecheș, R.M. and Ungureanu, M.I. 2012. The Saga of the Romanian Health Care Reform. *The Lancet* 379(9829):e52

Chubarova T. 2004. Public Health Management and Policy Education and Training: Russia. In *Health Care Delivery Systems: Opportunities for Public Management Education in Central and Eastern Europe* edited by A. Rosenbaum, J. Nemeč and K. Tolo. Bratislava: NISPAcee Press. Pages 170-184

Chubarova, T. 2008. Providing Medical Services: Economic Problems. *Studies on Russian Economic Development* 6:98-109 (Чубарова Т.В. Обеспечение населения медицинскими услугами: экономические проблемы. Проблемы прогнозирования. 2008, № 6. С. 98-109)

Cockerham, W. 1999. *Health and Social Change in Russia and Eastern Europe.* New York: Routledge

Comisia Prezidențială pentru analiza și elaborarea politicilor din domeniul sănătății publice din România (Presidential Commission for the Analysis and Elaboration of Public Health Policies in Romania). 2008. *Un sistem sanitar centrat pe nevoile cetățeanului (A Citizens' Need-centered Health System).* Bucharest. <www.presidency.ro/static/ordine/COMISIASANATATE/UN_SISTEM_SANITAR_CENTRAT_PE_NEVOILE_CETATEANULUI.pdf>

Constitutional Court of the Republic of Macedonia. 2010. *Decision No.185/2009-0-1* (27 January)

Coombes, D. and T. Verheijen. 1997. *Public Management Reform: Comparative Experiences from East and West.* Bratislava: European Commission

Coulter, F., C. Heady, C. Lawson and S. Smith. 1997. Social Security Reform for Economic Transition: The Case of the Czech Republic. *Journal of Public Economics* 65:313-326

Cullis, J. 1979. *The Economics of Health*. London: Martin Robertson

Cullis, J. and P. Jones. 1992. *Public Finance and Public Choice*. London: McGraw-Hill

Cutler, D.M. 2002. Health Care and the Public Sector. In *Handbook of Public Economics* edited by A.J. Auerbach and M. Feldstein. Volume 4:2143-2243. Amsterdam: Elsevier

Cutler, T. 2007. A Necessary Complexity: History and Public Management Reform. *History and Policy* (<www.historyandpolicy.org>)

Darmopilová, Z. and J. Špalek. 2008. Brokering Health Policy: The Case of Czech Republic Health Care Reform. In *Public Policy and Administration: Challenges and Synergies*. Bratislava: NISPAcee. Pages 1-25

Darmopilová, Z. and J. Špalek. 2009. Czech Health Care Reform (2006-2010) from the point of view of interest group´s support. *Acta Aerarii Publici* 5(1):22. Banská Bystrica: Univerzita Mateja Bela

Darmopilová, Z. and J. Špalek. 2009. Role of Interest Groups in Brokering Health Policy: The Case of Czech Health-Care Reform. *NISPAcee Journal of Public Administration and Policy* 2(1):43-76

Daskalovski, Zhidas. 2002. Language and Identity: The Ohrid Framework Agreement and Liberal Notion of Language and Identity. *Journal of Ethnopolitics and Minority Issues in Europe* 3:1-32 <www.ecmi.de/jemie/download/Focus1-2002Daskalovski.pdf>

Daskalovski, Z. 2004. Democratic Consolidation and the 'Stateness' Problem: The Case of Macedonia. The Global Review of Ethnopolitics 3(2):52-66 <www.ethnopolitics.org/ethnopolitics/archive/volume_III/issue_2/daskalovski.pdf>

D'Auria, F., A. Pagano, M. Ratto and J. Varga. 2009. *A Comparison of Structural Reform Scenarios across the EU Member States* – Simulation-based analysis using the QUEST model with endogenous growth <http://ec.europa.eu/economy_finance/publications/publication16461_en.pdf>

Davis, C. 1993. Russia´s Health Reform: Complicated Question. *Transition* 4:1–3.

Davis, C. 2001. The Health Sector: Illness, Medical Care and Mortality. In *Russia's Post-Communist Economy* edited by B. Granville and P. Oppenheimer. Oxford: Oxford University Press. Pages 475-538

Delcheva, E. 2011. Disbalances in Health Expenditures in Bulgaria. *Scripta Scientifica Medica* 43(4):292-293

Deletant, D. 1999. Romania under Communist Rule. Bucharest: Center for Romanian Studies

Demirchyan, A. and M. Thompson. 2008. Determinants of Self-related Health in Women: A Population-based Study in Armavir Marz, Armenia, 2001 & 2004. *International Journal for Equity in Health* 7:25

Dimova, A., M. Popov and M. Rohova. 2007. *Health Care Reform in Bulgaria: An Analysis.* Sofia: Open Society Institute

Dolea, C., Nolte, E. and M. McKee. 2002. Changing Life Expectancy in Romania after the Transition. *Journal of Epidemiology and Community Health* 56:444-449

Donev, D. 1999. Health Insurance System in the Republic of Macedonia. *Croatian Medical Journal* 40(2):175-180 <www.cmj.hr/1999/40/2/10234059.htm>

Donev, Doncho. 2009. Health Insurance System and the Provider Reform Payment in the Republic of Macedonia. *Italian Journal of Public Health* 6(1):30-39 <www.ijph.it/pdf//19/30.pdf>

Dopolnilno zdravstveno zavarovanje in zdravstvena reforma (Additional Health Insurance and Health Reform). 2011. Ljubljana: Slovenian Insurance Association

Dózsa, C. 2008. 2006-2007-es Évek az Egészségügyben: Reformtervek és Programok Kavalkádja (Health Care in 2006–2007: An Abundance of Reform Plans and Programs). In *Magyarország politikai évkönyve 2007-ről* (*Political Yearbook of Hungary – 2007*) edited by Péter Sándor and László Vass. Budapest: Demokrácia Kutatások Magyar Központja Közhasznú Alapítvány (Hungarian Centre for Democracy Studies). Pages 889-914

Dragomiristeanu, A. *et al.* 2008. Migrația medicilor din România (The Migration of Medical Doctors from Romania). *Revista Medica* <http://medicalnet.ro/2011/content/view/498/31/>

Dunn, W.D., K. Staronova and S. Pushkarev. 2006. *Implementation: The Missing Link in PA Reforms in Central and Eastern Europe.* Bratislava: NISPAcee

Economic Science in Modern Russia. 2007. Special issue. Moscow: VININI (Экономическая наука современной России. Экспресс выпуск.Москва: ВИНИТИ. 2007)

Egészségjelentés. 2010. Jelentés egy Egészségben Elmaradott Országból (Healthcare Report 2010 – Report from a Country Low in Health). prepared by József Vitrai, Márta Bakacs, Attila Juhász, Csilla Kaposvári and Csilla Nagy. Budapest: Egészség Monitor <www.egeszsegmonitor.hu/dok/Osszefoglalo_Egeszsegjelentes_2010.pdf>

Eržen, I. 2009. *Novi zakon o zdravstveni dejavnosti z vidika upravljanja zdravstvenega varstva* (The New Law on Healthcare from the Perspective of Health Care Management). Portorož: Days of Slovenian Public Administration

European Health for All Data Base (HFA-DB). 2011. Copenhagen: World Health Organization, Regional Office for Europe <http://data.euro.who.int/hfadb/>

European Health Report. 2002. Copenhagen: World Health Organization

Eurostat. 2011. Brussels: European Commission <http://epp.eurostat.ec.europa.eu/portal/page/portal/statistics/themes>

Eurostat. 2012. <http://epp.eurostat.ec.europa.eu/portal/page/portal/national_accounts/data/main_tables>

Exter, den A. and J. Sándor. 2002. Editors. *Frontiers of European Health Law Yearbook 2002.* Rotterdam: Erasmus University Press

Fallenbuch, Z.M. 1991. Economic Reform and Changes in the Welfare System in Poland. In *Economic Reforms and Welfare Systems in the USSR, Poland and Hungary.* Basingstoke and London: Macmillan. Pages 110-131

Fărcăşanu, D. 2010. Population Perception on Corruption, Informal Payments and Introduction of Co-payments in the Public Health System in Romania. *Management in Health* 14:8-13

Feldstein, P.J. 1993. *Health Care Economics.* Albany: Delmar Publishers

Feschieva, N., S. Popova and A. Kerekovska. 2011. Population Aging and Public Health: Challenges and Policies for the EU and Bulgaria. In *Public Health and Health Care in Greece and Bulgaria: The Challenge of the Cross-border Collaboration in Times of Financial Crisis* edited by John Kyriopoulos and Donka Dimitrova. Athens: Papazissis Publishers. Pages 325-333

Florescu, S., C. Mihăescu Pinţia, M. Gălăon and V. Constantinescu. 2012. Perspectives of Romanian Healthcare Consumers on Patient Co-payments. *Management in Health* 16(2):33-39

Freddi, G. and J.W. Björkman. 1989. Editors. *Controlling Medical Professionals: The Comparative Politics of Health Governance.* London: Sage Publications

Füzesi, Z., G. Ivády, Z. Kovácsy and K. Orbán. 2005. Hungarian Healthcare Reforms in the 1990s. In *Decentralization in Healthcare: Analyses and Experiences in Central and Eastern Europe in the 1990s* edited by George Shakarishvili. Budapest: Local Government and Public Service Reform Initiative, Open Society Institute. Pages 273-312

Gaál, Péter. 2004. *Health Care Systems in Transition: Hungary.* Copenhagen: WHO Regional Office for Europe on behalf of the European Observatory on Health Systems and Policies

Gaál, P., P. Belli, M. McKee and M. Szocsk. 2006. Informal Payments for Health Care: Definitions, Distinctions, and Dilemmas. *Journal of Health Politics Policy and Law* 31(2):251-293

Gălan, A., Olsavszky V. and C. Vlădescu. 2011. Emergent Challenge of Health Professional Emigration: Romania's Accession to the EU (pp. 449-478). In *Health Professional Mobility and Health Systems. Evidence from 17 European Countries* edited by Wismar *et al.* Copenhagen: European Observatory on Health Systems and Policies

Gallai, S. 2000. The Hungarian Electoral System. In *Hungary and India: Aspects of Political Systems* edited by Vinay Kumar Malhotra. New Delhi: Creative Books. Pages 89-100

Gallai, S. 2003a. Politikai Rendszerváltás Magyarországon (Political Regime Change in Hungary). In *Politika és Politikatudomány* (*Politics and Political Science*) edited by Sándor Gallai and Gábor Török. Budapest: Aula Kiadó. Pages 225-237

Gallai, S. 2003b. Magyarország Politikai Intézményrendszere (Structure of Hungary's Political Institutions). In *Politika és Politikatudomány* (*Politics and Political Science*) edited by Sándor Gallai and Gábor Török. Budapest: Aula Kiadó. Pages 347-394

Gallai, S. and T. Lánczi. 2006. Személyre Szabott Kormányzás – A Második Gyurcsány-kormány Anatómiája (Personalized Governance – The Anatomy of the Second Gyurcsány-Government). In *Parlamenti Választás 2006* (*Parliamentary Elections 2006*) edited by Gergely Karácsony. Demokrácia Kutatások Magyar Központja Közhasznú Alapítvány – BCE Politikatudományi Intézet (Hungarian Centre for Democracy Studies –Institute of Political Science, CUB). Pages 293-334

Gedeon, P. 1995. Hungary: Social Policy in Transition. *East European Politics and Societies* 9:433-458

Gewertz, K. 2005. Armenia's Remarkable Alphabet. *Harvard University Gazette.* <www.news.harvard.edu/gazette/2005/11.03/09-mashtots.html>

Gjorgjev, D. *et al.* 2006. The Former Yugoslav Republic of Macedonia: Health System Review. *Health Systems in Transition.* Copenhagen: World Health Organization

Government of the Slovak Republic. 1992. *Programmatic Declaration of the Government of the Slovak Republic.* Document submitted for debate in the Slovak National Council, No. 2477/92/A

Government of the Slovak Republic. 2002. *Programmatic Declaration of the Government of the Slovak Republic.* Daily SME, 5 November

Gregorič Rogelj, E. 2008. *Javno zasebno partnerstvo kot možna oblika investiranja v zdravstvene zavode* (Public-Private Partnership as a Way of Investing in Healthcare Institutions). Master Thesis. Ljubljana: Faculty of Social Sciences

Gregorič Rogelj, E. 2009. *Javno zasebno partnerstvo v zdravstvu z vidika razvojnih možnosti in potreb slovenskega zdravstva* (Public-Private Partnership in Healthcare in Terms of Development Potential and Needs in Slovenian Healthcare). Portorož: Days of Slovenian Public Administration 2009

Gregorič Rogelj, E. 2011. *Poslovni podatki* (Business Data). Ljubljana: Ministry of Health of Republic of Slovenia

Gregorič Rogelj, E. (2012). *Nadgrajevanje zdravstvenega sistema* (Upgrading the Healthcare System). Ljubljana: Faculty of Administration, <www.fu.uni-lj.si/horizont/novice/mag.Gregoric-Rogelj.pptx>

Griffin, K., T. Kelly, T. McKinley, B. Asatryan, L. Barkhudaryan and A. Yeghiazarian. 2002. *Growth, Inequality and Poverty in Armenia.* UNDP. <www.ipc-undp.org/publications/reports/Armenia.pdf>

Grigorieva, N. 2007. Understanding Modern European Social Policy: From Minimal Standards to Social Quality. *Problems of Modern State Governance in Russia* 7 (12). Moscow: Nauchnyi Expert. (Григорьева Н.С. К вопросу о понимании современной европейской социальной политики: от минимальных стандартов к социальному качеству. Проблемы современного государственного управления в России. Выпуск № 7 (12). Москва: Научный эксперт, 2007)

Grigorieva, N. 2008. Citizens and Society in Health Care Reforms. In *Modern Health Care: Possibilities and Limits* edited by N. Grigorieva. Moscow: Moscow State University. Pages 106-115. (Григорьева Н.С.. Гражданин и общество в контексте реформы здравоохранения. В кн. ;oFСовременное здравоохранение: возможности и пределы настоящего;cF. Под ред. Н.С.Григорьевой. М: МГУ. 2008. С. 106-115)

Guerschanik Calvo, S. 2010. *The Global Financial Crisis of 2008-10: A View from Social Sectors.* Human Development Research Paper 2010/18. New York: UNDP

Hakobyan, T., M. Nazaretyan, T. Makarova, M. Aristakesyan, H. Margaryants and E. Nolte. 2006. Armenia: Health System Review. *Health Systems in Transition* 8(6):1-180

Hall, D. and E. Lobina. 2005. *The Relative Efficiency of Public and Private Sector Water.* London: Public Sector International Research Unit, Business School, University of Greenwich

Háva, P. and M. Rokosová. 2005. Health Care Systems in Transitions. Czech Republic. *WHO – European Observatory on Health Systems and Policies* 7(1):109

Hayrapetyan, S. and A. Khanjyan. 2004. *Healthcare in Armenia: Challenges and Prospects.* Armenian International Policy Research Group. Working Paper #04/13 <www.aiprg.net/UserFiles/File/wp/jan2004/13.pdf>

HCL. 2005. *Health Care Law.* Official Gazette of the Republic of Macedonia 38/91, 46/93, 55/95, 10/04, 84/05

HCL. 2012. Health Care Law. Official Gazette of the Republic of Macedonia 43/2012.

Health for All Data Base. 2003. Geneva: World Health Organization

Healthgrouper.com 2012a. Special reports: Job Satisfaction among Physicians in Macedonia <http://healthgrouper.com/en/page/Press_release_Physicians_Satisfaction>.

Healthgrouper.com 2012b. Short reports: <http://healthgrouper.com/en/page/Capitation-and-expenses>

HFA (Health for All). 2009. *European Health for All Database.* Copenhagen: World Health Organization Regional Office for Europe, 2009 <www.euro.who.int/hfadb>

HIF (Health Insurance Fund). 2007. *Annual Report of the Health Insurance Fund 2007.* <www.fzo.org.mk/WBStorage/Files/gIzvestaj07.pdf>

HIF. 2008. *Annual Report of the Health Insurance Fund 2007* [in Macedonian] <www.fzo.org.mk/default.asp?ItemID=C349CD3739E3124B8D3C4C71C64F2121>

HIF. 2009. *Annual Report of the Health Insurance Fund 2008* [in Macedonian] <www.fzo.org.mk/WBStorage/Files/gIzvestaj08.pdf>

HIF. 2009. *Health Insurance Fund. DRG Results and Reports.* [in Macedonian] <www.fzo.org.mk/default.asp?ItemID=321A8D9BF62E77479E0158EA9CBEFDEA>

HIF. 2009. *Monthly Reports Disbursement of the Health Insurance Fund Budget* [in Macedonian] <www.fzo.org.mk/WBStorage/Files/Mesecen%20Izvestaj_Noemvri2009.pdf>

HIF. 2010. *Health Insurance Fund. Reference Pricing of Services with Co-payment* [in Macedonian] <www.fzo.org.mk>

HIL. 2000. Health Insurance Law 2000. *Official Gazette of the Republic of Macedonia* 25/00

HIL. 2003. Health Insurance Law. *Official Gazette of the Republic of Macedonia*, 25/2000, 34/2000, 96/2000, 50/2001, 11/2002, 31/2003

Health Systems Development Program (HSDP). 2007. Poletti, T., D. Balabanova, O. Ghazaryan, M. Kamal-Yanni, H. Kocharyan, K. Arakelyan and M. Hakobyan. *Options for Scaling-up Community-based Health Insurance for Rural Communities in Armenia*. London: London School of Hygiene and Tropical Medicine. <www.cspn.am/files/resources/Oxfam-resource/445_Oxfam-GB-Armenia--CBHI.pdf>

Herczeg, J. 2002. A Magyar Egészségügy Privatizációjának Sajátosságai (Peculiarities of Privatization in the Hungarian Health Care System). *Gazdaság és Társadalom* 1:91-113

Heuer, O. 2002. Editor. *Betegjogok Magyarországon – Szabályok és Gyakorlat* (*Patient Rights in Hungary – Rules and Practice*). Budapest: Társaság a Szabadságjogokért (The Hungarian Civil Liberties Union)

Hill, M. and P. Hupe. 2002. *Implementing Public Policy: Governance in Theory and in Practice*. London: Sage Publications

Hislope, R. 2003. Between a Bad Peace and a Good War: Insights and Lessons from the Almost-war in Macedonia. *Ethnic and Racial Studies* 26(1):129-151

Holt, E. 2010. Romania mulls over fast food tax. *The Lancet* 375(9720):1070

Holt, E. 2011. Hungary to introduce broad range of fat taxes. *The Lancet* 378(9793):755

Holt, E. 2012. Romania redrafts health-care law after violent protests. *The Lancet* 379:505

Hovhannisyan, S., E. Tragakes, S. Lessof, H. Aslanian and A. Mkrtchyan. 2001. *Healthcare Systems in Transition: Armenia*. Copenhagen: European Observatory on Healthcare Systems. <www.euro.who.int/document/e73698.pdf>

Hovhannisyan S. 2004. Healthcare in Armenia. *British Medical Journal* 2:329-522. <www.bmj.com/cgi/content/full/329/7465/522>

Hovsepyan, A. and A. Khudaverdyan. 2006. *Public Sector Reforms in Armenia 1999-2005: Achievements and Challenges*. AIPRG Working Paper No. 06/03 <www.aiprg.net/UserFiles/File/wp/jan2006/wp03-06.pdf>

Information Agency Regnum. 2011. <http://regnum.ru/new/fd-abroad/armenia/1364780.html>

Institute for Public Health. 2009. *Health Map of the Republic of Macedonia 2007*. Skopje: Institute for Public Health

Institute of Public Health. 2010. <www.ivz.si/index.php?akcija=kategorija&k=69>

International IDEA. 2007. *Political Parties in Central and Eastern Europe: In Search of Consolidation*. <www.idea.int/publications/pp_c_and_e_europe/index.cfm>

International Monetary Fund (IMF*). 2010. World Economic Outlook: Rebalancing Growth.* Washington, DC

International Monetary Fund (IMF). *2011. World Economic Outlook: Slowing Growth, Rising Risks*. Washington, DC

Ivanovska, L. and I. Ljuma. 1999. Health Sector Reform in the Republic of Macedonia. *Croatian Medical Journal* 40:181-9 <www.cmj.hr/1999/40/2/10234060.htm>

Jovanovska, J. 2010. Hospitals Drown in Debts Again. *Utrinski Vesnik* (24 March)

Keber, D. 2003. *Utrjevanje vrednot in vzpodbujanje sprememb* (Consolidating Values and Promoting Changes). Zdravstvena reforma 2003. Uvodnik, <http://vestnik.szd.si/st3-2/st3-2-57-58.htm> (accessed 22 March 2011)

Kerekovska, A., N. Feschieva, K. Dokova and N. Usheva. 2007. Health Status of the Bulgarian Population: Social Determinants, Recent Dynamics and Policy Implications. *Scripta Scientifica Medica* 40

Klein, R. 1992. NHS Reforms. *British Medical Journal* 25:36-51

Knavs, N. 2011. *Zdravstvena reforma: jasna meja med obveznim in prostovoljnimi zavarovanji* (Healthcare Reform: a Clear Boundary Between Compulsory and Voluntary Insurances). Dnevnik.si, <www.dnevnik.si/novice/slovenija/1042423288>

Kolesnikov, S. 2010. Legal Aspects of PPP in Health Care. *Health Management* 1(26):16-23 (Колесников С.И. Правовое обеспечение государственно-частного партнерства в здравоохранении // Управление здравоохранением, 2010 № 1(26). С. 16-23)

Kornai, J. 2009. The Soft Budget Constraint Syndrome in the Hospital Sector. *Society and Economy* 31:5-31

Körösényi, A. 2001. Parlamentáris Vagy "Elnöki" Kormányzás? Az Orbán-kormány Összehasonlító Perspektívából (Parliamentary or "Presidential" Governance?" The Orbán-Government from a Comparative Perspective). *Századvég, Új folyam* 22:3-38

Körösényi, A., C. Tóth and G. Török. 2003. *A Magyar Politikai Rendszer* (*The Hungarian political system*). Budapest: Osiris

Kovač, K. Aleksandra. 2011. *Zdravstvena reforma: povišanje prispevne stopnje ob enaki bruto plači?* (Healthcare Reform: Increase in Contribution Rate at Equal Gross Salary?) Ljubljana: MMC RTV Slovenija<www.rtvslo.si/zdravje/zdravstvena-reforma-povisanje-prispevne-stopnje-ob-enaki-bruto-place/251057>

Kranjec, M. 2007. *Nekateri strateški problemi slovenskega zdravstva* (Some Strategic Problems of Slovenian Healthcare). 7. Seja Strateškega sveta za gospodarski razvoj. Ljubljana: Government of the Republic of Slovenia

Krebs, V. and A. Slaný. 2009. Solidarita a Ekvivalence v Sociálních Systémech (Solidarity and Equivalence in Social Systems). Praha: Výzkumný Ústav Práce a Sociálních Věcí. 178 s. Neuveden

Kurtán, S. 2003. Politikai Kultúra (Political Culture). In *Politika és Politikatudomány* (*Politics and Political Science*) edited by Sándor Gallai and Gábor Török. Budapest: Aula. Pages147-157

Kuvikova, H., M. Murgas and J. Nemec. 1995. *Ekonomia Zdravotnictva* (Health Economics). Banska Bystrica: Phoenix

Kuzuzovlev, O., O. Goncharova. 2008. State and Problems of Private Health Care: A Case of Moscow Region. *Medical Science and Practice.* № 1. Pages 28-34 (Кузовлев О.П., Гончарова О.В. Состояние и проблемы частного здравоохранения России на примере Московского региона // Медицинская наука и практика. 2008. № 1. С. 28-34)

Lánczi, A. 2007. What is Post-communism? *Society and Economy* 29:65-85

Langenbrunner, J. 2003. *Healthcare Financing: Issues, Reforms, the Unfinished Agenda.* Washington DC: The World Bank <http://siteresources.worldbank.org/INTECAREGTOPHEANUT/Resources/HNPinECA_Dec2003_Ch5.pdf>

Law no. 95/2006 regarding Reform in Health Care, Section VII, Quality Assurance in Romania. <www.cdep.ro/pls/legis/legis_pck.htp_act_text?idt=72105>

Lawson, C. and J. Nemec. 2003. The Political Economy of Slovak and Czech Health Policy. *International Political Science Review* 24:219-236

Lazarevik, V. and D. Donev. 2012a. The Public Hospital System in Macedonia. In *Health Reforms in South East Europe* edited by William Bartlett, Jadranka Bozikov and Bernd Rechel. Basingstoke: Palgrave Macmillan

Lazarevik, Vladimir 2012b. Administrative Workload of GPs in the Republic of Macedonia: An Urgent Call for Change. *Macedonian Journal of Medical Sciences* June <www.mjms.ukim.edu.mk/Online/MJMS_OnlineFirst/MJMS.1857-5773.2012-0227v.pdf>

Lazarevik, V., M. Risteska and V. Simonovska. 2009. The Impact of Social Assistance Programs on Reducing Inequities in Health Care among Vulnerable Groups in the Republic of Macedonia. *Macedonian Journal of Medical Sciences* 2:73-78 <www.mjms.ukim.edu.mk/Online/MJMS_2009_2_1/MJMS.1857-5773.2009-0033.pdf>

Lazarevik, V. 2010. Policy Interventions to Tackle Inequities in Health: Patient Rights and Reference Pricing of Pharmaceuticals. *Macedonian Journal of Medical Sciences* 3:57-60 <www.mjms.ukim.edu.mk/Online/MJMS_2010_3_1/MJMS.1857-5773.2010-0079.pdf>

Legicon, Center for Urban and Regional Sociology. 2005. *Report on Informal Payments in the Romanian Health-care Sector.* Bucharest: Center for Urban and Regional Sociology

Levada Center. 2011. <www.levada.ru/community.html> (Левада-Центр, 2011)

Lijphart, A. 1992. Democratization and Constitutional Choices in Czechoslovakia, Hungary and Poland, 1989-1991. *Journal of Theoretical Politics* 4:207-223

Lewis, M. 2000. *Who is Paying for Healthcare in Eastern Europe and Central Asia?* World Bank. Washington, DC <www.sec.lt/pages/alfdiskusijos/pages/discuss3/docs/Who+Is+Paying+text.pdf>

Lewis, M. and Musgrove P. 2008. Governance Issues in Health Financing. *International Encyclopedia of Public Health* 3:81-88

Macedonian Informative Agency (MIA). 2010. *What were Constitutional Court's Motives to Pass Two Contradictory Rulings on HIF in Six Months* <www.mia.cdom.mk/default.aspx?vId=71716063&1Id=2>

Macroeconomic. 1999. *Peculiarities and Stages of Economic Reforms in Armenia 1991-1998: Main Characteristic Changes.* Yerevan: National Statistical Service of the Republic of Armenia <http://armstat/am/file/article/tntbar_91-98eng_1.pdf>

Malý, I. 1998. *Problem optimalni alokace zdroju ve zdravotnictvi (The Problem of the Optimal Allocation of Resources in Health Care).* Brno: Masarykova Univerzita

Malý, I., M. Pavlík and V. Krůtilová. 2012. Aktuální Problémy Tvorby a Implementace Zdravotní Politiky z Pohledu Region (Regional Point of View on Health Policy Implementation: Current Issues). In *Dopady Vybraných Veřejných Politik na Regionální Rozvoj v České a Slovenské Republice.* První. Brno: Masarykova Univerzita. Pages 139-149

Marcheva, A. 2010. *Human Resources in the Health System in Bulgaria.* Svistov: Zenov Academy

Mazmanian, D.A. and P.A. Sabatier. 1989. *Implementation and Public Policy.* Washington DC: University Press

McPake, Barbara. 2002. The Globalization of Health Sector Reform Policies: Is Lesson Drawing Part of the Process? In *Health Policy in a Globalizing World* edited by Kelly Lee, Kent Buse and Suzanne Fustukian: Cambridge: Cambridge University Press. Pages 120-139

Menon, Sonia. 2006. Decentralization and Health Care in the Republic of Macedonia. *International Journal of Health Planning and Management* 21:3-21

Mihályi, P. and L. Molnár. 2006. Az Egészségügyi Reform Első Szakasza (The First Stage of Health Reform). In *Magyarország Politikai Évkönyve 2006-ról* (*Political Yearbook of Hungary - 2006*) edited by Péter Sándor, Ágnes Tolnai and László Vass. Budapest: Demokrácia Kutatások Magyar Központja Alapítvány (Hungarian Centre for Democracy Studies). Pages 409-464

Millard, F. 1994. Developments in Polish Health Care. In *Societies in Transition: East-Central Europe Today* edited by S. Ringen and C Wallace. Aldershot: Avebury. Pages 73–89

Miller, V.L., A.B. Grodeland and T.Y. Koschechkina. 1998. *Are the People Victims or Accomplices?* Budapest: Open Society Institute/Local Government Initiative

Ministry of Health. 2007. *Planul strategic pentru 2008-2010* (Strategic plan for 2008-2010). Bucharest <http://vechi.ms.ro/pagina.php?id=119>

Misovski, J. 2001. Book: *Comments on the Law on Health Insurance with Bylaws.* Skopje. Ministry of Health

MoH (Ministry of Health) 2001. *Health Sector Transition Project:. Strategy for Financing and Future Organization of Primary Health Care* (policy paper)

MoH. 2006. *Health Sector Transition Project: Strategic Health Summit 2006*: Conclusions <www.moh-hsmp.gov.mk/index.php?id=67>

MoH. 2007a. *Health Sector Management Project: Formulation of a Co-payment Policy under Social Health Insurance, Final Report* <www.moh-hsmp.gov.mk/uploads/media/Co-Payment_Policy_-_Final_Report_by_Karl_Karol.pdf>

MoH. 2007b. *Health Sector Management Project. Consultancy on Health Care Providers Legislation* <www.moh-hsmp.gov.mk/uploads/media/Consultancy_on_health_care_providers_legislation.pdf>

MoH. 2007c. *Health Sector Transition Project. Health Management and Leadership Training Manual* [in Macedonian]. <www.moh-hsmp.gov.mk/fileadmin/user_upload/Priracnik%20za%20menagment%20i%20liderstvo.PDF>

MoH. 2008. *Information for the Implementation of the Health Care Law in the Transformation of Primary Health Care*

Molnár, A. 2001. A Magyar Betegjogi Szabályozás a Nemzetközi Rendelkezések Tükrében (The Hungarian Regulation of Patient Rights in the Light of International Directives). *Lege Artis Medicina* 8-9:597-610

Monitorul Oficial (Official Monitor). Order no. 1199/26.07.2011 regarding the introduction of RO DRG classification <http://legestart.ro?Ordinul-1199-2011-introducerea-utilizarea-clasificarii-RO-DRG-v-1(NTg5ODEy).htm>

Mossialos, E., A. Dixon, J. Figuera and J Kutazin. 2002. *Funding Health Care: Options for Europe*. European Observatory on Health Systems and Policies

Nadgradnja zdravstvenega sistema do leta 2020: korak naprej (Upgrading the Healthcare System by 2020: a Step Forward). 2011. Ljubljana: Ministry of Health of Republic of Slovenia

Nadgradnja zdravstvenega sistema (Upgrading the Healthcare System). (2012). Ljubljana: Government of the Republic of Slovenia. <www.vlada.si/si/teme_in_projekti/izhod_iz_krize/strukturni_ukrepi/nadgradnja_zdravstvenega_sistema/>

Národná správa o ľudskom rozvoji Slovenská republika 2001-2002 (National Report on Human Development in Slovakia). 2003. Bratislava: UNDP and INEKO

National Institute of Public Health. 2011. *Raportul stării de sănătate 2010* (2010 Health status report). Bucharest <www.insp.gov.ro/cnepss/wp-content/themes/PressBlue/pdf/Raport%20stare%20sanatate.%20Indicatori%20ECHI.pdf>

National Policy on Population Health Protection of RA. 2002. Yerevan: Ministry of Health of the Republic of Armenia. Document No.502 (2 August)

Nemec, J., B. Meričková and J. Štrangfeldová. 2010. The Ownership Form of Hospitals from the Viewpoints of Economic Theory and Slovak Practice. In *Ekonomie a management* 13(2):19-31

Obvezno zdravstveno zavarovanje v Sloveniji: danes za jutri (Compulsory Health Insurance in Slovenia: Today for Tomorrow). 2007. Ljubljana: Health Insurance Institute of Slovenia

Official Gazette of the Republic of Macedonia (OG). 2008a. No. 142. *Law for Contributions of Mandatory Social Insurance*

OG. 2008b. No. 7. Law for Concessions and Other Forms of Public Private Partnerships

Ohanian, C. 2007. *Armenian Cultural Values and the Issue of European Integration*. Yerevan: International Center for Human Development (ICHD). <http://news.am/rus/news/45386.html>

Okma, K.G.H. and L. Crivelli. 2010. Editors. *Six Countries, Six Reform Models: The Healthcare Reform Experience*. Singapore: World Scientific Publishing

Open Society Institute. 2005. *Mediating Romani Health Policy and Program Opportunities*. New York: Open Society Institute

Open Society Institute. 2008. *The Illegal Payment in Health Care*. Sofia: Open Society Institute

Orenstein, M. 1995. Transitional Social Policy in the Czech Republic and Poland. *Sociological Review* 3:179-196

Organization for Economic Cooperation and Development (OECD). 2012. *StatExtracts: Health*. Paris. <http://stats.oecd.org/Index.aspx?>

Orviska, M. and J. Hudson. 2003. Tax Evasion, Civic Duty and the Law Abiding Citizen. *European Journal of Political Economy* 19:83-102

Pavel, J. 2007. *Ekonomické aspekty veřejných zakázek*. Praha: Oeconomica

Pavlík, M. 2008. *Implementace veřejné politiky*. Brno: Masaryk University

Pavlík, M. 2010. *Zdravotní Politika z Pohledu Vlády – Analýza Implementačního Deficitu* (Health Policy from the Cabinet Point of View – Analysis of Implementation Deficit). Brno: Masarykova Univerzita. 158 s. 1. vydání.

Pažitný, P. and R. Zajač. 2001. *Stratégia reformy zdravotníctva – reálnej reformy pre občana (Strategy of Health Care Reform)*. Bratislava: M.E.S.A. 10 (think-tank)

Pažitný, P., T. Szalay, A. Szalayová and H. Maďarová. 2006. Zdravotníctvo (Health Care). In *Slovensko 2005*. Bratislava: Institute for Public Affairs

Pažitný, P., T. Szalay and A. Szalayová. 2008. Zdravotníctvo (Health Care). In *Slovensko 2007*. Bratislava: Institute for Public Affairs

Pew Research Center. 2009. Two Decades after the Wall's Fall: End of Communism Cheered but Now with More Reservations. Pew Global Attitudes Project <http://pewglobal.org/files/pdf/267.pdf>

Planning and Development Cooperative International (PADCO). 2000. Armenia Social Transition Report No. 5: *Legal Analysis: Issues Related to Organization and Delivery of Healthcare in Armenia*. <www.aecom.com>

PADCO. 2002. Armenia Social Transition Report No. 86: *Recommendations on How to Reduce Informal Payments for Medical Services in Armenia.* <www.padco.aecom.com>

Poslovno poročilo ZZZS za leto 2001 (HIIS 2001 Annual Report). 2002. Ljubljana: Health Insurance Institute of Slovenia

Poslovno poročilo ZZZS za leto 2005 (HIIS 2005 Annual Report). 2006. Ljubljana: Health Insurance Institute of Slovenia

Poslovno poročilo ZZZS za leto 2009 (HIIS 2009 Annual Report). 2010. Ljubljana: Health Insurance Institute of Slovenia

Poslovno poročilo ZZZS za leto 2010 (HIIS 2010 Annual Report). 2011. Ljubljana: Health Insurance Institute of Slovenia

Poslovno poročilo ZZZS za leto 2011 (HIIS 2011 Annual Report). 2012. Ljubljana: Health Insurance Institute of Slovenia

Pražáková, V. and K. Dušek. 2011. Outcome of Regulatory Fees in Health Care. *Journal of Nursing, Social Studies and Public Health* 1-2:60-72

Prva statistična objava (First Statistical Publication). 2009. *Izdatki sektorja država po namenih, Slovenija, 2000-2007.* Statistical Office of the Republic of Slovenia <www.stat.si/novica_prikazi.aspx?id=2120>

Prva statistična objava (First Statistical Publication). 2011. *Izdatki in viri financiranja za zdravstvo, Slovenija, 2003-2009.* Statistical Office of the Republic of Slovenia <www.stat.si/novica_prikazi.aspx?id=3975>

Prva statistična objava (First Statistical Publication). 2012. *Izdatki in viri financiranja zdravstvenega varstva, Slovenija, 2003-2010.* Statistical Office of the Republic of Slovenia <www.stat.si/novica_prikazi.aspx?id=4776>

Public Opinion Foundation (FOM). 2010. *Situation in Health Care: Sociological Survey.* (Фонд ;оFОбщественное мнение;cF (ФОМ). 25.02.2010. Ситуация в здравоохранении)

Qushqyan, Harutyun. 2010. Interview with the Minister of Health of the Government of the Republic of Armenia. Pan Armenian Network. <www.armtown.com/news/ru/pan/20100316/44278> (in Russian <www.armtown.com/news/ru/noa/20100226/42208549/>)

Radičová, I. and M. Potůček. 1997. Two Social Policies Out of One: The Czech and Slovak Example. Paper presented at the 19th meeting of the International Sociological Association Research Committee on Welfare state Challenge, Marginalization and Poverty. Copenhagen

Radin, D. 2009. Too Ill to Find the Cure? Corruption, Institutions, and Health Care Sector Performance in the New Democracies of Central and Eastern Europe and Former Soviet Union. *East European Politics & Societies 23* (1):105-125

Řeháková, B. 2001. Změny Hodnot v České Republice a Inglehartova Hodnotová Typologie (Changing Values in the Czech Republic and the Inglehart Value Typology). *Sociální studia* 6:47-71

Rimashevskaya, N. 2007. Editor. *Health and Health Care in Gender Perspective*. Moscow: Social Project Agency. (Здоровье и здравоохранение в гендерном измерении. Под общ. ред. Н.М.Римашевской. М.: Агентство ;oFСоциальный проект;cF. 2007)

Rimashevskaya, N., L. Migranov and E. Molchanova. 2011. Factors that Affect Population Health Status in Russia. *Population Studies*. № 1. Pages 38-49 (Римашевская Н.М., Мигранова Л.А. Молчанова Е.В. Факторы, влияющие на состояние здоровья населения России. Народонаселение. 2011. № 1. С. 38-49)

România – sectorul de sănătate. Studiu de politică sectorială. (Romania – Health Sector. Sectorial Policy Study). ECHSD <http://siteresources.worldbank.org/INTROMANIAINROMANIAN/Resources/HealthSectorPolicyNoteRomanian.pdf>

Rosenbaum, A., J. Nemec and K. Tolo. 2004. *Health Care Delivery Systems*. Bratislava: NISPAcee

Rosstat Survey. 2008. Influence of Behavioral Factors on Population Health Status. *Demoscope Weekly*, Numbers 379-380 (10-14 June 2009)

Russian Statistical Agency (RSA). 2009. *Health Care in Russia*. Moscow: Russian Statistical Agency (Здравоохранение в России. Стат.сб./Росстат. М. 2009)

Saltman, R.B. and J. Figueras. 1998. Analyzing the Evidence on European Health Care Reforms. *Health Affairs* 17:85-108

Saltman, R., R. Busse and J. Figueras. 2004. Editors. *Social Health Insurance Systems in Western Europe*. Berkshire / New York: Open University Press / McGraw-Hill Education

Saric, M. and V.G. Rodwin. 1993. The Once and Future Health System in Former Yugoslavia: Myths and Realities. *Journal of Public Health Policy* 14:220-237

Sartori, G. 1976. *Parties and Party Systems*. Cambridge: Cambridge University Press

Sándor, P. and L. Vass. 2007. *Magyarország Politikai Évkönyve 1988–2006* (*Political Yearbook of Hungary 1988-2006*) DVD. Budapest: Demokrácia Kutatások Magyar Központja Alapítvány (Hungarian Centre for Democracy Studies)

Savedoff, W.D. 2007. What Should a Country Spend on Health Care? *Health Affairs* 26:962-970

SEEurope.NET. 2010. *Agreements on Procurement of Modern Medical Equipment in Public Health* Signed in Vreme (23 February)

Selimyan, G. and L. Danielian. 2005. *Public Health Management and Policy Education and Training: Armenia*. <www.my-world-guide.com/upload/File/Reports/Armenia/Public_Health_Education.pdf>

Setnikar-Cankar, S. and J. Seljak. 2006. Ekonomika zdravstva: izkušnje drugih držav in raziskava Fakulteta za upravo (Healthcare Economics: Experiences of Other Countries and the Research of the Faculty of Administration). In *Značilnosti Javnega sektorja v Sloveniji in ugotavljanje njegove učinkovitosti* (Characteristics of the Public Sector in Slovenia and Determination of its Effectiveness) edited by Stanka Setnikar-Cankar and Maja Klun. Upravna misel. Ljubljana: Faculty of Administration. Pages 147-195

Shakarashvili, G. 2005. *Decentralization in Healthcare*. Budapest: Open Society Institute – Local Government Initiative

Shishkin, S.1999. *Problems of Transition from Tax-Based System of Healthcare Finance to Mandatory Health Insurance in Russia*. Croatian Medical Journal.40:195-201. Cited in Balabanova *et al.* 2004

Shkolnikov, V., E. Andreeva and T. Maleva. 2000. Editors. *Inequality and Mortality in Russia*. Moscow: Carnegie Center (Неравенство и смертность в России. Под ред. В. Школьникова, Е.Андреева, Т.Малевой.Моск. Центр Карнеги. М: 2000)

Shuhrcke, M., L. Rocco and M. McKee. *Health: Vital Investment for Economic Development in Eastern Europe and Central Asia*. 2007. Geneva: World Health Organization

Sinfield A. 2005. The Goals of Social Policy: Context and Change. *The Changing Face of Welfare: Consequences and Outcomes from a Citizenship Perspective*. Bristol: Policy Press

Sinkó, E. 2008. Az Egészségbiztosítási Rendszer Átalakításának Menete (The Reorganization Process of the Social Insurance System). In *Magyarország Politikai Évkönyve 2007-ről* (*Political Yearbook of Hungary* 2007) edited by Péter Sándor and László Vass. Budapest: Demokrácia Kutatások Magyar Központja Közhasznú Alapítvány (Hungarian Centre for Democracy Studies). Pages 805-846

SKUPR (Working Group for a Reform). 1990. *Návrh Reformy Péče o Zdraví* (Health Reform Proposal). Praha: MZSV

Slaveski, Trajko. 1997. Privatization in the Republic of Macedonia. *Eastern European Economics* 35:31-51

Socialni razgledi 2009 (2009 Social Monitor). 2010. Ljubljana: Institute of Macroeconomic Analysis and Development

Sociologický ústav AV ČR . 2006. Oddělení Studia Sociální Struktury: *Názory Veřejnosti na Problémy Zdravotnictví a Jeho Financování* (Public Opinion on Health Care System Issues and Financing). <www.soc.cas.cz/dowload/151/Tiskov%C3%A1%20 zpr%C3%A1va.pdf>

Staines, V. 1999. *A Health Sector Strategy for the Europe and Central Asia Region*. Washington DC: The World Bank

State Statistical Office. 2007. *Statistical Yearbook of the Republic of Macedonia. 2006*. Skopje: State Statistical Office

State Statistical Office. 2009a. *Statistical Yearbook of the Republic of Macedonia 2009*. Skopje: State Statistical Office.

State Statistical Office. 2012. *Key indicators*. Skopje: State Statistical Office. <www.stat.gov.mk/OblastOpsto_en.aspx?id=2>

State Statistical Office. 2010. *Household Survey 2009*. Skopje: State Statistical Office

Statistical Yearbook of Armenia. 2010. Yerevan: National Statistical Service of the Republic of Armenia. <http://armstat.am>

Statistični letopis 2009 (Statistical Yearbook 2009). 2009. Ljubljana: Statistical Office of the Republic of Slovenia

Statistični letopis 2010 (Statistical Yearbook 2009). 2010. Ljubljana: Statistical Office of the Republic of Slovenia

Stratégia reformy zdravotnictva (Health Care Reforms Strategy). 2003. Ministry of Health, Slovak Republic

Štrangfeldová, J. 2008. *Komparácia liečebnej a ekonomickej efektívnosti v štátnych a súkromných zdravotníckych zariadeniach*. Banská Bystrica: Matej Bel University

Strategia națională de raționalizare a spitalelor (National Strategy for Hospital Rationalization). 2011. Bucharest: Ministry of Health. <www.ms.ro/?pag=207>

Stiglitz, J. 1986. *Economics of the Public Sector*, second edition. London: Princeton University Press

Suhrcke, M., L. Rocco, M. McKee, S. Mazzuco, D. Urban and A. Steinherr. 2007. *Economic Consequences of Non-Communicable Diseases and Injuries in the Russian Federation*. Copenhagen: World Health Organization on behalf of the European Observatory on Health Systems and Policies

Szajkowski, Bogdan. 1999. *Elections and Electoral Politics in Macedonia: Transitions*. Brussel: Institut de Sociologie, ULB. XL(1-2) :55-82 <dev.ulb.ac.be/cevipol/dossiers_fichiers/szajkowski-1999-1-2.pdf>

Szalay, T., P. Pazitny, A. Szalayova, S. Frisova, K. Morvay, M. Petrovic and E. van Ginneken. Slovakia: Health system review. Health systems in transition. 2011, 13(2). Copenhagen, World Health Organization on behalf of the European Observatory on Health Systems and Policies

Szilvásy, G. 2003. A Közigazgatás a Negyedik Ciklus Után (Public Administration after the Fourth Cycle). In *Magyarország Politikai Évkönyve 2002-ről* (*Political Yearbook of Hungary - 2002*) edited by Péter Sándor and László Vass. Budapest: Demokrácia Kutatások Magyar Központja Alapítvány (Hungarian Centre for Democracy Studies). Pages 79-95

Tajnikar, M. 2009. Predavanje 1. *Osnove ekonomike zdravstvenega varstva* (Basics of Healthcare Economics). Ljubljana: Faculty of Economics <www.ef.uni-lj.si/predmeti32/_struktura/izpis.asp?vrsta=2&id=192337> (accessed 14 March 2011)

Tajnikar, M. and P. Došenovič Bonča. 2010. *Kritična analiza organiziranosti zdravstva v Sloveniji* (A Critical Analysis of the Organisation of Healthcare in Slovenia). Ljubljana: Faculty of Economics

Temesi, I. 2000. Local Government in Hungary. In *Decentralization: Experiments and Reforms* edited by Horváth M. Tamás. Budapest: Local Government Initiative Books, Open Society Institute. Volume 1:344-384

TEMPO-online. 2011. Bucharest: Romanian National Institute of Statistics <https://statistici.insse.ro/shop/>

Tőkés, R. 1998. *A Kialkudott Forradalom. Gazdasági Reform, Társadalmi Átalakulás és Politikai Hatalomutódlás 1957-1990 (Hungary's Negotiated Revolution: Economic Reform, Social Change and Political Succession 1957-1990)*. Budapest: Kossuth Kiadó

Tonoyan, T. 2004. *Healthcare System Armenia: Past, Present and Prospects*. <www.ww.tu-berlin.de/diskussionspapiere/2004/dp11-2004.pdf>

Tonoyan, T. 2005. *Poverty, Inequality and Health: A Case Study of Armenia*. <www.econstor.eu/bitstream/10419/22149/1/NO_124.pdf>

Torosyan, A., P. Romaniuk and K. Krajewski-Siuda. 2008. The Armenian Healthcare System: Recent Changes and Challenges. *Public Health* 8:83-190

United Nations. *World Population Prospects: The 2008 Revision Population Database*. <http://esa.un.org/unpp/>

United Nations Development Program (UNDP). 2003. *National Human Development Report Slovak Republic 2001-2002*. Bratislava: UNDP

UNDP. 2010. *Poverty and Social Impact Analysis of the Global Economic Crisis*. Synthesis Report of 18 Country Studies. <www.undp.org/poverty/topics2_social_impact_assessment.shtml>

UNICEF. 2003. *Social Monitor*. <www.aegis.com/files/unicef/socialmonitor2002.pdf>

US Agency for International Development (USAID). 2005. *Armenian Political Party Assessment*. <www.usaid.gov/.../political_party_assessment>

USAID. 2010. *Health in Armenia*. <www.usaid.gov/locations/europe_eurasia/health/countries/docs/country_profile_armenia.pdf>

USAID. 2008. Primary Healthcare Reform Project. *How Great Is the Burden of Household Health Expenditure in Armenia*. <www.phcr.am/upload/files/PHCR_article_Access_and_Affordability_Analysis_Eng.pdf>

Van den Noord, P. and B. Cournède. 2006. *Short-term Pain for Long-term Gain: The Impact of Structural Reform on Fiscal Outcomes in EMU*. <www.bancaditalia.it/studiricerche/convegni/atti/fiscal_ind/Fiscal/10.pdf>

Vekov, T. 2009. Health Reform in Bulgaria 1999-2009. *Results, Opinions and Recommendations*. Siela

Vekov, T. 2011. On Informal Payments by Patients (2008-2011): Bulgaria. *European Journal of Public Health* 20(1):42

Vepřek, J., P. Vepřek and J. Janda. 2002. *Zpráva o léčení českého zdravotnictví aneb Zdravotnická reforma včera, dnes a zítra* (Report on Healing the Czech Health Care System or Health Reform – Yesterday, Today and Tomorrow). Praha: Grada Publishing

Vlach, J., E. Sičáková and J. Nemeč. 2004. *Monitoring verejného obstarávania vo vybraných nemocniciach SR*. Bratislava: Transparency International Slovakia

Vlădescu, C., G. Scîntee and V. Olsavszky. 2008. Romania: Health System Review: *Health Systems in Transition* 10(3):137-158 European Observatory on Health Systems and Policies

Verhoeven, M., V. Gunnarsson and S. Lugaresi. 2007. *The Health Sector in the Slovak Republic: Efficiency and Reform*. Washington DC: IMF Working Paper WP/07/226

VMRO-DPMNE. *Rebirth in 100 steps: Political Program for the Parliamentary Elections in 2006*. <www.vmro-dpmne.org.mk>

Wagstaff, A. 2009. *Social Health Insurance vs Tax Financed Health Systems-Evidence from the OECD*. PRWP 4821: Washington DC: The World Bank

Whyte, A. 2004. *Landscape Analysis of Donor Trends in International Development*. New York: The Rockefeller Foundation

Wilensky, H.L. 2002. *Rich Democracies, Political Economy, Public Policy, and Performance*. Berkeley: University of California Press

World Bank. 1993. *World Development Report 1993: Investing in Health*. New York: Oxford University Press

World Bank. 1996. *Staff Appraisal Report*. <www.wds.worldbank.org/external/default/WDSContentServer/WDSP/IB/1996/05/24/000009265_3961214123024/Rendered/PDF/multi0page.pdf>

World Bank. 2001. *Transition – The First Ten Years: Analysis and Lessons for Eastern Europe and the Former Soviet Union*. <http://siteresources.worldbank.org/ECAEXT/Resources/complete.pdf

World Bank. 2003. *Implementation Completion Report*. <www.wds.worldbank.org/external/default/WDSContentServer/WDSP/IB/2003/06/30/000112742_20030630111113/Rendered/PDF/25735.pdf>

World Bank. 2005. *Macedonia Poverty Assessment for 2002-2003*. <www.wds.worldbank.org/servlet/WDSContentServer/WDSP/IB/2005/12/21/000090341_20051221144229/Rendered/PDF/343240MK.pdf>

World Bank. 2007. *Staff Estimates based on Multi-Topic Household Survey*. Sofia: World Bank

World Bank. 2010. *From Rags to Riches: Armenia's Healthcare is Modernizing*. <www.worldbank.org.am/WBSITE/EXTERNAL/COUNTRIES/ECAEXT/ARMENIAEXTN/0,,contentMDK:22703458~menuPK:3949610~pagePK:1497618~piPK:217854~theSitePK:301579,00.html>

World Bank. 2011a. *Armenia: Program Snapshot*. <www.worldbank.org.am/WBSITE/EXTERAL/COUNTRIES/ECAEXT/ARMENIAEXTN/0,,contentMDK:20628754~menuPK:301586~pagePK:141137~piPK:141127~theSitePK:301579,00.html>

World Bank. 2011b. *Republic of Armenia: Fiscal Consolidation and Recovery*. Report No. 62587-AM. 2:47-56>

World Bank. 2012. *Data and Statistics for Macedonia*. <www.worldbank.org.mk/WBSITE/EXTERNAL/COUNTRIES/ECAEXT/MACEDONIAEXTN/0,,contentMDK:20179336~

menuPK:304498~pagePK:1497618~piPK:217854~theSitePK:304473,00.html> World Bank. 2005. *Dying Too Young: Addressing Premature Mortality and Ill Health Due to Non-Communicable Diseases and Injuries in the Russian Federation*. Moscow: World Bank

World Bank. 2012. <http://data.worldbank.org/country/romania>

World Development Indicators. 2007. <http://devdata.worldbank.org/wdi2006>

World Food Program (WFP). 2010. *Armenia*. <http://home.wfp.org/stellent/groups/public/documents;op_reports/wfp228588.pdf>

World Health Organization (WHO). 1946. *Constitution of the World Health Organization*. Geneva: World Health Organization

WHO. 2005. *Highlights on Health in Armenia*. Copenhagen: Regional Office for Europe <www.euro.who.int?_data/assets/pdf_file/0007/103201/E88387.pdf>

WHO. 2006. *World Health Report 2007: A Safer Future: Global Public Health Security in the 21st Century*. Geneva: World Health Organization

WHO. 2009. *World Health Statistics 2009. Health Expenditure* <www.who.int/whosis/whostat/EN_WHS09_Table7.pdf>

WHO. 2009. *Health for All Database*. Copenhagen: World Health Organization Regional Office for Europe.

WHO and Ministry of Health. 2009. *Mental Health System in Armenia*. A report of the assessment of the mental health system in Armenia using the World Health Organization ? Assessment Instrument for Mental Health Systems (WHO-AIMS). Yerevan, Armenia. <www.who.int/mental_health/armenia_who_aims_report.pdf>

WHO. 2010. *European Health for All Database* (HFA-DB). Copenhagen: World Health Organization Regional Office for Europe

WHO. 2012. *Global Health Expenditure Atlas*. Geneva. World Health Organization

WHO. 2012. *European Health for All Database* (HFA-DB). Copenhagen: World Health Organization Regional Office for Europe

WHOSIS. 2010. <http://apps.who.int/whosis/data/Search.jsp>

World Health Report. 2001. Geneva: World Health Organization

World Health Statistics. 2010. Geneva: World Health Organization

Yeghiyan, G. 2010. *Improving Financial Risk Protection in Armenian Healthcare System*. Yerevan: Precise Health Research LLC. <http://phrcro.com/risk_protection.pdf>

Zajac, R. and P. Pažitný. 2000. Zdravotníctvo (Health Care). In *Slovensko 2000*. Bratislava: Institute for Public Affairs

Zajac, R. and P. Pažitný. 2001. Zdravotníctvo (Health Care). In *Slovensko 2001*. Bratislava: Institute for Public Affairs

Zajac, R. and P. Pažitný. 2002. Zdravotníctvo (Health Care). In *Slovensko 2002*. Bratislava: Institute for Public Affairs

Zdravotnícka ročenka (Health Statistics Yearbook) 1990-2008. Bratislava: Ústav zdravotníckych informácií a štatistiky

Websites

<www.government.gov.sk>	
<www.uzis.sk>	
<www.ivo.sk>	
<www.health.gov.sk>	
<www.finance.gov.sk>	
<www.pewglobal.org>	
<www.statistics.gov.sk>	
<www.transparency.sk>	
<www.lpr.sk>	
<www.aop.sk>	
<www.udzs.sk>	
<www.volby.cz>	Election Results (Czech Statistical Office)
<www.uzis.cz>	Institute of Health Statistics of the Czech Republic
<www.czso.cz>	Czech Statistical Office
<www.imf.org>	International Monetary Fund
<www.minfin.government.bg>	Ministry of Finance (Bulgaria)
<www.mh.government.bg>	Ministry of Health (Bulgaria)
<www.nchi.bg>	National Center for Health Information (Bulgaria)
<www.nhif.bg>	National Health Insurance Fund (Bulgaria)
<www.mh.government.bg>	National Health Strategy (Bulgaria)
<www.nsi.bg>	National Statistical Institute (Bulgaria)

Association of Companies and Health Insurance Funds, Czech Republic <http://szpcr.cz/reforma/100204_strategie_SZPCR.pdf>

Christian Democrats (KDU-ČSL): 2006 Election Program <www.kdu.cz/default.asp?page=510&idr=10149%IDC1=15076>

Civic Democratic Party (ODS): 2006 Election Program www.ods.cz/volby/2006/program.php

Communist Party of Czechoslovakia (KSČM): 2006 Election Program <www.kscm.cz/article.asp?thema=3783&item=35527>

Czech Social Democratic Party (ČSSD): 2006 Election Program <www.cssd.cz/nas-program/volebni-program>

Green Party (SZ): 2006 Election Program <www.zeleni.cz/155/clanek/6-socialni-politika-stejna-prava-stejne-sance/#6.5>

About the Authors

James Warner Björkman is Professor Emeritus of Public Policy and Administration at the Institute of Social Studies, The Hague, The Netherlands, and past Chair of the International Political Science Association's Research Committee on Comparative Health Policy. Educated at the University of Minnesota (BA 1966) and Yale University (MPhil 1969, PhD 1976), he was Professor of Public Administration and Development at Leiden University during 1990-2008 and episodically Visiting Professor at the International Centre for the Promotion of Enterprise in Ljubljana (Slovenia), the University of Namibia (Windhoek), Ritsumeikan University (Japan) and Stellenbosch University (South Africa). Previously faculty member at the University of Wisconsin-Madison and Executive Director of the International Institute of Comparative Government in Lausanne (Switzerland), he held appointments in Sweden (Linköping University), England (Essex University), India (Institute of Economic Growth), Pakistan (Institute of Development Economics) and Yale University. During 1987-1990 he directed the American Studies Research Centre, Hyderabad, India, and during 1996-1999 he was Deputy Rector of the Institute of Social Studies. He has published 15 books and more than 80 journal articles and reviews.

Juraj Nemec is Professor of Public Finance and Public Management at Matej Bel University in Banska Bystrica (Slovakia) and at Masaryk University in Brno (Czech Republic). His fields of interest are public economics and public finance, public administration reforms, health care policy, economics and management, and public procurement. He co-authored the first Slovak monographs on health economics (1995) and health management (1998), published scientific evaluations of health policy and health reforms in Slovakia and in the region, and participated in Phare and World Bank programs that supported health reforms in Slovakia. As author, co-author or editor, he has published more than 60 books and 300 articles. He is editor-in-chief of the *NISPAcee Journal in Public Administration and Public Policy*, vice-chair of the International Research Society for Public Management, member of the Board of Management of the International Association of Schools and Institutes of Administration, and vice-chair of the European Accreditation Committee for Public Administration.

Razvan M. Chereches is Executive Director of the Center for Health Policy and Public Health, Institute for Social Research, Faculty of Political, Administrative and Communication Sciences at Babes-Bolyai University in Cluj, Romania. Focused on health and mental health care, he serves as expert-evaluator for the European Union's Executive Agency for Health and Consumer Affairs as well as for Romania's National Commission for the Accreditation of Hospitals.

Tatiana Chubarova is Head, Center for Economic Theory of the Social Sector, Institute of Economy, at the Russian Academy of Sciences, and teaches at the Moscow School of Economics, Moscow State University, and Moscow State Institute of International Relations. Educated at the latter (MS 1986), she holds a Candidate of Science Degree in International Economy from the Russian Academy of Sciences and a PhD (Social Policy) from the London School of Economics and Political Science. She is Executive Secretary of *Upravliniye Zdravookhraneniem* (a health management journal), member of the New Economic Association (Russia) and the International Political Science Association, and author or co-author of four books as well as contributor to numerous journals. Her professional interests span health and social policy in comparative perspective, the organization and financing of health care, and gender issues.

Zuzana Darmopilová is Lecturer at the Faculty of Economics of Masaryk University in Brno and the Czech Technical University in Prague (Czech Republic). Educated at Masaryk University (MA 2003; PhD 2010), she teaches Public Economics and Economics of Health Care at economic, medical and technical faculties of Masaryk University, Charles University and the Czech Technical University. She served as Visiting Professor at Université de Rennes I (France) and has published a book concerning the influence of interest groups in health care reforms.

Branko Dimeski is Assistant Professor, Faculty of Administration and Information Systems Management, St Kliment Ohridski University, Bitola, Macedonia. Formerly research assistant in the Department of Political Science and Criminal Justice, Appalachian State University (2003-2005) and teaching assistant at St Kliment Ohridski University (2005-2009), he graduated in international economy from St Kliment Ohridski University in 2003, earned a Master of Public Administration at Appalachian State University in 2005 and a PhD in public administration from St. Kliment Ohridski in 2009. His dissertation – Principles of New Public Management in Local Governments in the Republic of Macedonia – is a study of reforms in local municipalities. His professional interests include local government, public sector reforms and health system reforms.

Nevyana Feschieva, (PhD 1982) is Associate Professor in Public Health. Before her academic career she was a general practitioner and neurologist. With specialization in epidemiology, public health and medical sociology from the UK (Cambridge University) and The Netherlands (Erasmus University, Maastricht University), she was a founder of the Faculty of Public Health at the Medical University of Varna and of the specialty of Health Care Management. During 1990-2000 she was Head, Department of Social Medicine and Health Care Organization, and in 2001 became the first Dean of Public Health. As a principal investigator for international research projects, supervisor for PhD students and visiting lecturer in all Faculties of Public Health in Bulgaria, Feschieva has over 200 publications in Bulgarian and international journals. Since 1999 she has been President of "Public Health 99" and is a member of the editorial boards of three scientific journals.

Sándor Gallai is Associate Professor at Corvinus University in Budapest and Director-General of the Institute for Public Policy Research (a government think-tank). With an MA degree in economics and a PhD in political science from the Budapest University of Economic Sciences, he teaches political science and public policy. His research interests include issues of Central and Eastern European transition, Hungarian politics and public policy-making in Hungary.

Natalia S. Grigorieva is Professor of Sociology and Head, Centre for Comparative Social Policy and Social Administration, School of Public Administration, Lomonosov Moscow State University. She is Editor-in-Chief of the journal *Health Management*, advisor to the Committee for Health Care Policy of the Duma (federal assembly of the Russian Federation) and expert member of the UN Gender Theme Group. In the field of comparative social policy with specialist interest in health care policy, she has published over 150 research monographs, reports, book chapters, articles and pamphlets in Russian. Her latest monographs are *From Tradition to Innovation: Modern Health Care Reforms* (with V. Sadovnichi and T. Chubarova), 2012, and *Modern Health Care: Health Policy, Health Economics, Health Management* (with T. Chubarova), 2013. Publications in English include Health Care in the Commonwealth of Independent States, *Routledge International Encyclopedia of Women*, 2001; Health Status in Russia: The Role of the State in Economic Growth and Socio-economic Reforms, *Human Development Report of the Russian Federation*, 2002-2003; Public Health Policy and Gender-Based Approaches, 2003; and Family Strategies of Modern Russian Youth, *Work Family Conflict Resolution*, International Labor Organization's Office for Eastern Europe and Central Asia, 2009.

Blasko Kasapinov, MD, MPH, has been associated with the National Institute of Public Health in Skopje since 2006 as a researcher in the Department for Social Medicine and since 2008 as a lecturer in the Institute of Social Medicine at the Medical Faculty. His work is focused on research of the national health system, analysis of health data and public health preventive programs. With experience in governmental and international non-governmental agencies, he teaches undergraduate and postgraduate students at the Medical Faculty in Skopje in social medicine, health systems organization, management, health economics and health policy.

Todorka Kostadinova is Professor of Strategic Management, Department of Health Economics and Management, Dean of the Faculty of Public Health, and Vice Rector of the

Medical University in Varna, Bulgaria. With a Master's degree in economics from the University of Economics in Varna and a PhD in management administration from the University of National and World Economy in Sofia, she has been faculty member at George Washington University (2005-2008), guest lecturer in Health Care Management at the University of Bern, Switzerland (2006) and at the Medical University of Vienna's Summer School (2008-2010), and member of the Research Network at the University of California, Berkeley (2008-2011). Kostadinova served as a parliamentary secretary and deputy minister of health in Bulgaria (2009-2010), Associate Editor of the *International Journal of Integrated Care* and Vice Editor-in-Chief of the Bulgarian journal *Health Economics and Management*. Her academic publications include over 100 articles and reviews.

Vladimir Lazarevik is founder and CEO of <www.healthgrouper.com>. He was Deputy Minister of Health in the government of the Republic of Macedonia (2006-2008), member of the Standing Committee of the Regional Committee of the World Health Organization Europe (2007-2010) and Executive President for its 60th session. With a Masters of Public Health from the Braun School of Public Health and Community Medicine, Hebrew University, Jerusalem, Israel, Lazarevik has a faculty position at the Institute of Social Medicine, Faculty of Medicine, in Skopje, where he teaches undergraduate and postgraduate students in medicine. He has published over 20 journal articles and numerous commentaries on health system reforms.

Ivan Maly is Associate Professor of Public Economics at the Faculty of Economics and Administration, and Deputy Rector at Masaryk University in Brno. He graduated from its Faculty of Law (MA 1986) and, based on studies at Antwerp University's Faculty of Saint Ignatius (1990) and during a Soros Open Society fellowship at the University of California in Berkeley (1993), he defended his doctoral thesis on Health Care Financing at the University of Economics in Prague in 1993. He began his career in 1988 as a lecturer at Masaryk University and successively taught at the South Bohemian University in Jindřichův Hradec, Military University in Vyškov and other universities. In 1998 he earned his *Habilitation* in public economics. Since then he has served as Head of Department, Vice-Dean and Dean of the Faculty of Economics and Administration, and is in charge of the development of three new study programs including the PhD Program in Public Economics. He has published five books and more than ten journal articles.

George Manliev is Lecturer on Public Sector Economics at the Technical University and at the University of National and World Economy, both in Sofia (Bulgaria). He studied at Roma University (Sapienza), Leicester University (UK), Maastricht University (The Netherlands) and George Mason University, Washington DC (USA). He has published articles and books related to fiscal policy, asymmetric information, new public sector management, and fiscal efficiency in education and health.

Lianna Mkhitaryan works as Project Manager at the Tufenkian Hospitality Company in Yerevan, Armenia. She has a diploma in engineering from Yerevan State Engineering University (1984), an engineer-researcher diploma from Moscow Power Engineering University (1993), and holds an MBA from the American University of Armenia (2000). She started her career as engineer designer on industrial enterprise in Yerevan. Since 2005 she has been involved in research and technical assistance projects funded by the World Bank, the Asian Development Bank, the Open Society Institute, the Local Government Initiative (Open Society Institute-Budapest) and the Eurasia Foundation. Her areas of expertise include applied research in public policy with special focus on public services delivery, land management, land and real asset acquisition, and resettlement.

Dance Gudeva-Nikovska has an MD from the Faculty of Medicine, University of Saints Cyril and Methodius in Skopje and a Masters in Public Health in 2003 from the Braun School of Public Health and Community Medicine, Hebrew University, Jerusalem, Israel. Since 2008 Gudeva-Nikovska has been at the Department of Social Medicine, Faculty of Medicine, and responsible for teaching and practical training of undergraduate medical and dentistry students. She also teaches research methods and development of research protocols for students enrolled in Master of Public Health program. Her research covers a range of topics in public health and health policy: socio-economic differences in health, behavior and access to health care; analysis of governance in public health institutions; community injuries; monitoring the performance of health institutions in the Republic of Macedonia; and cost-benefit analysis on the prevention of absenteeism from work.

Marek Pavlík is Assistant Professor at the Faculty of Economics and Administration of Masaryk University, Brno (Czech Republic). Educated at Masaryk University (MA 2003, PhD 2009), he teaches courses focused on public policy, health policy and economics, and the economics and policy of sport. He published a book on aspects of implementation in health policy.

Veronika Petkovšek, MSc, is an Assistant in the Department of Public Sector Economics at the Faculty of Administration, University of Ljubljana, Slovenia, where she is involved in the Centre for the Development of Pedagogic Excellence. Her areas of research include public sector economics in health reform, public procurement, and measurements of the efficiency and effectiveness of the public sector. She is also active in cross-border cooperation between Slovenia, Austria, and Italy.

Stanka Setnikar-Cankar, PhD, is Professor of Public Sector Economics and a Dean of the Faculty of Administration, University of Ljubljana. She is the author of many articles and books on public sector economics and editor-in-chief of the magazine *International Public Administration Review* (previously *Administration*). Formerly member of the NISPAcee Steering Committee, she is a member of the Program Committee of annual conference of Public Administration in Slovenia, the International Association of Schools and Institutes of Administration, and the European Group for Public Administration. She heads research projects in the fields of Public Sector Reform, Public Sector Reform in Health Care, Effectiveness Measurement in Public Administration, and Cross-border Cooperation in the European Union and between Slovenia, Austria and Italy.

Milena Krasimirova Vladimirova is chief expert in the Office of Public Health Policy, Department of Health System Performance, National Center of Public Health and Analyses, Sofia, Bulgaria. With a Master's degree in Public Finance from the University of National and World Economy in Sofia and an MA in Social Work and Health Management from Veliko Tarnovo University, her professional interests focus on new public management in hospital marketing, patient satisfaction and quasi-markets as well as gender equality and women' health. She has published broadly in patient safety and quality of life.